AF854306

EMPLOYEE'S RECEIPT

I acknowledge receipt of the 2020 Emergency Response Guidebook detailing emergency response procedures developed jointly by Transport Canada, the U. S. Department of Transportation, and the Secretariat of Communication and Transport of Mexico with the assistance of many interested parties from government and industry including the collaboration of CIQUIME of Argentina.

EMPLOYEE'S SIGNATURE DATE

COMPANY

COMPANY REPRESENTATIVE'S SIGNATURE

NOTE: This receipt shall be read and signed by the employee. A responsible company supervisor shall countersign the receipt and place it in the employee's personnel file.

REMOVABLE PAGE - PULL SLOWLY FROM TOP RIGHT CORNER

HOW TO USE THIS GUIDEBOOK

RESIST RUSHING IN!
APPROACH INCIDENT FROM UPWIND, AND UPHILL AND/OR UPSTREAM
STAY CLEAR OF ALL SPILLS, VAPORS, FUMES, SMOKE, AND POTENTIAL HAZARDS

WARNING: DO NOT USE THIS FLOWCHART if more than one hazardous material/dangerous good is involved. Immediately call the appropriate emergency response agency telephone number listed on the inside back cover of this guidebook.

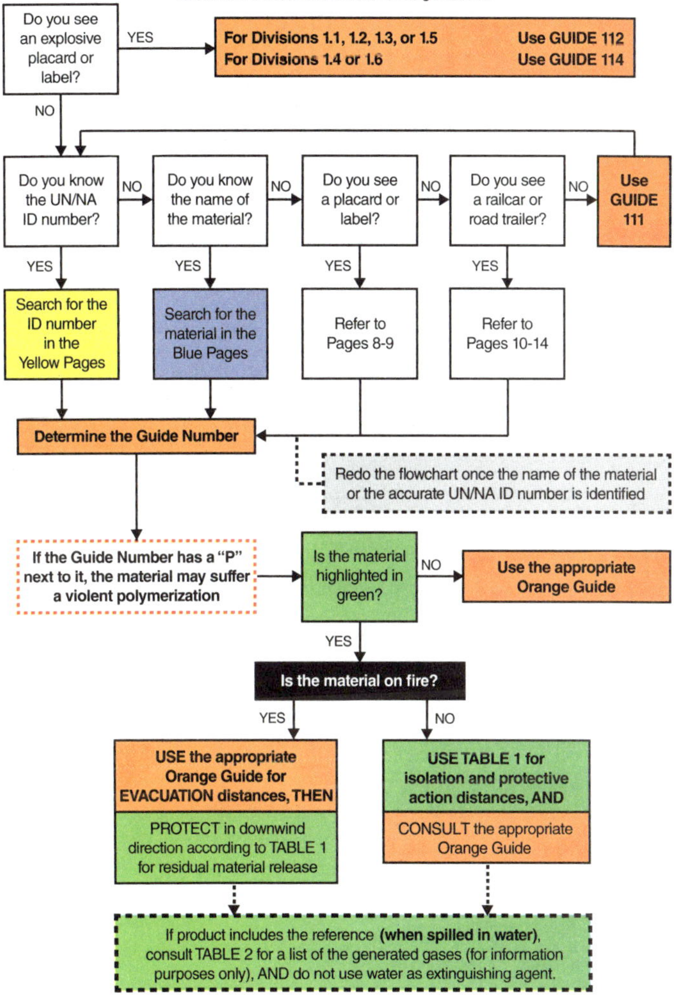

BEFORE AN EMERGENCY - BECOME FAMILIAR WITH THIS GUIDEBOOK!

First responders must be trained in the use of this guidebook.

LOCAL EMERGENCY TELEPHONE NUMBERS

Please populate this page with emergency telephone numbers for local assistance:

HAZMAT CONTRACTORS

RAIL COMPANIES

FEDERAL/STATE/PROVINCIAL AGENCIES

OTHERS

TABLE OF CONTENTS

SAFETY PRECAUTIONS

RESIST RUSHING IN!

APPROACH CAUTIOUSLY FROM *UPWIND, UPHILL* AND/OR *UPSTREAM*:

- Stay clear of ***Vapor, Fumes, Smoke and Spills.***
- Keep vehicle at a safe distance from the scene.

SECURE THE SCENE:

- Isolate the area and protect yourself and others.

IDENTIFY THE HAZARDS USING ANY OF THE FOLLOWING:

- Placards
- Container labels
- Shipping papers
- Rail Car and Road Trailer Identification Chart
- Safety Data Sheets (SDS)
- Knowledge of persons on scene
- Consult applicable guide page

ASSESS THE SITUATION:

- Is there a fire, a spill or a leak?
- What are the weather conditions?
- What is the terrain like?
- Who/what is at risk: people, property or the environment?
- What actions should be taken – evacuation, shelter-in-place or dike?
- What resources (human and equipment) are required?
- What can be done immediately?

OBTAIN HELP:

- Advise your headquarters to notify responsible agencies and call for assistance from qualified personnel.

RESPOND:

- Enter only when wearing appropriate protective gear.
- Rescue attempts and protecting property must be weighed against you becoming part of the problem.
- Establish a command post and lines of communication.
- Continually reassess the situation and modify response accordingly.
- Consider safety of people in the immediate area first, including your own safety.

ABOVE ALL: Do not assume that gases or vapors are harmless because of lack of a smell – odorless gases or vapors may be harmful. Use **CAUTION** when handling empty containers because they may still present hazards until they are cleaned and purged of all residues.

NOTIFICATION AND REQUEST FOR TECHNICAL INFORMATION

Follow the steps outlined in your organization's standard operating procedures and/or local emergency response plan for obtaining qualified assistance. Generally, the notification sequence and requests for technical information beyond what is available in this guidebook should occur in the following order:

1. **NOTIFY YOUR ORGANIZATION/AGENCY:**
   - Based on information provided, this will set in motion a series of events. Actions may range from dispatching additional trained personnel to the scene, to activating the local emergency response plan.
   - Ensure that local fire and police departments have been notified.

2. **CALL THE EMERGENCY RESPONSE TELEPHONE NUMBER ON THE SHIPPING PAPER**
   - If shipping paper is not available, use guidance under next section "**NATIONAL ASSISTANCE**".

3. **NATIONAL ASSISTANCE**
   - Contact the appropriate emergency response agency listed on the inside back cover of this guidebook.
   - Provide as much information about the hazardous material/dangerous good and the nature of the incident.
   - The agency will provide immediate advice on handling the early stages of the incident.
   - The agency will also contact the shipper or manufacturer of the material for more detailed information if necessary.
   - The agency will request on-scene assistance when necessary.

4. **PROVIDE AS MUCH OF THE FOLLOWING INFORMATION AS POSSIBLE:**
   - Your name, call-back telephone number, fax number
   - Location and nature of problem (spill, fire, etc.)
   - Name and identification number of material(s) involved
   - Shipper/consignee/point-of-origin
   - Carrier name, rail car or truck number
   - Container type and size
   - Quantity of material transported/released
   - Local conditions (weather, terrain)
   - Proximity to schools, hospitals, waterways, etc.
   - Injuries and exposures
   - Local emergency services that have been notified

HAZARD CLASSIFICATION SYSTEM

The hazard class of hazardous materials/dangerous goods is indicated either by its class (or division) number or name. Placards are used to identify the class or division of a material. The hazard class or division number must be displayed in the lower corner of a placard and is required for both primary and subsidiary hazard classes and divisions, if applicable. For other than Class 7 placards, text indicating a hazard (for example, "CORROSIVE") is not required. Text is shown only in the U.S. The hazard class or division number and subsidiary hazard classes or division numbers placed in parentheses (when applicable), must appear on the shipping paper after each proper shipping name.

Class 1 - Explosives

Division 1.1	Explosives which have a mass explosion hazard
Division 1.2	Explosives which have a projection hazard but not a mass explosion hazard
Division 1.3	Explosives which have a fire hazard and either a minor blast hazard or a minor projection hazard or both, but not a mass explosion hazard
Division 1.4	Explosives which present no significant hazard
Division 1.5	Very insensitive explosives with a mass explosion hazard
Division 1.6	Extremely insensitive articles which do not have a mass explosion hazard

Class 2 - Gases

Division 2.1	Flammable gases
Division 2.2	Non-flammable, non-toxic* gases
Division 2.3	Toxic* gases

Class 3 - Flammable liquids (and Combustible liquids [U.S.])

Class 4 - Flammable solids; Substances liable to spontaneous combustion; Substances which, on contact with water, emit flammable gases

Division 4.1	Flammable solids, self-reactive substances and solid desensitized explosives
Division 4.2	Substances liable to spontaneous combustion
Division 4.3	Substances which in contact with water emit flammable gases

Class 5 - Oxidizing substances and Organic peroxides

Division 5.1	Oxidizing substances
Division 5.2	Organic peroxides

Class 6 - Toxic* substances and Infectious substances

Division 6.1	Toxic* substances
Division 6.2	Infectious substances

Class 7 - Radioactive materials

Class 8 - Corrosive substances

Class 9 - Miscellaneous hazardous materials/dangerous goods and articles

* The words "poison" or "poisonous" are synonymous with the word "toxic".

INTRODUCTION TO THE TABLE OF MARKINGS, LABELS AND PLACARDS

USE THIS TABLE ONLY WHEN THE ID NUMBER OR PROPER SHIPPING NAME IS NOT AVAILABLE.

The next two pages display the placards used on transport vehicles carrying hazardous materials/dangerous goods with the applicable reference GUIDE circled. Follow these steps:

1. **Approach scene from upwind, uphill and/or upstream at a safe distance to safely identify and/or read the placard or orange panel. Use binoculars if available.**
2. **Match the vehicle placard(s) with one of the placards displayed on the next two pages.**
3. **Consult the circled guide number associated with the placard. Use that guide information for now. For example:**
   - Use GUIDE 127 for a FLAMMABLE (Class 3) placard 

   - Use GUIDE 153 for a CORROSIVE (Class 8) placard 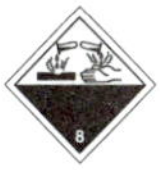

   - Use GUIDE 111 when the DANGER or DANGEROUS placard is displayed or the nature of the spilled, leaking or burning material is not known. Also use this GUIDE when the presence of hazardous materials/dangerous goods is suspected but no placards can be seen.

   If multiple placards point to more than one guide, initially use the most conservative guide (i.e., the guide requiring the greatest degree of protective actions).
4. **Guides associated with the placards provide the most significant risk and/or hazard information.**
5. **When specific information, such as ID number or proper shipping name, becomes available, the more specific Guide recommended for that material must be consulted.**
6. **A single asterisk (*) on orange placards represents an explosive's compatibility group letter. The asterisk must be replaced with the appropriate compatibility group letter. Refer to the Glossary (page 375).**
7. **Double asterisks (**) on orange placards represent the division of the explosive. The double asterisks must be replaced with the appropriate division number.**

TABLE OF MARKINGS, LABELS, AND PLACARDS

USE THIS TABLE ONLY IF MATERIALS CANNOT BE SPECIFICALLY IDENTIFIED BY

111

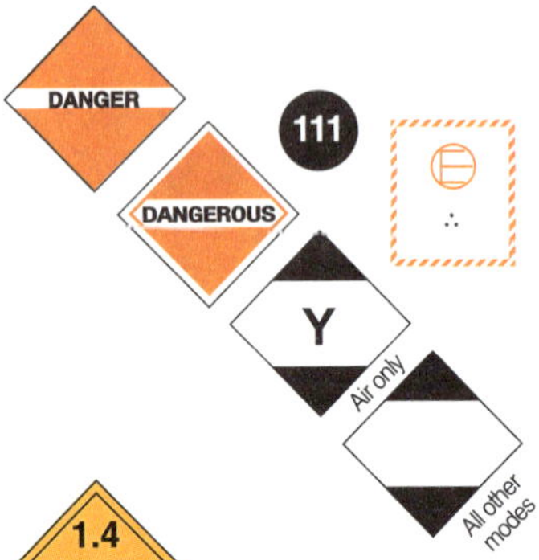

112

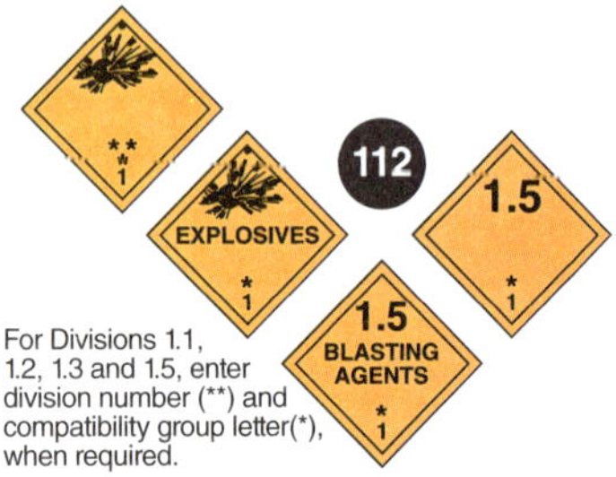

For Divisions 1.1, 1.2, 1.3 and 1.5, enter division number (**) and compatibility group letter(*), when required.

114

For Divisions 1.4 and 1.6, enter compatibility group letter(*), when required.

118

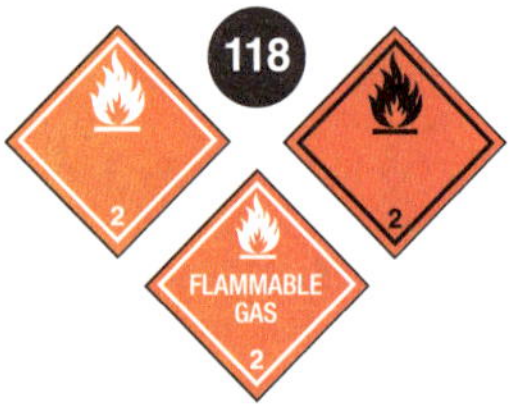

123

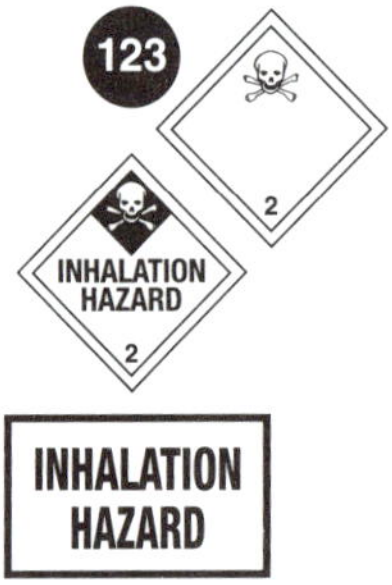

120

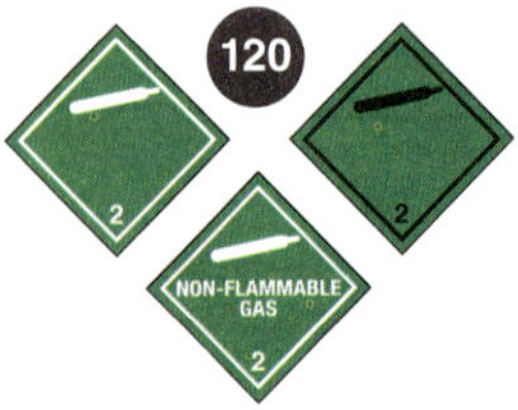

122

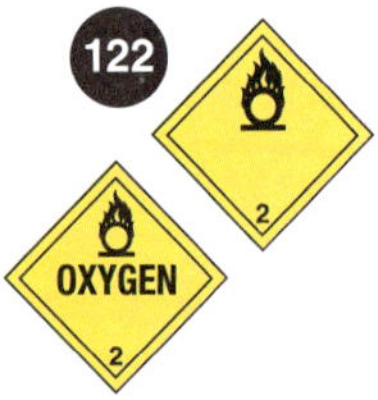

127

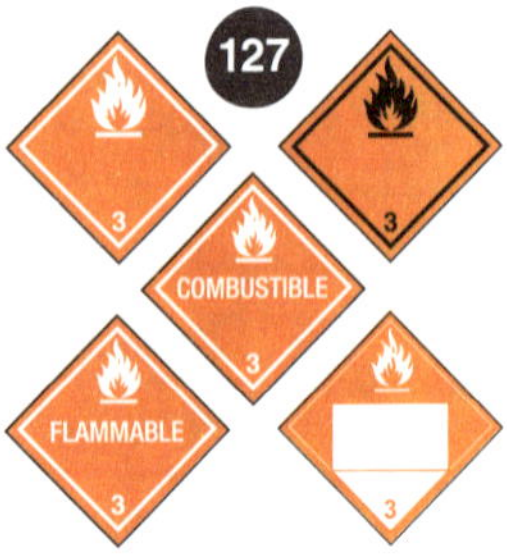

125

128

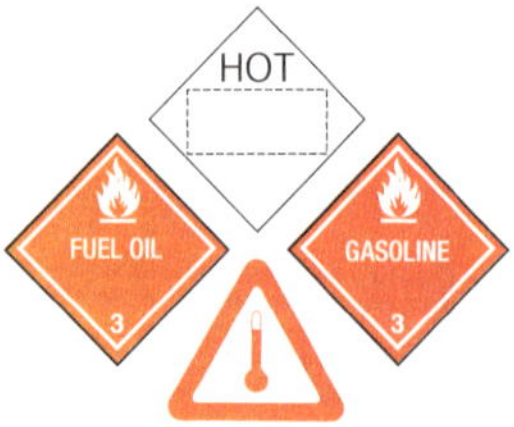

AND INITIAL RESPONSE GUIDE TO USE ON-SCENE

USING THE SHIPPING PAPER, NUMBERED PLACARD, OR ORANGE PANEL NUMBER

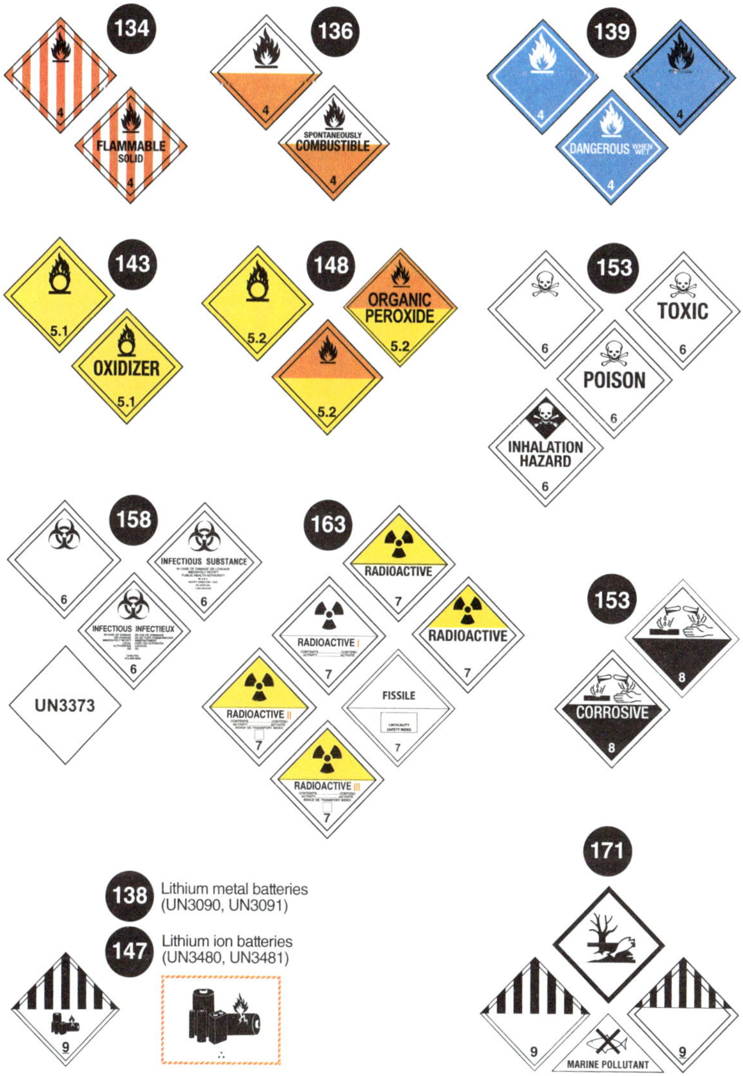

RAIL CAR IDENTIFICATION CHART

CAUTION: Emergency response personnel must be aware that rail tank cars vary widely in construction, fittings and purpose. Tank cars could transport products that may be solids, liquids or gases. The products may be under pressure. It is essential that products be identified by consulting shipping papers or train consist or contacting dispatch centers before emergency response is initiated. The information stenciled on the sides or ends of tank cars, as illustrated below, may be used to identify the product utilizing:

a. the commodity name shown;
b. the other information shown, especially reporting marks and car number which, when supplied to a dispatch center, will facilitate the identification of the product.

The recommended guides should be considered as last resort if the material cannot be identified by any other means.

117 Pressure tank car

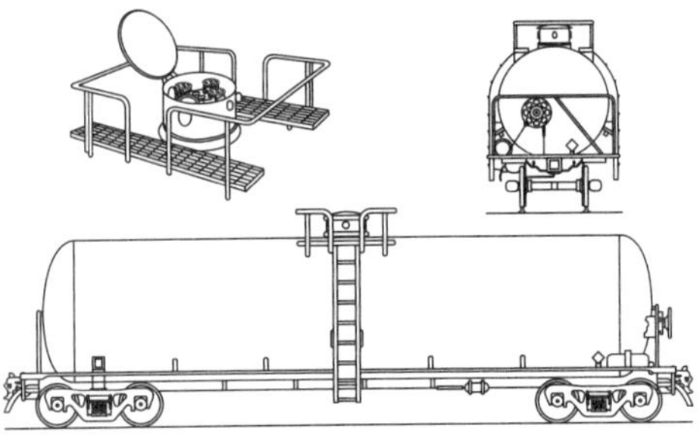

- For flammable, non-flammable, toxic and/or liquefied compressed gases
- Protective housing
- No bottom fittings
- Pressures usually above 40 psi

131 Non-pressure / low pressure tank car

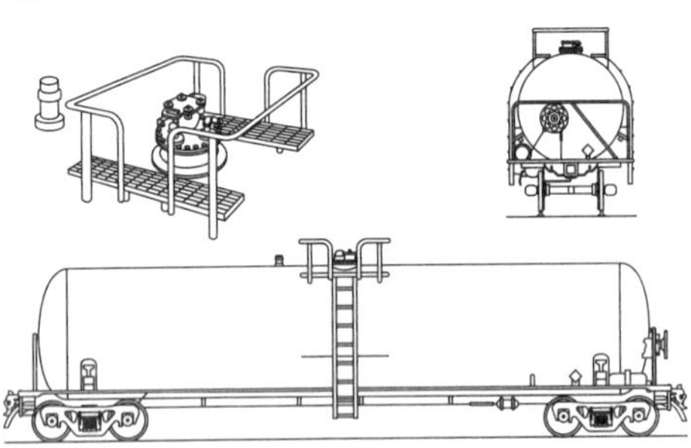

- Known as **general service tank car**
- For variety of hazardous and non-hazardous materials
- Fittings and valves normally visible at the top of the tank
- Some may have bottom outlet valve
- Pressures usually below 25 psi

RAIL CAR IDENTIFICATION CHART

128 Non-pressure / low pressure tank car (TC117, DOT117)

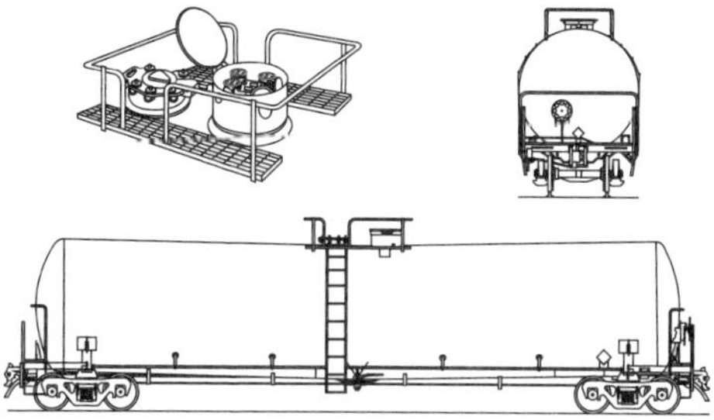

- For flammable liquids (e.g.,
- Petroleum crude oil, ethanol)
- Protective housing separate from manway
- Bottom outlet valve
- Pressures usually below 25 psi

111 Box car

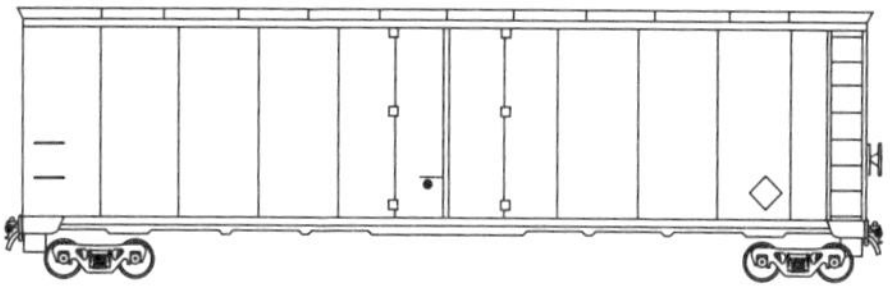

- For general freight that carry bulk or non-bulk packages
- May transport hazardous materials/dangerous goods in small packages or "tote bins"
- Single or double sliding door

140 Hopper car

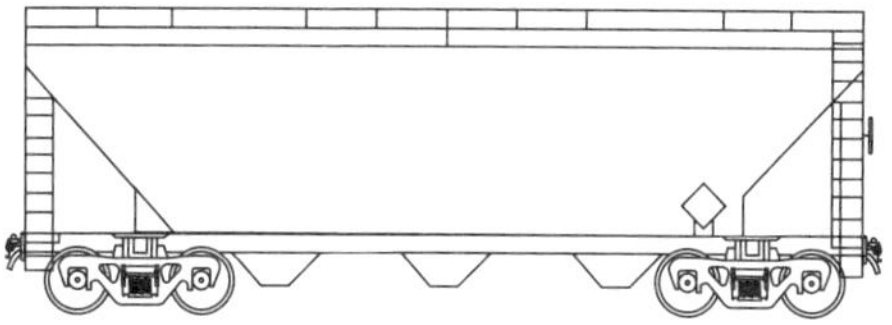

- For bulk commodities and bulk cargo (e.g., coal, ore, cement and solid granular materials)
- Bulk lading discharged by gravity through the hopper bottom doors when doors opened

COMMON MARKINGS ON RAIL CARS: reporting marks and car number, load limit (pounds or kilograms), empty weight of car, placard, tank qualification and pressure relief device information, car specification, and commodity name.

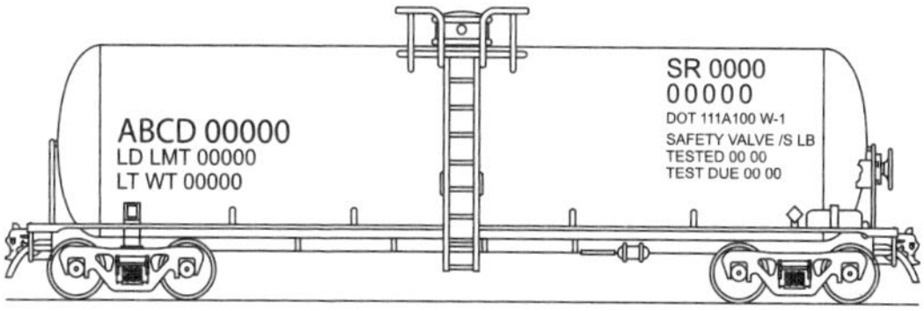

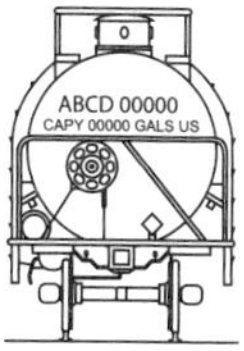

ROAD TRAILER IDENTIFICATION CHART

CAUTION: This chart depicts only the most general shapes of road trailers and cargo transport units. Emergency response personnel must be aware that there are many variations of road trailers, not illustrated below, that are used for shipping chemical products. Many intermodal tanks that transport liquids, solids, liquefied compressed gases, and refrigerated liquefied gases have similar silhouettes. The suggested guides are for the most hazardous products that may be transported in these trailer types.

WARNING: Road trailers may be jacketed, the cross-section may look different than shown and external ring stiffeners would be invisible.

NOTE: An emergency shut-off valve is commonly found at the front of the tank, near the driver door.

The recommended guides should be considered as last resort if the material cannot be identified by any other means.

MAWP: Maximum Allowable Working Pressure.

117 MC331, TC331, SCT331

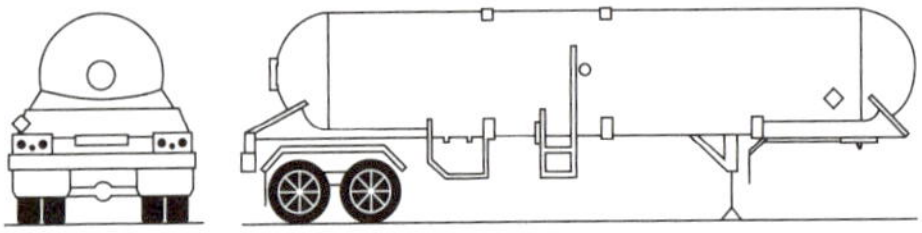

- For liquefied compressed gases (e.g., LPG, ammonia)
- Rounded heads
- Design pressure between 100-500 psi

117 MC338, TC338, SCT338, TC341, CGA341

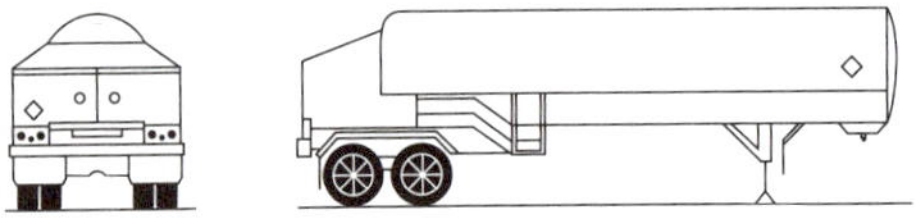

- For refrigerated liquefied gases (cryogenic liquids)
- Similar to a "giant thermo-bottle"
- Fitting compartments located in a cabinet at the rear of the tank
- MAWP between 25-500 psi

131 DOT406, TC406, SCT306, MC306, TC306

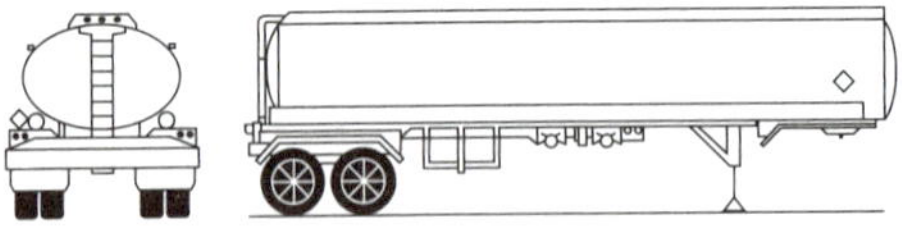

- For flammable liquids (e.g., gasoline, diesel)
- Elliptical cross-section
- Rollover protection at the top
- Bottom outlet valves
- MAWP between 3-15 psi

ROAD TRAILER IDENTIFICATION CHART

137 DOT407, TC407, SCT307, MC307, TC307

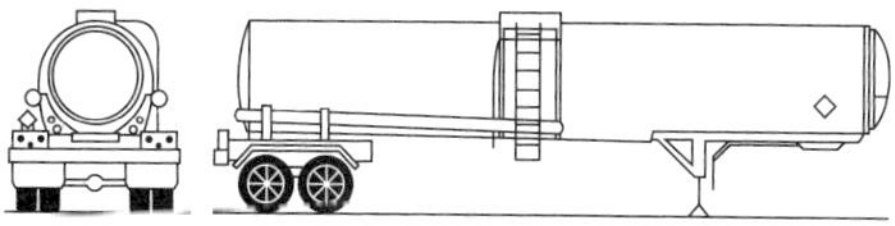

- For toxic, corrosive, and flammable liquids
- Circular cross-section
- May have external ring stiffeners
- MAWP of at least 25 psi

137 DOT412, TC412, SCT312, MC312, TC312

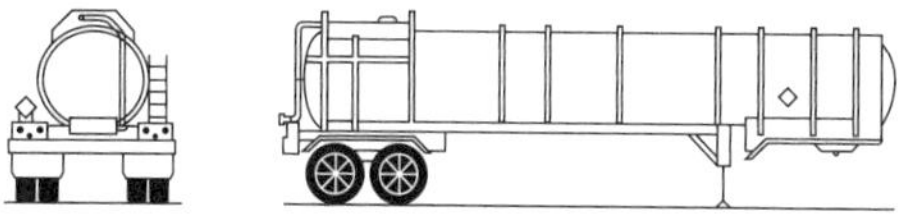

- Usually for corrosive liquids
- Circular cross-section
- External ring stiffeners
- Tank diameter is relatively small
- MAWP of at least 15 psi

112 TC423

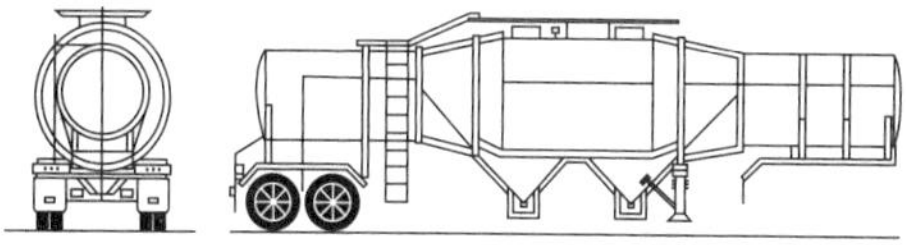

- For emulsion and water-gel explosives
- Hopper-style configuration
- MAWP between 5-15 psi

117 Compressed Gas/Tube Trailer

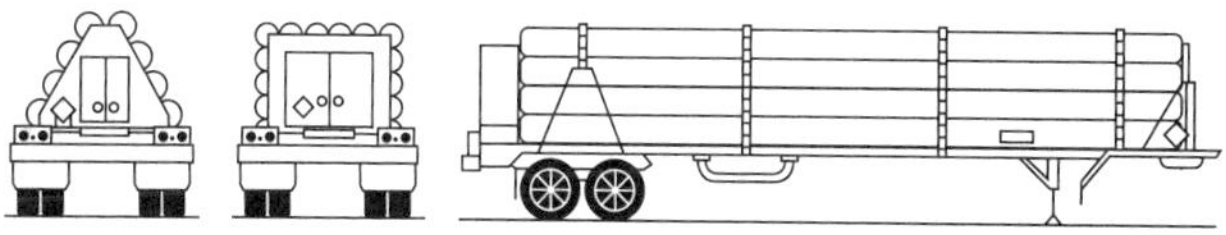

ROAD TRAILER IDENTIFICATION CHART

134 Dry Bulk Cargo Trailer

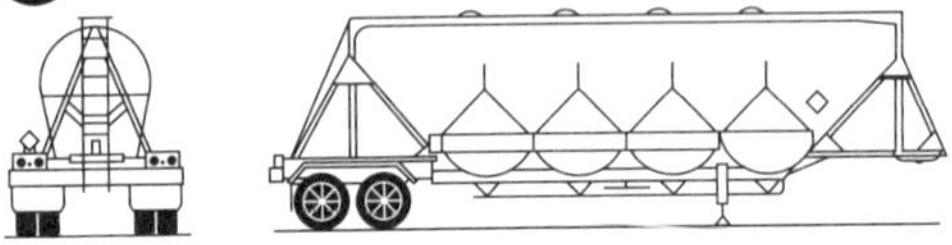

137 Vacuum Tanker

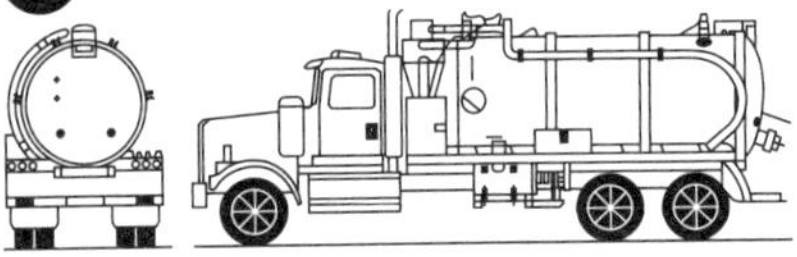

111 Mixed Cargo

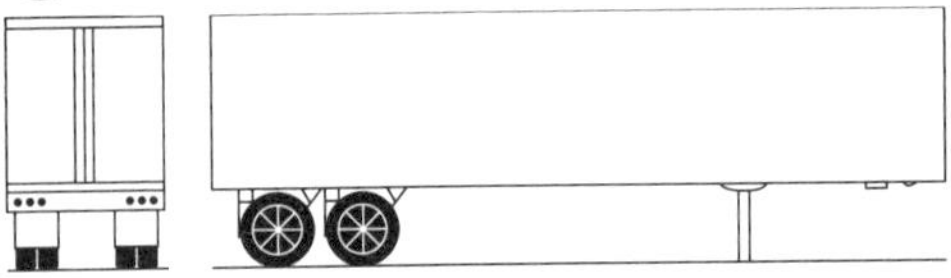

111 Intermodal Freight Container

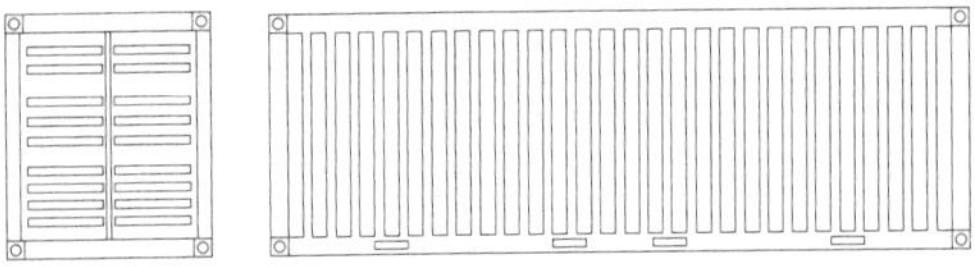

117 Intermodal Tank

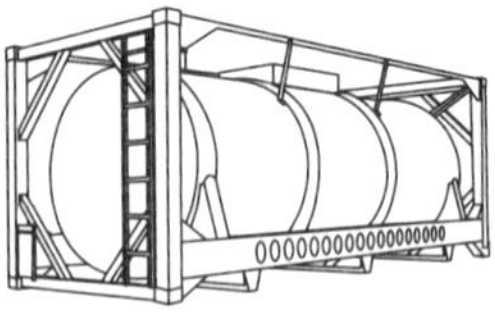

NOTES

GLOBALLY HARMONIZED SYSTEM OF CLASSIFICATION AND LABELING OF CHEMICALS (GHS)

(May be found on means of containment during transport)

The Globally Harmonized System of Classification and Labeling of Chemicals (GHS) is an international guideline published by the United Nations. The GHS aims to harmonize the classification and labeling systems for all sectors involved in the life cycle of a chemical (production, storage, transport, workplace use, consumer use and presence in the environment).

The GHS has nine symbols used to convey specific physical, health and environmental hazard information. These symbols are part of a pictogram that is diamond shaped and includes the GHS symbol in black on a white background with a red frame. The pictogram is part of the GHS label, which also includes the following information:

- **Signal word**
- **Hazard statement**
- **Precautionary statements**
- **Product identifier**
- **Supplier identification**

GHS pictograms are similar in shape to transport labels; however, transport labels have backgrounds of different colors.

The elements of the GHS that address signal words and hazard statements are not expected to be adopted in the transport sector. For substances and mixtures covered by the UN Recommendations on the Transport of Dangerous Goods, Model Regulations, the transport labels for physical hazards will have precedence. In transport, a GHS pictogram for the same (or lesser) hazard as the one reflected by the transport label or placard should not be present, but it could exist on the package.

Examples of GHS labeling:

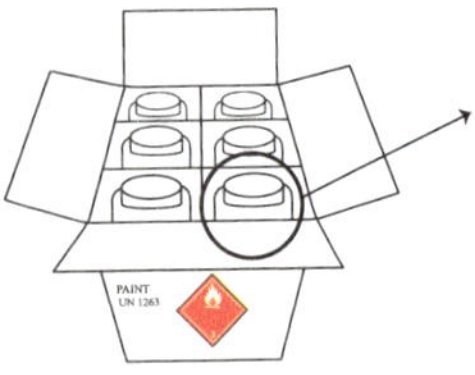

Outer Packaging: Box with flammable liquid transport label

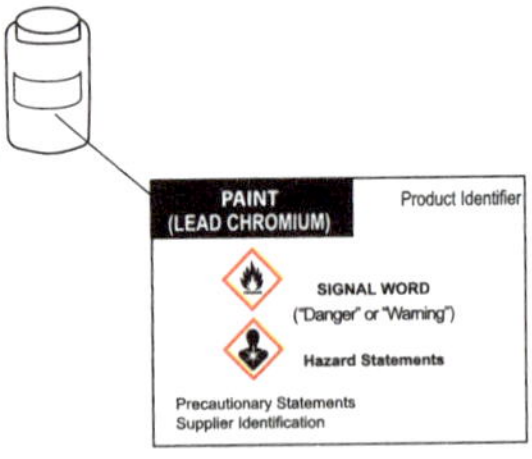

Inner Packaging: Plastic bottle with GHS hazard warning label

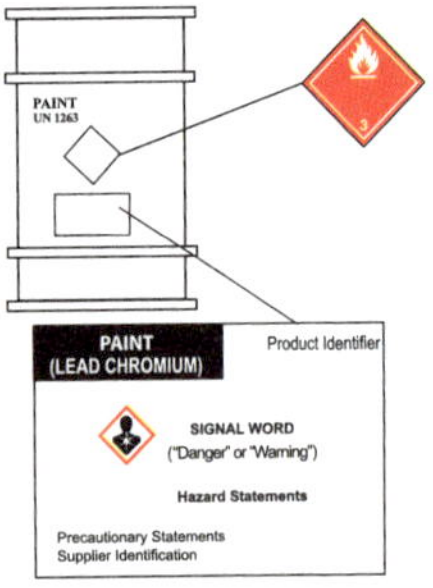

Single Packaging: 200 L (55 US gallons) drum with a flammable liquid transport label combined with GHS hazard warning label

In some cases, such as on drums or international bulk containers (IBCs), which must address information for all sectors, the GHS label may be found in addition to the required transport labels and placards. Both types of labels (GHS and transport) will differ in a way that will make them easy to identify during an emergency.

GHS Pictograms	Physical hazards	GHS Pictograms	Health and Environmental hazards
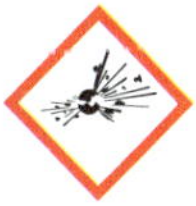	Explosive; Self-reactive; Organic peroxide		Skin corrosion; Serious eye damage
	Flammable; Pyrophoric; Self-reactive; Organic peroxide; Self-heating; Emits flammable gases when in contact with water		Acute toxicity (harmful); Skin sensitizer; Irritant (skin and eye); Narcotic effect; Respiratory tract irritant; Hazardous to ozone layer (environment)
	Oxidizer		Respiratory sensitizer; Mutagen; Carcinogen; Reproductive toxicity; Target organ toxicity; Aspiration hazard
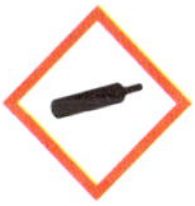	Gas under pressure	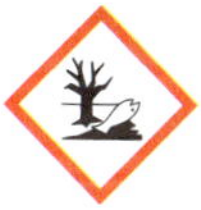	Hazardous to aquatic environment
	Corrosive to metals		Acute toxicity (fatal or toxic)

HAZARD IDENTIFICATION NUMBERS DISPLAYED ON SOME INTERMODAL CONTAINERS

Hazard identification numbers, utilized under European and some South American regulations, may be found in the top half of an orange panel on some intermodal bulk containers. The 4-digit ID number is in the bottom half of the orange panel.

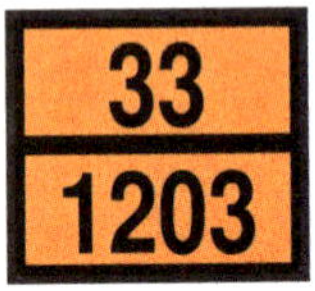

The hazard identification number in the top half of the orange panel consists of two or three digits. In general, the digits indicate the following hazards:

2 - Emission of gas due to pressure or chemical reaction

3 - Flammability of liquids (vapors) and gases or self-heating liquid

4 - Flammability of solids or self-heating solid

5 - Oxidizing (fire-intensifying) effect

6 - Toxicity or risk of infection

7 - Radioactivity

8 - Corrosivity

9 - Risk of spontaneous violent reaction

NOTE: The risk of spontaneous violent reaction within the meaning of digit 9 includes the possibility, due to the nature of a substance, of a risk of explosion, disintegration and polymerization reaction followed by the release of considerable heat or flammable and/or toxic gases.

- Doubling of a digit indicates an intensification of that particular hazard (i.e., 33, 66, 88).
- Where the hazard associated with a substance can be adequately indicated by a single digit, the digit is followed by a zero (i.e., 30, 40, 50).
- A hazard identification number prefixed by the letter "X" indicates that the substance will react dangerously with water (i.e., X88).

HAZARD IDENTIFICATION NUMBERS DISPLAYED ON SOME INTERMODAL CONTAINERS

The hazard identification numbers listed below have the following meanings:

20	Asphyxiant gas or gas with no subsidiary hazard
22	Refrigerated liquefied gas, asphyxiant
223	Refrigerated liquefied gas, flammable
225	Refrigerated liquefied gas, oxidizing (fire intensifying)
23	Flammable gas
238	Gas, flammable corrosive
239	Flammable gas which can spontaneously lead to violent reaction
25	Oxidizing (fire-intensifying) gas
26	Toxic gas
263	Toxic gas, flammable
265	Toxic gas, oxidizing (fire-intensifying)
268	Toxic gas, corrosive
28	Gas, corrosive
30	Flammable liquid (flash-point between 23°C and 60°C, inclusive), or flammable liquid or solid in the molten state with a flash-point above 60°C, heated to a temperature equal to or above its flash point, or self-heating liquid
323	Flammable liquid which reacts with water, emitting flammable gases
X323	Flammable liquid which reacts dangerously with water, emitting flammable gases
33	Highly flammable liquid (flash-point below 23°C)
333	Pyrophoric liquid
X333	Pyrophoric liquid which reacts dangerously with water
336	Highly flammable liquid, toxic
338	Highly flammable liquid, corrosive
X338	Highly flammable liquid, corrosive, which reacts dangerously with water
339	Highly flammable liquid which can spontaneously lead to violent reaction
36	Flammable liquid (flash-point between 23°C and 60°C, inclusive), slightly toxic, or self-heating liquid, toxic
362	Flammable liquid, toxic, which reacts with water, emitting flammable gas
X362	Flammable liquid, toxic, which reacts dangerously with water, emitting flammable gases
368	Flammable liquid, toxic, corrosive
38	Flammable liquid (flash-point between 23°C and 60°C, inclusive), slightly corrosive or self-heating liquid, corrosive
382	Flammable liquid, corrosive, which reacts with water, emitting flammable gases
X382	Flammable liquid, corrosive, which reacts dangerously with water, emitting flammable gases
39	Flammable liquid, which can spontaneously lead to violent reaction
40	Flammable solid, or self-reactive substance, or self-heating substance, or polymerizing substance

HAZARD IDENTIFICATION NUMBERS DISPLAYED ON SOME INTERMODAL CONTAINERS

423	Solid which reacts with water, emitting flammable gases, or flammable solid which reacts with water, emitting flammable gases, or self-heating solid which reacts with water, emitting flammable gases
X423	Solid which reacts dangerously with water, emitting flammable gases, or flammable solid which reacts dangerously with water, emitting flammable gases, or self-heating solid which reacts dangerously with water, emitting flammable gases
43	Spontaneously flammable (pyrophoric) solid
X432	Spontaneously flammable (pyrophoric) solid which reacts dangerously with water, emitting flammable gases
44	Flammable solid, in the molten state at an elevated temperature
446	Flammable solid, toxic, in the molten state at an elevated temperature
46	Flammable or self-heating solid, toxic
462	Toxic solid which reacts with water, emitting flammable gases
X462	Solid which reacts dangerously with water, emitting toxic gases
48	Flammable or self-heating solid, corrosive
482	Corrosive solid which reacts with water, emitting flammable gases
X482	Solid which reacts dangerously with water, emitting corrosive gases

50	Oxidizing (fire-intensifying) substance
539	Flammable organic peroxide
55	Strongly oxidizing (fire-intensifying) substance
556	Strongly oxidizing (fire-intensifying) substance, toxic
558	Strongly oxidizing (fire-intensifying) substance, corrosive
559	Strongly oxidizing (fire-intensifying) substance which can spontaneously lead to violent reaction
56	Oxidizing substance (fire-intensifying), toxic
568	Oxidizing substance (fire-intensifying), toxic, corrosive
58	Oxidizing substance (fire-intensifying), corrosive
59	Oxidizing substance (fire-intensifying), which can spontaneously lead to violent reaction

60	Toxic or slightly toxic substance
606	Infectious substance
623	Toxic liquid, which reacts with water, emitting flammable gases
63	Toxic substance, flammable (flash-point between 23°C and 60°C, inclusive)
638	Toxic substance, flammable, (flash-point between 23°C and 60°C, inclusive), corrosive
639	Toxic substance, flammable, (flash-point not above 60°C) which can spontaneously lead to violent reaction
64	Toxic solid, flammable or self-heating
642	Toxic solid which reacts with water, emitting flammable gases
65	Toxic substance, oxidizing (fire-intensifying)
66	Highly toxic substance

HAZARD IDENTIFICATION NUMBERS DISPLAYED ON SOME INTERMODAL CONTAINERS

663	Highly toxic substance, flammable (flash-point not above 60°C)
664	Highly toxic solid, flammable or self-heating
665	Highly toxic substance, oxidizing (fire-intensifying)
668	Highly toxic substance, corrosive
X668	Highly toxic substance, corrosive, which reacts dangerously with water
669	Highly toxic substance which can spontaneously lead to violent reaction
68	Toxic substance, corrosive
69	Toxic or slightly toxic substance which can spontaneously lead to violent reaction
70	Radioactive material
768	Radioactive material, toxic, corrosive
78	Radioactive material, corrosive
80	Corrosive or slightly corrosive substance
X80	Corrosive or slightly corrosive substance which reacts dangerously with water
823	Corrosive liquid which reacts with water, emitting flammable gases
83	Corrosive or slightly corrosive substance, flammable (flash-point between 23°C and 60°C, inclusive)
X83	Corrosive or slightly corrosive substance, flammable (flash-point between 23°C and 60°C, inclusive), which reacts dangerously with water
839	Corrosive or slightly corrosive substance, flammable (flash-point between 23°C and 60°C, inclusive), which can spontaneously lead to violent reaction
X839	Corrosive or slightly corrosive substance, flammable (flash-point between 23°C and 60°C, inclusive), which can spontaneously lead to violent reaction and which reacts dangerously with water
84	Corrosive solid, flammable or self-heating
842	Corrosive solid which reacts with water, emitting flammable gases
85	Corrosive or slightly corrosive substance, oxidizing (fire-intensifying)
856	Corrosive or slightly corrosive substance, oxidizing (fire-intensifying) and toxic
86	Corrosive or slightly corrosive substance, toxic
88	Highly corrosive substance
X88	Highly corrosive substance which reacts dangerously with water
883	Highly corrosive substance, flammable (flash-point between 23°C and 60°C, inclusive)
884	Highly corrosive solid, flammable or self-heating
885	Highly corrosive substance, oxidizing (fire-intensifying)
886	Highly corrosive substance, toxic
X886	Highly corrosive substance, toxic, which reacts dangerously with water
89	Corrosive or slightly corrosive substance which can spontaneously lead to violent reaction
90	Environmentally hazardous substance; miscellaneous dangerous substances
99	Miscellaneous dangerous substance carried at an elevated temperature

PIPELINE TRANSPORTATION

In North America, hazardous materials/dangerous goods are commonly transported through millions of miles of pipelines and related structures. Products transported include natural gas, natural gas liquids, crude oil, gasoline, diesel fuel, anhydrous ammonia, carbon dioxide, jet fuel, and other commodities. Although most pipelines are buried, often there are aboveground structures and markers indicating the presence of pipelines. First responders should be aware of the pipelines in their jurisdictions, the products they transport, and the operators responsible for those pipelines. Proactive relationships can be beneficial in the safe and effective management of pipeline emergencies.

Types of Pipelines

Natural Gas Pipelines

Natural Gas Transmission Pipelines

Large-diameter, steel pipelines transport flammable natural gas (toxic and non-toxic) at very high pressures ranging from 200 to 1,500 psi*. Natural gas in transmission pipelines is odorless — generally *not odorized* with mercaptan (the "rotten egg" smell); however, natural gas containing hydrogen sulfide (H_2S) will have a distinct "rotten egg" odor.

Natural Gas Distribution Pipelines

Natural gas is delivered directly to customers via distribution pipelines. These pipelines are typically smaller-diameter, lower-pressure pipelines constructed of steel, plastic, or cast iron. Natural gas in distribution pipelines *is odorized* with mercaptan (the "rotten egg" smell).

Natural Gas-Gathering and Natural Gas Well Production Pipelines

Natural gas-gathering/well production pipelines collect "raw" natural gas from wellheads and transport the product to gas-processing and/or gas-treating plants. These gathering pipelines carry natural gas mixed with some quantity of natural gas liquids, water, and, in some areas, contaminants such as toxic hydrogen sulfide (H_2S). Natural gas in these pipelines is *not odorized* with mercaptan (the "rotten egg" smell); however, natural gas that contains hydrogen sulfide (H_2S) will have a distinct "rotten egg" odor.

Hazardous Liquid and Highly Volatile Liquid Pipelines

Hazardous Liquid Pipelines

Crude oil, refined petroleum products (e.g. gasoline, kerosene, jet fuel or diesel) and hazardous liquids (e.g. anhydrous ammonia or ethanol) are often transported by pipelines.

Many liquid petroleum pipelines transport different types of liquid petroleum in the same pipeline. To do so, the pipeline operator sends different products in "batches." For example, an operator could send gasoline for several hours, and then switch to jet fuels, before switching to diesel fuel.

* Data from http://naturalgas.org/naturalgas/transport/

Highly Volatile Liquid (HVL) Pipelines

HVL pipelines transport hazardous liquids which will form a vapor cloud when released to the atmosphere and which have a vapor pressure exceeding 276 KPa (40 psia) at 37.8°C (100°F). An example of an HVL is liquid propane.

Pipeline Markers

Since pipelines are usually buried underground, pipeline markers are used to indicate their presence in an area along the pipeline route. Of the three types of pipelines typically buried underground — distribution, gathering, and transmission — only transmission pipelines are marked with the following above-ground markers used to indicate their route.

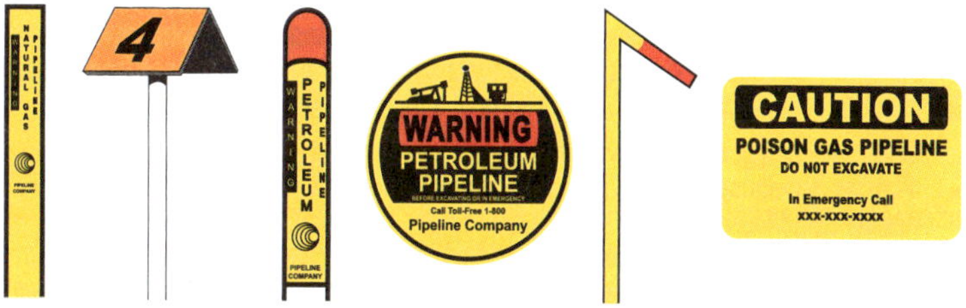

Markers warn that a transmission pipeline is located in the area, identify the product transported in the line, and provide the name and telephone number of the pipeline operator to call. Markers and warning signs are located at frequent intervals along natural gas and liquid transmission pipeline rights-of-way, and are located at prominent points such as where pipelines intersect streets, highways, railways, or waterways.

Pipeline markers only indicate the presence of a pipeline—they do not indicate the exact location of the pipeline. Pipeline locations within a right-of-way may vary along its length and there may be multiple pipelines located in the same right-of-way.

NOTE:

- Markers for pipelines transporting materials containing dangerous levels of hydrogen sulfide (H_2S) may have markers that say: "Sour" or "Poison."
- Natural gas distribution pipelines are not marked with above-ground signs.
- Gathering/production pipelines are often not marked with above-ground signs.

Other Important Considerations

- If no flames are present, do not introduce ignition sources such as open flames, running vehicles, or electrical equipment (cell phones, pagers, two-way radios, lights, garage door openers, fans, door bells, etc.).
- Abandon any equipment used in or near the area of the pipeline release.
- If there is no risk to your safety or the safety of others, move far enough away from any noise coming from the pipeline to allow for normal conversation.
- Pipelines often are close to other public utilities, railroads, and highways; these can be impacted by pipeline releases or may be potential ignition sources.
- Natural gas can migrate underground from the source of a release to other areas via the path of least resistance (including through sewers, water lines, and geologic formations).

Considerations for Establishing Protective Action Distances

- Type of product
  - If you know the material involved, identify the three-digit guide number by looking up the name in the alphabetical list (blue-bordered pages), then using the three-digit guide number, consult the recommendations in the assigned guide.
- Pressure and diameter of pipe (the pipeline operator can tell you this if you don't already know it)
- Timing of valve closure by the pipeline operator (quickly for automated valves; longer for manually operated valves)
- Dissipation time of the product in the pipeline once valves are closed
- Ability to conduct atmospheric monitoring and/or air sampling
- Weather (wind direction, etc.)
- Local variables such as topography, population density, demographics, and fire suppression methods available
- Nearby building construction material/density
- Natural and man-made barriers (such as highways, railroads, rivers, etc.)

U.S. Pipeline Resources

U.S. Pipeline Locations: The National Pipeline Mapping System (NPMS) *https://www.npms.phmsa.dot.gov* indicates the general locations of hazardous liquids and natural gas transmission pipelines found within the U.S. The pipelines depicted in the NPMS are within 500 feet of their actual locations. Emergency responders may apply for an NPMS web viewer account that will allow access to more detailed information than is available to the general public. The NPMS does not contain gathering/production or natural gas distribution pipelines.

U.S. Pipeline Emergency Response Training: Where appropriate, reference pipeline emergencies training materials produced by the Pipeline and Hazardous Materials Safety Administration. Your state or jurisdiction also may provide training on how to handle the response to a pipeline incident.

Other Resources:

Pipeline Association for Public Awareness
https://www.pipelineawareness.org/

U.S. DOT, Pipeline and Hazardous Materials Safety Administration
https://www.phmsa.dot.gov/safety-awareness/pipeline/safety-awareness-overview

Pipeline Emergency Responders Initiative (PERI)
https://www.phmsa.dot.gov/pipeline/peri/pipeline-emergency-responders-initiative-peri

Canadian Pipeline Resources

Canadian Pipeline Locations: The Canadian Energy Pipeline Association (CEPA) provides the general locations of natural gas and liquid pipelines found within Canada.

https://www.cepa.com

INTRODUCTION TO YELLOW PAGES

For entries highlighted in green follow these steps:

- **IF THERE IS NO FIRE**:
  - Go directly to **Table 1** (green-bordered pages)
  - Look up the ID number and name of material
  - Identify initial isolation and protective action distances
  - Also consult the appropriate Orange Guide

- **IF A FIRE IS INVOLVED**:
  - Use the appropriate Orange Guide for **EVACUATION** distances
  - Also protect in downwind direction according to Table 1 for residual material release

Note 1: If the name in **Table 1** is shown with **(when spilled in water)**, these materials produce large amounts of Toxic Inhalation Hazard (TIH) (PIH in the US) gases when spilled in water. Some Water Reactive materials are also TIH materials themselves (e.g., UN1746 (Bromine trifluoride), UN1836 (Thionyl chloride)). In these instances, two entries are provided in **Table 1** for land-based and water-based spills. If a water-reactive material only has one entry in Table 1 for **(when spilled in water)** and the product is NOT spilled in water, Table 1 and Table 2 do not apply. You will find safe distances in the appropriate orange-bordered guide.

Note 2: **Explosives** are not individually listed by their ID number because in an emergency situation, the response will be based only on the division of the explosive, not on the individual explosive.

For divisions 1.1, 1.2, 1.3 and 1.5, refer to GUIDE 112.

For divisions 1.4 and 1.6, refer to GUIDE 114.

Note 3: Chemical warfare agents do not have an assigned ID number because they are not commercially transported. In an emergency situation, the assigned orange guide will provide guidance for the initial response. Also consult "Criminal or Terrorist Use of Chemical, Biological and Radiological Agents", pp. 368 to 372.

ID No.	Guide No.	Name of Material
—	**117**	AC
—	**154**	Adamsite
—	**112**	Ammonium nitrate-fuel oil mixtures
—	**158**	Biological agents
—	**112**	Blasting agent, n.o.s.
—	**153**	Buzz
—	**153**	BZ
—	**159**	CA
—	**125**	CG
—	**125**	CK
—	**153**	CN
—	**153**	CS
—	**154**	CX
—	**151**	DA
—	**153**	DC
—	**154**	DM
—	**125**	DP
—	**151**	ED
—	**112**	Explosives, division 1.1, 1.2, 1.3 or 1.5
—	**114**	Explosives, division 1.4 or 1.6
—	**153**	GA
—	**153**	GB
—	**153**	GD
—	**153**	GF
—	**153**	H
—	**153**	HD
—	**153**	HL
—	**153**	HN-1
—	**153**	HN-2
—	**153**	HN-3

ID No.	Guide No.	Name of Material
—	**153**	L (Lewisite)
—	**153**	Lewisite
—	**152**	MD
—	**153**	Mustard
—	**153**	Mustard Lewisite
—	**152**	PD
—	**119**	SA
—	**153**	Sarin
—	**153**	Soman
—	**153**	Tabun
—	**153**	Thickened GD
—	**153**	Toxins
—	**153**	VX
1001	**116**	Acetylene, dissolved
1002	**122**	Air, compressed
1003	**122**	Air, refrigerated liquid (cryogenic liquid)
1005	**125**	Ammonia, anhydrous
1005	**125**	Anhydrous ammonia
1006	**120**	Argon
1006	**120**	Argon, compressed
1008	**125**	Boron trifluoride
1008	**125**	Boron trifluoride, compressed
1009	**126**	Bromotrifluoromethane
1009	**126**	Refrigerant gas R-13B1
1010	**116P**	Butadienes, stabilized
1010	**116P**	Butadienes and hydrocarbon mixture, stabilized
1010	**116P**	Hydrocarbon and butadienes mixture, stabilized
1011	**115**	Butane
1012	**115**	Butylene

ID No.	Guide No.	Name of Material
1013	**120**	Carbon dioxide
1013	**120**	Carbon dioxide, compressed
1014	**122**	Carbon dioxide and Oxygen mixture, compressed
1014	**122**	Oxygen and Carbon dioxide mixture, compressed
1015	**126**	Carbon dioxide and Nitrous oxide mixture
1015	**126**	Nitrous oxide and Carbon dioxide mixture
1016	**119**	Carbon monoxide
1016	**119**	Carbon monoxide, compressed
1017	**124**	Chlorine
1018	**126**	Chlorodifluoromethane
1018	**126**	Refrigerant gas R-22
1020	**126**	Chloropentafluoroethane
1020	**126**	Refrigerant gas R-115
1021	**126**	1-Chloro-1,2,2,2-tetrafluoroethane
1021	**126**	Refrigerant gas R-124
1022	**126**	Chlorotrifluoromethane
1022	**126**	Refrigerant gas R-13
1023	**119**	Coal gas
1023	**119**	Coal gas, compressed
1026	**119**	Cyanogen
1027	**115**	Cyclopropane
1028	**126**	Dichlorodifluoromethane
1028	**126**	Refrigerant gas R-12
1029	**126**	Dichlorofluoromethane
1029	**126**	Refrigerant gas R-21
1030	**115**	1,1-Difluoroethane
1030	**115**	Refrigerant gas R-152a
1032	**118**	Dimethylamine, anhydrous
1033	**115**	Dimethyl ether
1035	**115**	Ethane
1035	**115**	Ethane, compressed
1036	**118**	Ethylamine
1037	**115**	Ethyl chloride
1038	**115**	Ethylene, refrigerated liquid (cryogenic liquid)
1039	**115**	Ethyl methyl ether
1039	**115**	Methyl ethyl ether
1040	**119P**	Ethylene oxide
1040	**119P**	Ethylene oxide with Nitrogen
1041	**115**	Carbon dioxide and Ethylene oxide mixture, with more than 9% but not more than 87% Ethylene oxide
1041	**115**	Ethylene oxide and Carbon dioxide mixture, with more than 9% but not more than 87% Ethylene oxide
1043	**125**	Fertilizer, ammoniating solution, with free Ammonia
1044	**126**	Fire extinguishers with compressed or liquefied gas
1045	**124**	Fluorine
1045	**124**	Fluorine, compressed
1046	**120**	Helium
1046	**120**	Helium, compressed
1048	**125**	Hydrogen bromide, anhydrous
1049	**115**	Hydrogen
1049	**115**	Hydrogen, compressed
1050	**125**	Hydrogen chloride, anhydrous
1051	**117P**	Hydrogen cyanide, anhydrous, stabilized
1051	**117P**	Hydrogen cyanide, stabilized
1052	**125**	Hydrogen fluoride, anhydrous

ID No.	Guide No.	Name of Material
1053	**117**	Hydrogen sulfide
1053	**117**	Hydrogen sulphide
1055	**115**	Isobutylene
1056	**120**	Krypton
1056	**120**	Krypton, compressed
1057	**115**	Lighter refills containing flammable gas
1057	**115**	Lighters containing flammable gas
1057	**128**	Lighters, non-pressurized, containing flammable liquid
1058	**120**	Liquefied gases, non-flammable, charged with Nitrogen, Carbon dioxide or Air
1060	**116P**	Methylacetylene and Propadiene mixture, stabilized
1060	**116P**	Propadiene and Methylacetylene mixture, stabilized
1061	**118**	Methylamine, anhydrous
1062	**123**	Methyl bromide
1063	**115**	Methyl chloride
1063	**115**	Refrigerant gas R-40
1064	**117**	Methyl mercaptan
1065	**120**	Neon
1065	**120**	Neon, compressed
1066	**120**	Nitrogen
1066	**120**	Nitrogen, compressed
1067	**124**	Dinitrogen tetroxide
1067	**124**	Nitrogen dioxide
1069	**125**	Nitrosyl chloride
1070	**122**	Nitrous oxide
1070	**122**	Nitrous oxide, compressed
1071	**119**	Oil gas
1071	**119**	Oil gas, compressed
1072	**122**	Oxygen
1072	**122**	Oxygen, compressed
1073	**122**	Oxygen, refrigerated liquid (cryogenic liquid)
1075	**115**	Butane
1075	**115**	Butylene
1075	**115**	Isobutane
1075	**115**	Isobutylene
1075	**115**	Liquefied petroleum gas
1075	**115**	LPG
1075	**115**	Petroleum gases, liquefied
1075	**115**	Propane
1075	**115**	Propylene
1076	**125**	Phosgene
1077	**115**	Propylene
1078	**126**	Dispersant gas, n.o.s.
1078	**126**	Refrigerant gas, n.o.s.
1079	**125**	Sulfur dioxide
1079	**125**	Sulphur dioxide
1080	**126**	Sulfur hexafluoride
1080	**126**	Sulphur hexafluoride
1081	**116P**	Tetrafluoroethylene, stabilized
1082	**119P**	Refrigerant gas R-1113
1082	**119P**	Trifluorochloroethylene, stabilized
1083	**118**	Trimethylamine, anhydrous
1085	**116P**	Vinyl bromide, stabilized
1086	**116P**	Vinyl chloride, stabilized
1087	**116P**	Vinyl methyl ether, stabilized
1088	**127**	Acetal

ID No.	Guide No.	Name of Material
1089	**129P**	Acetaldehyde
1090	**127**	Acetone
1091	**127**	Acetone oils
1092	**131P**	Acrolein, stabilized
1093	**131P**	Acrylonitrile, stabilized
1098	**131**	Allyl alcohol
1099	**131P**	Allyl bromide
1100	**131P**	Allyl chloride
1104	**129**	Amyl acetates
1105	**129**	Pentanols
1106	**132**	Amylamine
1107	**129**	Amyl chloride
1108	**128**	n-Amylene
1108	**128**	1-Pentene
1109	**129**	Amyl formates
1110	**127**	n-Amyl methyl ketone
1110	**127**	Methyl amyl ketone
1111	**130**	Amyl mercaptan
1112	**128**	Amyl nitrate
1113	**129**	Amyl nitrite
1114	**130**	Benzene
1120	**129**	Butanols
1123	**129**	Butyl acetates
1125	**132**	n-Butylamine
1126	**130**	1-Bromobutane
1126	**130**	n-Butyl bromide
1127	**130**	n-Butyl chloride
1127	**130**	Chlorobutanes
1128	**129**	n-Butyl formate
1129	**129P**	Butyraldehyde
1130	**128**	Camphor oil

ID No.	Guide No.	Name of Material
1131	**131**	Carbon bisulfide
1131	**131**	Carbon bisulphide
1131	**131**	Carbon disulfide
1131	**131**	Carbon disulphide
1133	**128**	Adhesives (flammable)
1134	**130**	Chlorobenzene
1135	**131**	Ethylene chlorohydrin
1136	**128**	Coal tar distillates, flammable
1139	**127**	Coating solution
1143	**131P**	Crotonaldehyde
1143	**131P**	Crotonaldehyde, stabilized
1144	**128**	Crotonylene
1145	**128**	Cyclohexane
1146	**128**	Cyclopentane
1147	**130**	Decahydronaphthalene
1148	**129**	Diacetone alcohol
1149	**128**	Butyl ethers
1149	**128**	Dibutyl ethers
1150	**130P**	1,2-Dichloroethylene
1152	**130**	Dichloropentanes
1153	**127**	Ethylene glycol diethyl ether
1154	**132**	Diethylamine
1155	**127**	Diethyl ether
1155	**127**	Ethyl ether
1156	**127**	Diethyl ketone
1157	**128**	Diisobutyl ketone
1158	**132**	Diisopropylamine
1159	**127**	Diisopropyl ether
1160	**132**	Dimethylamine, aqueous solution
1160	**132**	Dimethylamine, solution
1161	**129**	Dimethyl carbonate

ID No.	Guide No.	Name of Material
1162	**155**	Dimethyldichlorosilane
1163	**131**	Dimethylhydrazine, unsymmetrical
1164	**130**	Dimethyl sulfide
1164	**130**	Dimethyl sulphide
1165	**127**	Dioxane
1166	**127**	Dioxolane
1167	**128P**	Divinyl ether, stabilized
1169	**127**	Extracts, aromatic, liquid
1170	**127**	Ethanol
1170	**127**	Ethanol, solution
1170	**127**	Ethyl alcohol
1170	**127**	Ethyl alcohol, solution
1171	**127**	Ethylene glycol monoethyl ether
1172	**129**	Ethylene glycol monoethyl ether acetate
1173	**129**	Ethyl acetate
1175	**130**	Ethylbenzene
1176	**129**	Ethyl borate
1177	**130**	2-Ethylbutyl acetate
1178	**130**	2-Ethylbutyraldehyde
1179	**127**	Ethyl butyl ether
1180	**130**	Ethyl butyrate
1181	**155**	Ethyl chloroacetate
1182	**155**	Ethyl chloroformate
1183	**139**	Ethyldichlorosilane
1184	**131**	Ethylene dichloride
1185	**131P**	Ethyleneimine, stabilized
1188	**127**	Ethylene glycol monomethyl ether
1189	**129**	Ethylene glycol monomethyl ether acetate
1190	**129**	Ethyl formate
1191	**129**	Ethylhexaldehydes
1191	**129**	Octyl aldehydes
1192	**129**	Ethyl lactate
1193	**127**	Ethyl methyl ketone
1193	**127**	Methyl ethyl ketone
1194	**131**	Ethyl nitrite, solution
1195	**129**	Ethyl propionate
1196	**155**	Ethyltrichlorosilane
1197	**127**	Extracts, flavoring, liquid
1197	**127**	Extracts, flavouring, liquid
1198	**132**	Formaldehyde, solution, flammable
1198	**132**	Formalin (flammable)
1199	**153P**	Furaldehydes
1201	**127**	Fusel oil
1202	**128**	Diesel fuel
1202	**128**	Fuel oil
1202	**128**	Gas oil
1202	**128**	Heating oil, light
1203	**128**	Gasohol
1203	**128**	Gasoline
1203	**128**	Motor spirit
1203	**128**	Petrol
1204	**127**	Nitroglycerin, solution in alcohol, with not more than 1% Nitroglycerin
1206	**128**	Heptanes
1207	**130**	Hexaldehyde
1208	**128**	Hexanes
1208	**128**	Neohexane
1210	**129**	Ink, printer's, flammable
1210	**129**	Printing ink, flammable

ID No.	Guide No.	Name of Material
1210	**129**	Printing ink related material, flammable
1212	**129**	Isobutanol
1212	**129**	Isobutyl alcohol
1213	**129**	Isobutyl acetate
1214	**132**	Isobutylamine
1216	**128**	Isooctenes
1218	**130P**	Isoprene, stabilized
1219	**129**	Isopropanol
1219	**129**	Isopropyl alcohol
1220	**129**	Isopropyl acetate
1221	**132**	Isopropylamine
1222	**130**	Isopropyl nitrate
1223	**128**	Kerosene
1224	**127**	Ketones, liquid, n.o.s.
1228	**131**	Mercaptan mixture, liquid, flammable, poisonous, n.o.s.
1228	**131**	Mercaptan mixture, liquid, flammable, toxic, n.o.s.
1228	**131**	Mercaptans, liquid, flammable, poisonous, n.o.s.
1228	**131**	Mercaptans, liquid, flammable, toxic, n.o.s.
1229	**129**	Mesityl oxide
1230	**131**	Methanol
1230	**131**	Methyl alcohol
1231	**129**	Methyl acetate
1233	**130**	Methylamyl acetate
1234	**127**	Methylal
1235	**132**	Methylamine, aqueous solution
1237	**129**	Methyl butyrate
1238	**155**	Methyl chloroformate
1239	**131**	Methyl chloromethyl ether
1242	**139**	Methyldichlorosilane
1243	**129**	Methyl formate
1244	**131**	Methylhydrazine
1245	**127**	Methyl isobutyl ketone
1246	**127P**	Methyl isopropenyl ketone, stabilized
1247	**129P**	Methyl methacrylate monomer, stabilized
1248	**129**	Methyl propionate
1249	**127**	Methyl propyl ketone
1250	**155**	Methyltrichlorosilane
1251	**131P**	Methyl vinyl ketone, stabilized
1259	**131**	Nickel carbonyl
1261	**129**	Nitromethane
1262	**128**	Isooctane
1262	**128**	Octanes
1263	**128**	Paint (flammable)
1263	**128**	Paint related material (flammable)
1264	**129**	Paraldehyde
1265	**128**	Isopentane
1265	**128**	Pentanes
1266	**127**	Perfumery products, with flammable solvents
1267	**128**	Petroleum crude oil
1268	**128**	Petroleum distillates, n.o.s.
1268	**128**	Petroleum products, n.o.s.
1270	**128**	Oil, petroleum
1270	**128**	Petroleum oil
1272	**129**	Pine oil
1274	**129**	n-Propanol
1274	**129**	Propyl alcohol, normal
1275	**129P**	Propionaldehyde

ID No.	Guide No.	Name of Material
1276	**129**	n-Propyl acetate
1277	**132**	Propylamine
1278	**129**	1-Chloropropane
1278	**129**	Propyl chloride
1279	**130**	1,2-Dichloropropane
1280	**127P**	Propylene oxide
1281	**129**	Propyl formates
1282	**129**	Pyridine
1286	**127**	Rosin oil
1287	**127**	Rubber solution
1288	**128**	Shale oil
1289	**132**	Sodium methylate, solution in alcohol
1292	**129**	Ethyl silicate
1292	**129**	Tetraethyl silicate
1293	**127**	Tinctures, medicinal
1294	**130**	Toluene
1295	**139**	Trichlorosilane
1296	**132**	Triethylamine
1297	**132**	Trimethylamine, aqueous solution
1298	**155**	Trimethylchlorosilane
1299	**128**	Turpentine
1300	**128**	Turpentine substitute
1301	**129P**	Vinyl acetate, stabilized
1302	**127P**	Vinyl ethyl ether, stabilized
1303	**130P**	Vinylidene chloride, stabilized
1304	**127P**	Vinyl isobutyl ether, stabilized
1305	**155P**	Vinyltrichlorosilane
1305	**155P**	Vinyltrichlorosilane, stabilized
1306	**129**	Wood preservatives, liquid
1307	**130**	Xylenes

ID No.	Guide No.	Name of Material
1308	**170**	Zirconium suspended in a flammable liquid
1308	**170**	Zirconium suspended in a liquid (flammable)
1309	**170**	Aluminum powder, coated
1310	**113**	Ammonium picrate, wetted with not less than 10% water
1312	**133**	Borneol
1313	**133**	Calcium resinate
1314	**133**	Calcium resinate, fused
1318	**133**	Cobalt resinate, precipitated
1320	**113**	Dinitrophenol, wetted with not less than 15% water
1321	**113**	Dinitrophenolates, wetted with not less than 15% water
1322	**113**	Dinitroresorcinol, wetted with not less than 15% water
1323	**170**	Ferrocerium
1324	**133**	Films, nitrocellulose base
1325	**133**	Flammable solid, organic, n.o.s.
1325	**133**	Fusee (railway or highway)
1326	**170**	Hafnium powder, wetted with not less than 25% water
1327	**133**	Bhusa, wet, damp or contaminated with oil
1327	**133**	Hay, wet, damp or contaminated with oil
1327	**133**	Straw, wet, damp or contaminated with oil
1328	**133**	Hexamethylenetetramine
1330	**133**	Manganese resinate
1331	**133**	Matches, "strike anywhere"
1332	**133**	Metaldehyde
1333	**170**	Cerium, slabs, ingots or rods
1334	**133**	Naphthalene, crude

ID No.	Guide No.	Name of Material
1334	**133**	Naphthalene, refined
1336	**113**	Nitroguanidine, wetted with not less than 20% water
1336	**113**	Picrite, wetted with not less than 20% water
1337	**113**	Nitrostarch, wetted with not less than 20% water
1338	**133**	Phosphorus, amorphous
1338	**133**	Red phosphorus
1339	**139**	Phosphorus heptasulfide, free from yellow and white Phosphorus
1339	**139**	Phosphorus heptasulphide, free from yellow and white Phosphorus
1340	**139**	Phosphorus pentasulfide, free from yellow and white Phosphorus
1340	**139**	Phosphorus pentasulphide, free from yellow and white Phosphorus
1341	**139**	Phosphorus sesquisulfide, free from yellow and white Phosphorus
1341	**139**	Phosphorus sesquisulphide, free from yellow and white Phosphorus
1343	**139**	Phosphorus trisulfide, free from yellow and white Phosphorus
1343	**139**	Phosphorus trisulphide, free from yellow and white Phosphorus
1344	**113**	Picric acid, wetted with not less than 30% water
1344	**113**	Trinitrophenol, wetted with not less than 30% water
1345	**133**	Rubber scrap, powdered or granulated
1345	**133**	Rubber shoddy, powdered or granulated
1346	**170**	Silicon powder, amorphous
1347	**113**	Silver picrate, wetted with not less than 30% water
1348	**113**	Sodium dinitro-o-cresolate, wetted with not less than 15% water
1349	**113**	Sodium picramate, wetted with not less than 20% water
1350	**133**	Sulfur
1350	**133**	Sulphur
1352	**170**	Titanium powder, wetted with not less than 25% water
1353	**133**	Fabrics impregnated with weakly nitrated Nitrocellulose, n.o.s.
1353	**133**	Fibers impregnated with weakly nitrated Nitrocellulose, n.o.s.
1353	**133**	Fibres impregnated with weakly nitrated Nitrocellulose, n.o.s.
1354	**113**	Trinitrobenzene, wetted with not less than 30% water
1355	**113**	Trinitrobenzoic acid, wetted with not less than 30% water
1356	**113**	TNT, wetted with not less than 30% water
1356	**113**	Trinitrotoluene, wetted with not less than 30% water
1357	**113**	Urea nitrate, wetted with not less than 20% water
1358	**170**	Zirconium powder, wetted with not less than 25% water
1360	**139**	Calcium phosphide
1361	**133**	Carbon, animal or vegetable origin
1361	**133**	Charcoal
1362	**133**	Carbon, activated
1363	**135**	Copra
1364	**133**	Cotton waste, oily

ID No.	Guide No.	Name of Material
1365	**133**	Cotton
1365	**133**	Cotton, wet
1366	**135**	Diethylzinc
1369	**135**	p Nitrosodimethylaniline
1370	**135**	Dimethylzinc
1372	**133**	Fibers, animal or vegetable, burnt, wet or damp
1372	**133**	Fibres, animal or vegetable, burnt, wet or damp
1373	**133**	Fabrics, animal or vegetable or synthetic, n.o.s. with oil
1373	**133**	Fibers, animal or vegetable or synthetic, n.o.s. with oil
1373	**133**	Fibres, animal or vegetable or synthetic, n.o.s. with oil
1374	**133**	Fish meal, unstabilized
1374	**133**	Fish scrap, unstabilized
1376	**135**	Iron oxide, spent
1376	**135**	Iron sponge, spent
1378	**170**	Metal catalyst, wetted
1379	**133**	Paper, unsaturated oil treated
1380	**135**	Pentaborane
1381	**136**	Phosphorus, white, dry or under water or in solution
1381	**136**	Phosphorus, yellow, dry or under water or in solution
1381	**136**	White phosphorus, dry or under water or in solution
1381	**136**	Yellow phosphorus, dry or under water or in solution
1382	**135**	Potassium sulfide, anhydrous
1382	**135**	Potassium sulfide, with less than 30% water of crystallization
1382	**135**	Potassium sulphide, anhydrous
1382	**135**	Potassium sulphide, with less than 30% water of crystallization
1383	**135**	Aluminum powder, pyrophoric
1383	**135**	Pyrophoric alloy, n.o.s.
1383	**135**	Pyrophoric metal, n.o.s.
1384	**135**	Sodium dithionite
1384	**135**	Sodium hydrosulfite
1384	**135**	Sodium hydrosulphite
1385	**135**	Sodium sulfide, anhydrous
1385	**135**	Sodium sulfide, with less than 30% water of crystallization
1385	**135**	Sodium sulphide, anhydrous
1385	**135**	Sodium sulphide, with less than 30% water of crystallization
1386	**135**	Seed cake, with more than 1.5% oil and not more than 11% moisture
1387	**133**	Wool waste, wet
1389	**138**	Alkali metal amalgam, liquid
1390	**139**	Alkali metal amides
1391	**138**	Alkali metal dispersion
1391	**138**	Alkaline earth metal dispersion
1392	**138**	Alkaline earth metal amalgam, liquid
1393	**138**	Alkaline earth metal alloy, n.o.s.
1394	**138**	Aluminum carbide
1395	**139**	Aluminum ferrosilicon powder
1396	**138**	Aluminum powder, uncoated
1397	**139**	Aluminum phosphide
1398	**138**	Aluminum silicon powder, uncoated
1400	**138**	Barium
1401	**138**	Calcium

ID No.	Guide No.	Name of Material
1402	**138**	Calcium carbide
1403	**138**	Calcium cyanamide, with more than 0.1% Calcium carbide
1404	**138**	Calcium hydride
1405	**138**	Calcium silicide
1407	**138**	Caesium
1407	**138**	Cesium
1408	**139**	Ferrosilicon
1409	**138**	Metal hydrides, water-reactive, n.o.s.
1410	**138**	Lithium aluminum hydride
1411	**138**	Lithium aluminum hydride, ethereal
1413	**138**	Lithium borohydride
1414	**138**	Lithium hydride
1415	**138**	Lithium
1417	**138**	Lithium silicon
1418	**138**	Magnesium alloys powder
1418	**138**	Magnesium powder
1419	**139**	Magnesium aluminum phosphide
1420	**138**	Potassium, metal alloys, liquid
1421	**138**	Alkali metal alloy, liquid, n.o.s.
1422	**138**	Potassium sodium alloys, liquid
1422	**138**	Sodium potassium alloys, liquid
1423	**138**	Rubidium
1426	**138**	Sodium borohydride
1427	**138**	Sodium hydride
1428	**138**	Sodium
1431	**138**	Sodium methylate, dry
1432	**139**	Sodium phosphide
1433	**139**	Stannic phosphides
1435	**138**	Zinc ashes
1435	**138**	Zinc dross
1435	**138**	Zinc residue
1435	**138**	Zinc skimmings
1436	**138**	Zinc dust
1436	**138**	Zinc powder
1437	**138**	Zirconium hydride
1438	**140**	Aluminum nitrate
1439	**141**	Ammonium dichromate
1442	**143**	Ammonium perchlorate
1444	**140**	Ammonium persulfate
1444	**140**	Ammonium persulphate
1445	**141**	Barium chlorate, solid
1446	**141**	Barium nitrate
1447	**141**	Barium perchlorate, solid
1448	**141**	Barium permanganate
1449	**141**	Barium peroxide
1450	**140**	Bromates, inorganic, n.o.s.
1451	**140**	Caesium nitrate
1451	**140**	Cesium nitrate
1452	**140**	Calcium chlorate
1453	**140**	Calcium chlorite
1454	**140**	Calcium nitrate
1455	**140**	Calcium perchlorate
1456	**140**	Calcium permanganate
1457	**140**	Calcium peroxide
1458	**140**	Borate and Chlorate mixture
1458	**140**	Chlorate and Borate mixture
1459	**140**	Chlorate and Magnesium chloride mixture, solid
1459	**140**	Magnesium chloride and Chlorate mixture, solid
1461	**140**	Chlorates, inorganic, n.o.s.

ID No.	Guide No.	Name of Material
1462	**143**	Chlorites, inorganic, n.o.s.
1463	**141**	Chromium trioxide, anhydrous
1465	**140**	Didymium nitrate
1466	**140**	Ferric nitrate
1467	**143**	Guanidine nitrate
1469	**141**	Lead nitrate
1470	**141**	Lead perchlorate, solid
1471	**140**	Lithium hypochlorite, dry
1471	**140**	Lithium hypochlorite mixture
1471	**140**	Lithium hypochlorite mixtures, dry
1472	**143**	Lithium peroxide
1473	**140**	Magnesium bromate
1474	**140**	Magnesium nitrate
1475	**140**	Magnesium perchlorate
1476	**140**	Magnesium peroxide
1477	**140**	Nitrates, inorganic, n.o.s.
1479	**140**	Oxidizing solid, n.o.s.
1481	**140**	Perchlorates, inorganic, n.o.s.
1482	**140**	Permanganates, inorganic, n.o.s.
1483	**140**	Peroxides, inorganic, n.o.s.
1484	**140**	Potassium bromate
1485	**140**	Potassium chlorate
1486	**140**	Potassium nitrate
1487	**140**	Potassium nitrate and Sodium nitrite mixture
1487	**140**	Sodium nitrite and Potassium nitrate mixture
1488	**140**	Potassium nitrite
1489	**140**	Potassium perchlorate
1490	**140**	Potassium permanganate
1491	**144**	Potassium peroxide
1492	**140**	Potassium persulfate
1492	**140**	Potassium persulphate
1493	**140**	Silver nitrate
1494	**140**	Sodium bromate
1495	**140**	Sodium chlorate
1496	**143**	Sodium chlorite
1498	**140**	Sodium nitrate
1499	**140**	Potassium nitrate and Sodium nitrate mixture
1499	**140**	Sodium nitrate and Potassium nitrate mixture
1500	**141**	Sodium nitrite
1502	**140**	Sodium perchlorate
1503	**140**	Sodium permanganate
1504	**144**	Sodium peroxide
1505	**140**	Sodium persulfate
1505	**140**	Sodium persulphate
1506	**143**	Strontium chlorate
1507	**140**	Strontium nitrate
1508	**140**	Strontium perchlorate
1509	**143**	Strontium peroxide
1510	**143**	Tetranitromethane
1511	**140**	Urea hydrogen peroxide
1512	**140**	Zinc ammonium nitrite
1513	**140**	Zinc chlorate
1514	**140**	Zinc nitrate
1515	**140**	Zinc permanganate
1516	**143**	Zinc peroxide
1517	**113**	Zirconium picramate, wetted with not less than 20% water
1541	**155**	Acetone cyanohydrin, stabilized
1544	**151**	Alkaloids, solid, n.o.s. (poisonous)

ID No.	Guide No.	Name of Material
1544	**151**	Alkaloid salts, solid, n.o.s. (poisonous)
1545	**155**	Allyl isothiocyanate, stabilized
1546	**151**	Ammonium arsenate
1547	**153**	Aniline
1548	**153**	Aniline hydrochloride
1549	**157**	Antimony compound, inorganic, solid, n.o.s.
1550	**151**	Antimony lactate
1551	**151**	Antimony potassium tartrate
1553	**154**	Arsenic acid, liquid
1554	**154**	Arsenic acid, solid
1555	**151**	Arsenic bromide
1556	**152**	Arsenic compound, liquid, n.o.s.
1556	**152**	Methyldichloroarsine
1557	**152**	Arsenic compound, solid, n.o.s.
1558	**152**	Arsenic
1559	**151**	Arsenic pentoxide
1560	**157**	Arsenic chloride
1560	**157**	Arsenic trichloride
1561	**151**	Arsenic trioxide
1562	**152**	Arsenical dust
1564	**154**	Barium compound, n.o.s.
1565	**157**	Barium cyanide
1566	**154**	Beryllium compound, n.o.s.
1567	**134**	Beryllium powder
1569	**131**	Bromoacetone
1570	**152**	Brucine
1571	**113**	Barium azide, wetted with not less than 50% water
1572	**151**	Cacodylic acid
1573	**151**	Calcium arsenate

ID No.	Guide No.	Name of Material
1574	**151**	Calcium arsenate and Calcium arsenite mixture, solid
1574	**151**	Calcium arsenite and Calcium arsenate mixture, solid
1575	**157**	Calcium cyanide
1577	**153**	Chlorodinitrobenzenes, liquid
1578	**152**	Chloronitrobenzenes, solid
1579	**153**	4-Chloro-o-toluidine hydrochloride, solid
1580	**154**	Chloropicrin
1581	**123**	Chloropicrin and Methyl bromide mixture
1581	**123**	Methyl bromide and Chloropicrin mixture
1582	**119**	Chloropicrin and Methyl chloride mixture
1582	**119**	Methyl chloride and Chloropicrin mixture
1583	**154**	Chloropicrin mixture, n.o.s.
1585	**151**	Copper acetoarsenite
1586	**151**	Copper arsenite
1587	**151**	Copper cyanide
1588	**157**	Cyanides, inorganic, solid, n.o.s.
1589	**125**	Cyanogen chloride, stabilized
1590	**153**	Dichloroanilines, liquid
1591	**152**	o-Dichlorobenzene
1593	**160**	Dichloromethane
1593	**160**	Methylene chloride
1594	**152**	Diethyl sulfate
1594	**152**	Diethyl sulphate
1595	**156**	Dimethyl sulfate
1595	**156**	Dimethyl sulphate
1596	**153**	Dinitroanilines

ID No.	Guide No.	Name of Material
1597	**152**	Dinitrobenzenes, liquid
1598	**153**	Dinitro-o-cresol
1599	**153**	Dinitrophenol, solution
1600	**152**	Dinitrotoluenes, molten
1601	**151**	Disinfectant, solid, poisonous, n.o.s.
1601	**151**	Disinfectant, solid, toxic, n.o.s.
1602	**151**	Dye, liquid, poisonous, n.o.s.
1602	**151**	Dye, liquid, toxic, n.o.s.
1602	**151**	Dye intermediate, liquid, poisonous, n.o.s.
1602	**151**	Dye intermediate, liquid, toxic, n.o.s.
1603	**155**	Ethyl bromoacetate
1604	**132**	Ethylenediamine
1605	**154**	Ethylene dibromide
1606	**151**	Ferric arsenate
1607	**151**	Ferric arsenite
1608	**151**	Ferrous arsenate
1611	**151**	Hexaethyl tetraphosphate
1612	**123**	Compressed gas and hexaethyl tetraphosphate mixture
1612	**123**	Hexaethyl tetraphosphate and compressed gas mixture
1613	**154**	Hydrocyanic acid, aqueous solution, with less than 5% Hydrogen cyanide
1613	**154**	Hydrocyanic acid, aqueous solution, with not more than 20% Hydrogen cyanide
1613	**154**	Hydrogen cyanide, aqueous solution, with not more than 20% Hydrogen cyanide
1614	**152**	Hydrogen cyanide, stabilized (absorbed)
1616	**151**	Lead acetate

ID No.	Guide No.	Name of Material
1617	**151**	Lead arsenates
1618	**151**	Lead arsenites
1620	**151**	Lead cyanide
1621	**151**	London purple
1622	**151**	Magnesium arsenate
1623	**151**	Mercuric arsenate
1624	**154**	Mercuric chloride
1625	**141**	Mercuric nitrate
1626	**157**	Mercuric potassium cyanide
1627	**141**	Mercurous nitrate
1629	**151**	Mercury acetate
1630	**151**	Mercury ammonium chloride
1631	**154**	Mercury benzoate
1634	**154**	Mercury bromides
1636	**154**	Mercury cyanide
1637	**151**	Mercury gluconate
1638	**151**	Mercury iodide
1639	**151**	Mercury nucleate
1640	**151**	Mercury oleate
1641	**151**	Mercury oxide
1642	**151**	Mercury oxycyanide, desensitized
1643	**151**	Mercury potassium iodide
1644	**151**	Mercury salicylate
1645	**151**	Mercury sulfate
1645	**151**	Mercury sulphate
1646	**151**	Mercury thiocyanate
1647	**151**	Ethylene dibromide and Methyl bromide mixture, liquid
1647	**151**	Methyl bromide and Ethylene dibromide mixture, liquid
1648	**127**	Acetonitrile

ID No.	Guide No.	Name of Material
1649	**152**	Motor fuel anti-knock mixture
1650	**153**	beta-Naphthylamine, solid
1650	**153**	Naphthylamine (beta), solid
1651	**153**	Naphthylthiourea
1652	**153**	Naphthylurea
1653	**151**	Nickel cyanide
1654	**151**	Nicotine
1655	**151**	Nicotine compound, solid, n.o.s.
1655	**151**	Nicotine preparation, solid, n.o.s.
1656	**151**	Nicotine hydrochloride, liquid
1656	**151**	Nicotine hydrochloride, solution
1657	**151**	Nicotine salicylate
1658	**151**	Nicotine sulfate, solution
1658	**151**	Nicotine sulphate, solution
1659	**151**	Nicotine tartrate
1660	**124**	Nitric oxide
1660	**124**	Nitric oxide, compressed
1661	**153**	Nitroanilines
1662	**152**	Nitrobenzene
1663	**153**	Nitrophenols
1664	**152**	Nitrotoluenes, liquid
1665	**152**	Nitroxylenes, liquid
1669	**151**	Pentachloroethane
1670	**157**	Perchloromethyl mercaptan
1671	**153**	Phenol, solid
1672	**151**	Phenylcarbylamine chloride
1673	**153**	Phenylenediamines
1674	**151**	Phenylmercuric acetate
1677	**151**	Potassium arsenate
1678	**154**	Potassium arsenite
1679	**157**	Potassium cuprocyanide
1680	**157**	Potassium cyanide, solid
1683	**151**	Silver arsenite
1684	**151**	Silver cyanide
1685	**151**	Sodium arsenate
1686	**154**	Sodium arsenite, aqueous solution
1687	**153**	Sodium azide
1688	**152**	Sodium cacodylate
1689	**157**	Sodium cyanide, solid
1690	**154**	Sodium fluoride, solid
1691	**151**	Strontium arsenite
1692	**151**	Strychnine
1692	**151**	Strychnine salts
1693	**159**	Tear gas devices
1693	**159**	Tear gas substance, liquid, n.o.s.
1694	**159**	Bromobenzyl cyanides, liquid
1695	**131**	Chloroacetone, stabilized
1697	**153**	Chloroacetophenone, solid
1698	**154**	Diphenylamine chloroarsine
1699	**151**	Diphenylchloroarsine, liquid
1700	**159**	Tear gas candles
1700	**159**	Tear gas grenades
1701	**152**	Xylyl bromide, liquid
1702	**151**	1,1,2,2-Tetrachloroethane
1704	**153**	Tetraethyl dithiopyrophosphate
1707	**151**	Thallium compound, n.o.s.
1708	**153**	Toluidines, liquid
1709	**151**	2,4-Toluenediamine, solid
1709	**151**	2,4-Toluylenediamine, solid
1710	**160**	Trichloroethylene
1711	**153**	Xylidines, liquid

ID No.	Guide No.	Name of Material
1712	**151**	Zinc arsenate
1712	**151**	Zinc arsenate and Zinc arsenite mixture
1712	**151**	Zinc arsenite
1712	**151**	Zinc arsenite and Zinc arsenate mixture
1713	**151**	Zinc cyanide
1714	**139**	Zinc phosphide
1715	**137**	Acetic anhydride
1716	**156**	Acetyl bromide
1717	**155**	Acetyl chloride
1718	**153**	Acid butyl phosphate
1718	**153**	Butyl acid phosphate
1719	**154**	Caustic alkali liquid, n.o.s.
1722	**155**	Allyl chlorocarbonate
1722	**155**	Allyl chloroformate
1723	**132**	Allyl iodide
1724	**155**	Allyltrichlorosilane, stabilized
1725	**137**	Aluminum bromide, anhydrous
1726	**137**	Aluminum chloride, anhydrous
1727	**154**	Ammonium bifluoride, solid
1727	**154**	Ammonium hydrogendifluoride, solid
1728	**155**	Amyltrichlorosilane
1729	**156**	Anisoyl chloride
1730	**157**	Antimony pentachloride, liquid
1731	**157**	Antimony pentachloride, solution
1732	**157**	Antimony pentafluoride
1733	**157**	Antimony trichloride
1733	**157**	Antimony trichloride, liquid
1733	**157**	Antimony trichloride, solid
1736	**137**	Benzoyl chloride
1737	**156**	Benzyl bromide
1738	**156**	Benzyl chloride
1739	**137**	Benzyl chloroformate
1740	**154**	Hydrogendifluorides, solid, n.o.s.
1741	**125**	Boron trichloride
1742	**157**	Boron trifluoride acetic acid complex, liquid
1743	**157**	Boron trifluoride propionic acid complex, liquid
1744	**154**	Bromine
1744	**154**	Bromine, solution
1744	**154**	Bromine, solution (Inhalation Hazard Zone A)
1744	**154**	Bromine, solution (Inhalation Hazard Zone B)
1745	**144**	Bromine pentafluoride
1746	**144**	Bromine trifluoride
1747	**155**	Butyltrichlorosilane
1748	**140**	Calcium hypochlorite, dry
1748	**140**	Calcium hypochlorite mixture, dry, with more than 39% available Chlorine (8.8% available Oxygen)
1749	**124**	Chlorine trifluoride
1750	**153**	Chloroacetic acid, solution
1751	**153**	Chloroacetic acid, solid
1752	**156**	Chloroacetyl chloride
1753	**156**	Chlorophenyltrichlorosilane
1754	**137**	Chlorosulfonic acid (with or without sulfur trioxide)
1754	**137**	Chlorosulphonic acid (with or without sulphur trioxide)
1755	**154**	Chromic acid, solution
1756	**154**	Chromic fluoride, solid

ID No.	Guide No.	Name of Material
1757	**154**	Chromic fluoride, solution
1758	**137**	Chromium oxychloride
1759	**154**	Corrosive solid, n.o.s.
1759	**154**	Ferrous chloride, solid
1760	**154**	Chemical kit
1760	**154**	Compounds, cleaning liquid (corrosive)
1760	**154**	Compounds, tree or weed killing, liquid (corrosive)
1760	**154**	Corrosive liquid, n.o.s.
1760	**154**	Ferrous chloride, solution
1761	**154**	Cupriethylenediamine, solution
1762	**156**	Cyclohexenyltrichlorosilane
1763	**156**	Cyclohexyltrichlorosilane
1764	**153**	Dichloroacetic acid
1765	**156**	Dichloroacetyl chloride
1766	**156**	Dichlorophenyltrichlorosilane
1767	**155**	Diethyldichlorosilane
1768	**154**	Difluorophosphoric acid, anhydrous
1769	**156**	Diphenyldichlorosilane
1770	**153**	Diphenylmethyl bromide
1771	**156**	Dodecyltrichlorosilane
1773	**157**	Ferric chloride, anhydrous
1774	**154**	Fire extinguisher charges, corrosive liquid
1775	**154**	Fluoroboric acid
1776	**154**	Fluorophosphoric acid, anhydrous
1777	**137**	Fluorosulfonic acid
1777	**137**	Fluorosulphonic acid
1778	**154**	Fluorosilicic acid
1778	**154**	Hydrofluorosilicic acid

ID No.	Guide No.	Name of Material
1779	**153**	Formic acid
1779	**153**	Formic acid, with more than 85% acid
1780	**156**	Fumaryl chloride
1781	**156**	Hexadecyltrichlorosilane
1782	**154**	Hexafluorophosphoric acid
1783	**153**	Hexamethylenediamine, solution
1784	**156**	Hexyltrichlorosilane
1786	**157**	Hydrofluoric acid and Sulfuric acid mixture
1786	**157**	Hydrofluoric acid and Sulphuric acid mixture
1786	**157**	Sulfuric acid and Hydrofluoric acid mixture
1786	**157**	Sulphuric acid and Hydrofluoric acid mixture
1787	**154**	Hydriodic acid
1788	**154**	Hydrobromic acid
1789	**157**	Hydrochloric acid
1789	**157**	Muriatic acid
1790	**157**	Hydrofluoric acid
1791	**154**	Hypochlorite solution
1791	**154**	Sodium hypochlorite
1792	**157**	Iodine monochloride, solid
1793	**153**	Isopropyl acid phosphate
1794	**154**	Lead sulfate, with more than 3% free acid
1794	**154**	Lead sulphate, with more than 3% free acid
1796	**157**	Nitrating acid mixture with more than 50% nitric acid
1796	**157**	Nitrating acid mixture with not more than 50% nitric acid
1798	**157**	Aqua regia
1798	**157**	Nitrohydrochloric acid

ID No.	Guide No.	Name of Material
1799	**156**	Nonyltrichlorosilane
1800	**156**	Octadecyltrichlorosilane
1801	**156**	Octyltrichlorosilane
1802	**157**	Perchloric acid, with not more than 50% acid
1803	**153**	Phenolsulfonic acid, liquid
1803	**153**	Phenolsulphonic acid, liquid
1804	**156**	Phenyltrichlorosilane
1805	**154**	Phosphoric acid, solution
1806	**137**	Phosphorus pentachloride
1807	**137**	Phosphorus pentoxide
1808	**137**	Phosphorus tribromide
1809	**137**	Phosphorus trichloride
1810	**137**	Phosphorus oxychloride
1811	**154**	Potassium hydrogen difluoride, solid
1812	**154**	Potassium fluoride, solid
1813	**154**	Caustic potash, solid
1813	**154**	Potassium hydroxide, solid
1814	**154**	Caustic potash, solution
1814	**154**	Potassium hydroxide, solution
1815	**132**	Propionyl chloride
1816	**155**	Propyltrichlorosilane
1817	**137**	Pyrosulfuryl chloride
1817	**137**	Pyrosulphuryl chloride
1818	**157**	Silicon tetrachloride
1819	**154**	Sodium aluminate, solution
1823	**154**	Caustic soda, solid
1823	**154**	Sodium hydroxide, solid
1824	**154**	Caustic soda, solution
1824	**154**	Sodium hydroxide, solution
1825	**157**	Sodium monoxide

ID No.	Guide No.	Name of Material
1826	**157**	Nitrating acid mixture, spent, with more than 50% nitric acid
1826	**157**	Nitrating acid mixture, spent, with not more than 50% nitric acid
1827	**137**	Stannic chloride, anhydrous
1827	**137**	Tin tetrachloride
1828	**137**	Sulfur chlorides
1828	**137**	Sulphur chlorides
1829	**137**	Sulfur trioxide, stabilized
1829	**137**	Sulphur trioxide, stabilized
1830	**137**	Sulfuric acid
1830	**137**	Sulfuric acid, with more than 51% acid
1830	**137**	Sulphuric acid
1830	**137**	Sulphuric acid, with more than 51% acid
1831	**137**	Sulfuric acid, fuming
1831	**137**	Sulphuric acid, fuming
1832	**137**	Sulfuric acid, spent
1832	**137**	Sulphuric acid, spent
1833	**154**	Sulfurous acid
1833	**154**	Sulphurous acid
1834	**137**	Sulfuryl chloride
1834	**137**	Sulphuryl chloride
1835	**153**	Tetramethylammonium hydroxide, solution
1836	**137**	Thionyl chloride
1837	**157**	Thiophosphoryl chloride
1838	**137**	Titanium tetrachloride
1839	**153**	Trichloroacetic acid
1840	**154**	Zinc chloride, solution
1841	**171**	Acetaldehyde ammonia

ID No.	Guide No.	Name of Material
1843	**141**	Ammonium dinitro-o-cresolate, solid
1845	**120**	Carbon dioxide, solid
1845	**120**	Dry ice
1846	**151**	Carbon tetrachloride
1847	**153**	Potassium sulfide, hydrated, with not less than 30% water of crystallization
1847	**153**	Potassium sulphide, hydrated, with not less than 30% water of crystallization
1848	**153**	Propionic acid
1848	**153**	Propionic acid, with not less than 10% and less than 90% acid
1849	**153**	Sodium sulfide, hydrated, with not less than 30% water
1849	**153**	Sodium sulphide, hydrated, with not less than 30% water
1851	**151**	Medicine, liquid, poisonous, n.o.s.
1851	**151**	Medicine, liquid, toxic, n.o.s.
1854	**135**	Barium alloys, pyrophoric
1855	**135**	Calcium, pyrophoric
1855	**135**	Calcium alloys, pyrophoric
1856	**133**	Rags, oily
1857	**133**	Textile waste, wet
1858	**126**	Hexafluoropropylene
1858	**126**	Hexafluoropropylene, compressed
1858	**126**	Refrigerant gas R-1216
1859	**125**	Silicon tetrafluoride
1859	**125**	Silicon tetrafluoride, compressed
1860	**116P**	Vinyl fluoride, stabilized
1862	**130**	Ethyl crotonate
1863	**128**	Fuel, aviation, turbine engine
1865	**128**	n-Propyl nitrate
1866	**127**	Resin solution
1868	**134**	Decaborane
1869	**138**	Magnesium
1869	**138**	Magnesium, in pellets, turnings or ribbons
1869	**138**	Magnesium alloys, with more than 50% Magnesium, in pellets, turnings or ribbons
1870	**138**	Potassium borohydride
1871	**170**	Titanium hydride
1872	**140**	Lead dioxide
1873	**143**	Perchloric acid, with more than 50% but not more than 72% acid
1884	**157**	Barium oxide
1885	**153**	Benzidine
1886	**156**	Benzylidene chloride
1887	**160**	Bromochloromethane
1888	**151**	Chloroform
1889	**157**	Cyanogen bromide
1891	**131**	Ethyl bromide
1892	**151**	Ethyldichloroarsine
1894	**151**	Phenylmercuric hydroxide
1895	**151**	Phenylmercuric nitrate
1897	**160**	Perchloroethylene
1897	**160**	Tetrachloroethylene
1898	**156**	Acetyl iodide
1902	**153**	Diisooctyl acid phosphate
1903	**153**	Disinfectant, liquid, corrosive, n.o.s.
1905	**154**	Selenic acid
1906	**153**	Acid, sludge

ID No.	Guide No.	Name of Material
1906	**153**	Sludge acid
1907	**154**	Soda lime, with more than 4% Sodium hydroxide
1908	**154**	Chlorite solution
1910	**157**	Calcium oxide
1911	**119**	Diborane
1911	**119**	Diborane, compressed
1911	**119**	Diborane mixtures
1912	**115**	Methyl chloride and Methylene chloride mixture
1912	**115**	Methylene chloride and Methyl chloride mixture
1913	**120**	Neon, refrigerated liquid (cryogenic liquid)
1914	**130**	Butyl propionates
1915	**127**	Cyclohexanone
1916	**152**	2,2'-Dichlorodiethyl ether
1916	**152**	Dichloroethyl ether
1917	**129P**	Ethyl acrylate, stabilized
1918	**130**	Cumene
1918	**130**	Isopropylbenzene
1919	**129P**	Methyl acrylate, stabilized
1920	**128**	Nonanes
1921	**131P**	Propyleneimine, stabilized
1922	**132**	Pyrrolidine
1923	**135**	Calcium dithionite
1923	**135**	Calcium hydrosulfite
1923	**135**	Calcium hydrosulphite
1928	**138**	Methyl magnesium bromide in Ethyl ether
1929	**135**	Potassium dithionite
1929	**135**	Potassium hydrosulfite
1929	**135**	Potassium hydrosulphite

ID No.	Guide No.	Name of Material
1931	**171**	Zinc dithionite
1931	**171**	Zinc hydrosulfite
1931	**171**	Zinc hydrosulphite
1932	**135**	Zirconium scrap
1935	**157**	Cyanide solution, n.o.s.
1938	**156**	Bromoacetic acid, solution
1939	**137**	Phosphorus oxybromide, solid
1940	**153**	Thioglycolic acid
1941	**171**	Dibromodifluoromethane
1941	**171**	Refrigerant gas R-12B2
1942	**140**	Ammonium nitrate, with not more than 0.2% combustible substances
1944	**133**	Matches, safety
1945	**133**	Matches, wax "vesta"
1950	**126**	Aerosols
1951	**120**	Argon, refrigerated liquid (cryogenic liquid)
1952	**126**	Carbon dioxide and Ethylene oxide mixtures, with not more than 9% Ethylene oxide
1952	**126**	Ethylene oxide and Carbon dioxide mixtures, with not more than 9% Ethylene oxide
1953	**119**	Compressed gas, poisonous, flammable, n.o.s.
1953	**119**	Compressed gas, poisonous, flammable, n.o.s. (Inhalation Hazard Zone A)
1953	**119**	Compressed gas, poisonous, flammable, n.o.s. (Inhalation Hazard Zone B)
1953	**119**	Compressed gas, poisonous, flammable, n.o.s. (Inhalation Hazard Zone C)
1953	**119**	Compressed gas, poisonous, flammable, n.o.s. (Inhalation Hazard Zone D)

ID No.	Guide No.	Name of Material
1953	**119**	Compressed gas, toxic, flammable, n.o.s.
1953	**119**	Compressed gas, toxic, flammable, n.o.s. (Inhalation Hazard Zone A)
1953	**119**	Compressed gas, toxic, flammable, n.o.s. (Inhalation Hazard Zone B)
1953	**119**	Compressed gas, toxic, flammable, n.o.s. (Inhalation Hazard Zone C)
1953	**119**	Compressed gas, toxic, flammable, n.o.s. (Inhalation Hazard Zone D)
1954	**115**	Compressed gas, flammable, n.o.s.
1954	**115**	Dispersant gases, n.o.s. (flammable)
1954	**115**	Refrigerant gases, n.o.s. (flammable)
1955	**123**	Compressed gas, poisonous, n.o.s.
1955	**123**	Compressed gas, poisonous, n.o.s. (Inhalation Hazard Zone A)
1955	**123**	Compressed gas, poisonous, n.o.s. (Inhalation Hazard Zone B)
1955	**123**	Compressed gas, poisonous, n.o.s. (Inhalation Hazard Zone C)
1955	**123**	Compressed gas, poisonous, n.o.s. (Inhalation Hazard Zone D)
1955	**123**	Compressed gas, toxic, n.o.s.
1955	**123**	Compressed gas, toxic, n.o.s. (Inhalation Hazard Zone A)
1955	**123**	Compressed gas, toxic, n.o.s. (Inhalation Hazard Zone B)
1955	**123**	Compressed gas, toxic, n.o.s. (Inhalation Hazard Zone C)

ID No.	Guide No.	Name of Material
1955	**123**	Compressed gas, toxic, n.o.s. (Inhalation Hazard Zone D)
1955	**123**	Organic phosphate compound mixed with compressed gas
1955	**123**	Organic phosphate mixed with compressed gas
1955	**123**	Organic phosphorus compound mixed with compressed gas
1956	**126**	Compressed gas, n.o.s.
1957	**115**	Deuterium
1957	**115**	Deuterium, compressed
1958	**126**	1,2-Dichloro-1,1,2,2-tetrafluoroethane
1958	**126**	Refrigerant gas R-114
1959	**116P**	1,1-Difluoroethylene
1959	**116P**	Refrigerant gas R-1132a
1961	**115**	Ethane, refrigerated liquid
1961	**115**	Ethane-Propane mixture, refrigerated liquid
1961	**115**	Propane-Ethane mixture, refrigerated liquid
1962	**116P**	Ethylene
1962	**116P**	Ethylene, compressed
1963	**120**	Helium, refrigerated liquid (cryogenic liquid)
1964	**115**	Hydrocarbon gas mixture, compressed, n.o.s.
1965	**115**	Hydrocarbon gas mixture, liquefied, n.o.s.
1966	**115**	Hydrogen, refrigerated liquid (cryogenic liquid)
1967	**123**	Insecticide gas, poisonous, n.o.s.
1967	**123**	Insecticide gas, toxic, n.o.s.
1967	**123**	Parathion and compressed gas mixture

ID No.	Guide No.	Name of Material
1968	**126**	Insecticide gas, n.o.s.
1969	**115**	Isobutane
1970	**120**	Krypton, refrigerated liquid (cryogenic liquid)
1971	**115**	Methane
1971	**115**	Methane, compressed
1971	**115**	Natural gas, compressed
1972	**115**	Liquefied natural gas (cryogenic liquid)
1972	**115**	LNG (cryogenic liquid)
1972	**115**	Methane, refrigerated liquid (cryogenic liquid)
1972	**115**	Natural gas, refrigerated liquid (cryogenic liquid)
1973	**126**	Chlorodifluoromethane and Chloropentafluoroethane mixture
1973	**126**	Chloropentafluoroethane and Chlorodifluoromethane mixture
1973	**126**	Refrigerant gas R-502
1974	**126**	Chlorodifluorobromomethane
1974	**126**	Refrigerant gas R-12B1
1975	**124**	Dinitrogen tetroxide and Nitric oxide mixture
1975	**124**	Nitric oxide and Dinitrogen tetroxide mixture
1975	**124**	Nitric oxide and Nitrogen dioxide mixture
1975	**124**	Nitrogen dioxide and Nitric oxide mixture
1976	**126**	Octafluorocyclobutane
1976	**126**	Refrigerant gas RC-318
1977	**120**	Nitrogen, refrigerated liquid (cryogenic liquid)
1978	**115**	Propane
1982	**126**	Refrigerant gas R-14
1982	**126**	Refrigerant gas R-14, compressed
1982	**126**	Tetrafluoromethane
1982	**126**	Tetrafluoromethane, compressed
1983	**126**	1-Chloro-2,2,2-trifluoroethane
1983	**126**	Refrigerant gas R-133a
1984	**126**	Refrigerant gas R-23
1984	**126**	Trifluoromethane
1986	**131**	Alcohols, flammable, poisonous, n.o.s.
1986	**131**	Alcohols, flammable, toxic, n.o.s.
1987	**127**	Alcohols, n.o.s.
1987	**127**	Denatured alcohol
1988	**131P**	Aldehydes, flammable, poisonous, n.o.s.
1988	**131P**	Aldehydes, flammable, toxic, n.o.s.
1989	**129P**	Aldehydes, n.o.s.
1990	**171**	Benzaldehyde
1991	**131P**	Chloroprene, stabilized
1992	**131**	Flammable liquid, poisonous, n.o.s.
1992	**131**	Flammable liquid, toxic, n.o.s.
1993	**128**	Combustible liquid, n.o.s.
1993	**128**	Compounds, cleaning liquid (flammable)
1993	**128**	Compounds, tree or weed killing, liquid (flammable)
1993	**128**	Diesel fuel
1993	**128**	Flammable liquid, n.o.s.
1993	**128**	Fuel oil
1994	**136**	Iron pentacarbonyl

ID No.	Guide No.	Name of Material
1999	**130**	Asphalt
1999	**130**	Asphalt, cut back
1999	**130**	Tars, liquid
2000	**133**	Celluloid, in blocks, rods, rolls, sheets, tubes, etc., except scrap
2001	**133**	Cobalt naphthenates, powder
2002	**135**	Celluloid, scrap
2004	**135**	Magnesium diamide
2005	**135**	Magnesium diphenyl
2006	**135**	Plastics, nitrocellulose-based, self-heating, n.o.s.
2008	**135**	Zirconium powder, dry
2009	**135**	Zirconium, dry, finished sheets, strips or coiled wire
2010	**138**	Magnesium hydride
2011	**139**	Magnesium phosphide
2012	**139**	Potassium phosphide
2013	**139**	Strontium phosphide
2014	**140**	Hydrogen peroxide, aqueous solution, with not less than 20% but not more than 60% Hydrogen peroxide (stabilized as necessary)
2015	**143**	Hydrogen peroxide, aqueous solution, stabilized, with more than 60% Hydrogen peroxide
2015	**143**	Hydrogen peroxide, stabilized
2016	**151**	Ammunition, poisonous, non-explosive
2016	**151**	Ammunition, toxic, non-explosive
2017	**159**	Ammunition, tear-producing, non-explosive
2018	**152**	Chloroanilines, solid
2019	**152**	Chloroanilines, liquid
2020	**153**	Chlorophenols, solid
2021	**153**	Chlorophenols, liquid
2022	**153**	Cresylic acid
2023	**131P**	Epichlorohydrin
2024	**151**	Mercury compound, liquid, n.o.s.
2025	**151**	Mercury compound, solid, n.o.s.
2026	**151**	Phenylmercuric compound, n.o.s.
2027	**151**	Sodium arsenite, solid
2028	**153**	Bombs, smoke, non-explosive, with corrosive liquid, without initiating device
2029	**132**	Hydrazine, anhydrous
2030	**153**	Hydrazine, aqueous solution, with more than 37% Hydrazine
2031	**157**	Nitric acid, other than red fuming, with more than 65% nitric acid
2031	**157**	Nitric acid, other than red fuming, with not more than 65% nitric acid
2032	**157**	Nitric acid, red fuming
2033	**154**	Potassium monoxide
2034	**115**	Hydrogen and Methane mixture, compressed
2034	**115**	Methane and Hydrogen mixture, compressed
2035	**115**	Refrigerant gas R-143a
2035	**115**	1,1,1-Trifluoroethane
2036	**120**	Xenon
2036	**120**	Xenon, compressed
2037	**115**	Gas cartridges
2037	**115**	Receptacles, small, containing gas

ID No.	Guide No.	Name of Material
2038	**152**	Dinitrotoluenes, liquid
2044	**115**	2,2-Dimethylpropane
2045	**130**	Isobutyl aldehyde
2045	**130**	Isobutyraldehyde
2046	**130**	Cymenes
2047	**129**	Dichloropropenes
2048	**130P**	Dicyclopentadiene
2049	**130**	Diethylbenzene
2050	**128**	Diisobutylene, isomeric compounds
2051	**132**	2-Dimethylaminoethanol
2052	**128**	Dipentene
2053	**129**	Methylamyl alcohol
2053	**129**	Methyl isobutyl carbinol
2054	**132**	Morpholine
2055	**128P**	Styrene monomer, stabilized
2056	**127**	Tetrahydrofuran
2057	**128**	Tripropylene
2058	**129**	Valeraldehyde
2059	**127**	Nitrocellulose, solution, flammable
2067	**140**	Ammonium nitrate based fertilizer
2071	**140**	Ammonium nitrate based fertilizer
2073	**125**	Ammonia, solution, with more than 35% but not more than 50% Ammonia
2074	**153P**	Acrylamide, solid
2075	**153**	Chloral, anhydrous, stabilized
2076	**153**	Cresols, liquid
2077	**153**	alpha-Naphthylamine
2077	**153**	Naphthylamine (alpha)
2078	**156**	Toluene diisocyanate
2079	**154**	Diethylenetriamine
2186	**125**	Hydrogen chloride, refrigerated liquid
2187	**120**	Carbon dioxide, refrigerated liquid
2188	**119**	Arsine
2189	**119**	Dichlorosilane
2190	**124**	Oxygen difluoride
2190	**124**	Oxygen difluoride, compressed
2191	**123**	Sulfuryl fluoride
2191	**123**	Sulphuryl fluoride
2192	**119**	Germane
2193	**126**	Hexafluoroethane
2193	**126**	Hexafluoroethane, compressed
2193	**126**	Refrigerant gas R-116
2193	**126**	Refrigerant gas R-116, compressed
2194	**125**	Selenium hexafluoride
2195	**125**	Tellurium hexafluoride
2196	**125**	Tungsten hexafluoride
2197	**125**	Hydrogen iodide, anhydrous
2198	**125**	Phosphorus pentafluoride
2198	**125**	Phosphorus pentafluoride, compressed
2199	**119**	Phosphine
2200	**116P**	Propadiene, stabilized
2201	**122**	Nitrous oxide, refrigerated liquid
2202	**117**	Hydrogen selenide, anhydrous
2203	**116**	Silane
2203	**116**	Silane, compressed
2204	**119**	Carbonyl sulfide
2204	**119**	Carbonyl sulphide
2205	**153**	Adiponitrile

ID No.	Guide No.	Name of Material
2206	**155**	Isocyanate solution, poisonous, n.o.s.
2206	**155**	Isocyanate solution, toxic, n.o.s.
2206	**155**	Isocyanates, poisonous, n.o.s.
2206	**155**	Isocyanates, toxic, n.o.s.
2208	**140**	Bleaching powder
2208	**140**	Calcium hypochlorite mixture, dry, with more than 10% but not more than 39% available Chlorine
2209	**153**	Formaldehyde, solution (corrosive)
2209	**153**	Formalin (corrosive)
2210	**135**	Maneb
2210	**135**	Maneb preparation, with not less than 60% Maneb
2211	**171**	Polymeric beads, expandable
2212	**171**	Asbestos
2212	**171**	Asbestos, amphibole
2212	**171**	Asbestos, blue
2212	**171**	Asbestos, brown
2212	**171**	Blue asbestos
2212	**171**	Brown asbestos
2213	**133**	Paraformaldehyde
2214	**156**	Phthalic anhydride
2215	**156**	Maleic anhydride
2215	**156**	Maleic anhydride, molten
2216	**171**	Fish meal, stabilized
2216	**171**	Fish scrap, stabilized
2217	**135**	Seed cake, with not more than 1.5% oil and not more than 11% moisture
2218	**132P**	Acrylic acid, stabilized
2219	**129**	Allyl glycidyl ether
2222	**128**	Anisole
2224	**152**	Benzonitrile
2225	**156**	Benzenesulfonyl chloride
2225	**156**	Benzenesulphonyl chloride
2226	**156**	Benzotrichloride
2227	**130P**	n-Butyl methacrylate, stabilized
2232	**153**	Chloroacetaldehyde
2232	**153**	2-Chloroethanal
2233	**152**	Chloroanisidines
2234	**130**	Chlorobenzotrifluorides
2235	**153**	Chlorobenzyl chlorides, liquid
2236	**156**	3-Chloro-4-methylphenyl isocyanate, liquid
2237	**153**	Chloronitroanilines
2238	**129**	Chlorotoluenes
2239	**153**	Chlorotoluidines, solid
2240	**154**	Chromosulfuric acid
2240	**154**	Chromosulphuric acid
2241	**128**	Cycloheptane
2242	**128**	Cycloheptene
2243	**130**	Cyclohexyl acetate
2244	**129**	Cyclopentanol
2245	**128**	Cyclopentanone
2246	**128**	Cyclopentene
2247	**128**	n-Decane
2248	**132**	Di-n-butylamine
2249	**131**	Dichlorodimethyl ether, symmetrical
2250	**156**	Dichlorophenyl isocyanates
2251	**128P**	Bicyclo[2.2.1]hepta-2,5-diene, stabilized
2251	**128P**	2,5-Norbornadiene, stabilized

ID No.	Guide No.	Name of Material
2252	**127**	1,2-Dimethoxyethane
2253	**153**	N,N-Dimethylaniline
2254	**133**	Matches, fusee
2256	**130**	Cyclohexene
2257	**138**	Potassium
2258	**132**	1,2-Propylenediamine
2259	**153**	Triethylenetetramine
2260	**132**	Tripropylamine
2261	**153**	Xylenols, solid
2262	**156**	Dimethylcarbamoyl chloride
2263	**128**	Dimethylcyclohexanes
2264	**132**	N,N-Dimethylcyclohexylamine
2264	**132**	Dimethylcyclohexylamine
2265	**129**	N,N-Dimethylformamide
2266	**132**	Dimethyl-N-propylamine
2267	**156**	Dimethyl thiophosphoryl chloride
2269	**153**	3,3'-Iminodipropylamine
2270	**132**	Ethylamine, aqueous solution, with not less than 50% but not more than 70% Ethylamine
2271	**128**	Ethyl amyl ketone
2272	**153**	N-Ethylaniline
2273	**153**	2-Ethylaniline
2274	**153**	N-Ethyl-N-benzylaniline
2275	**129**	2-Ethylbutanol
2276	**132**	2-Ethylhexylamine
2277	**130P**	Ethyl methacrylate, stabilized
2278	**128**	n-Heptene
2279	**151**	Hexachlorobutadiene
2280	**153**	Hexamethylenediamine, solid
2281	**156**	Hexamethylene diisocyanate
2282	**129**	Hexanols
2283	**130P**	Isobutyl methacrylate, stabilized
2284	**131**	Isobutyronitrile
2285	**156**	Isocyanatobenzotrifluorides
2286	**128**	Pentamethylheptane
2287	**128**	Isoheptenes
2288	**128**	Isohexenes
2289	**153**	Isophoronediamine
2290	**156**	Isophorone diisocyanate
2291	**151**	Lead compound, soluble, n.o.s.
2293	**128**	4-Methoxy-4-methylpentan-2-one
2294	**153**	N-Methylaniline
2295	**155**	Methyl chloroacetate
2296	**128**	Methylcyclohexane
2297	**128**	Methylcyclohexanone
2298	**128**	Methylcyclopentane
2299	**155**	Methyl dichloroacetate
2300	**153**	2-Methyl-5-ethylpyridine
2301	**128**	2-Methylfuran
2302	**127**	5-Methylhexan-2-one
2303	**128**	Isopropenylbenzene
2304	**133**	Naphthalene, molten
2305	**153**	Nitrobenzenesulfonic acid
2305	**153**	Nitrobenzenesulphonic acid
2306	**152**	Nitrobenzotrifluorides, liquid
2307	**152**	3-Nitro-4-chlorobenzotrifluoride
2308	**157**	Nitrosylsulfuric acid, liquid
2308	**157**	Nitrosylsulphuric acid, liquid
2309	**128P**	Octadiene
2310	**131**	Pentane-2,4-dione
2311	**153**	Phenetidines

ID No.	Guide No.	Name of Material
2312	**153**	Phenol, molten
2313	**129**	Picolines
2315	**171**	Articles containing Polychlorinated biphenyls (PCB)
2315	**171**	PCB
2315	**171**	Polychlorinated biphenyls, liquid
2316	**157**	Sodium cuprocyanide, solid
2317	**157**	Sodium cuprocyanide, solution
2318	**135**	Sodium hydrosulfide, with less than 25% water of crystallization
2318	**135**	Sodium hydrosulphide, with less than 25% water of crystallization
2319	**128**	Terpene hydrocarbons, n.o.s.
2320	**153**	Tetraethylenepentamine
2321	**153**	Trichlorobenzenes, liquid
2322	**152**	Trichlorobutene
2323	**130**	Triethyl phosphite
2324	**128**	Triisobutylene
2325	**129**	1,3,5-Trimethylbenzene
2326	**153**	Trimethylcyclohexylamine
2327	**153**	Trimethylhexamethylenediamines
2328	**156**	Trimethylhexamethylene diisocyanate
2329	**130**	Trimethyl phosphite
2330	**128**	Undecane
2331	**154**	Zinc chloride, anhydrous
2332	**129**	Acetaldehyde oxime
2333	**131**	Allyl acetate
2334	**131**	Allylamine
2335	**131**	Allyl ethyl ether
2336	**131**	Allyl formate

ID No.	Guide No.	Name of Material
2337	**131**	Phenyl mercaptan
2338	**127**	Benzotrifluoride
2339	**130**	2-Bromobutane
2340	**130**	2-Bromoethyl ethyl ether
2341	**130**	1-Bromo-3-methylbutane
2342	**130**	Bromomethylpropanes
2343	**130**	2-Bromopentane
2344	**129**	Bromopropanes
2345	**130**	3-Bromopropyne
2346	**127**	Butanedione
2346	**127**	Diacetyl
2347	**130**	Butyl mercaptan
2348	**129P**	Butyl acrylates, stabilized
2350	**127**	Butyl methyl ether
2351	**129**	Butyl nitrites
2352	**127P**	Butyl vinyl ether, stabilized
2353	**132**	Butyryl chloride
2354	**131**	Chloromethyl ethyl ether
2356	**129**	2-Chloropropane
2357	**132**	Cyclohexylamine
2358	**128P**	Cyclooctatetraene
2359	**132**	Diallylamine
2360	**131P**	Diallyl ether
2361	**132**	Diisobutylamine
2362	**130**	1,1-Dichloroethane
2363	**129**	Ethyl mercaptan
2364	**128**	n-Propyl benzene
2366	**128**	Diethyl carbonate
2367	**130**	alpha-Methylvaleraldehyde
2367	**130**	Methyl valeraldehyde (alpha)
2368	**128**	alpha-Pinene

ID No.	Guide No.	Name of Material
2368	**128**	Pinene (alpha)
2370	**128**	1-Hexene
2371	**128**	Isopentenes
2372	**129**	1,2-Di-(dimethylamino)ethane
2373	**127**	Diethoxymethane
2374	**127**	3,3-Diethoxypropene
2375	**129**	Diethyl sulfide
2375	**129**	Diethyl sulphide
2376	**127**	2,3-Dihydropyran
2377	**127**	1,1-Dimethoxyethane
2378	**131**	2-Dimethylaminoacetonitrile
2379	**132**	1,3-Dimethylbutylamine
2380	**127**	Dimethyldiethoxysilane
2381	**131**	Dimethyl disulfide
2381	**131**	Dimethyl disulphide
2382	**131**	Dimethylhydrazine, symmetrical
2383	**132**	Dipropylamine
2384	**127**	Di-n-propyl ether
2385	**129**	Ethyl isobutyrate
2386	**132**	1-Ethylpiperidine
2387	**130**	Fluorobenzene
2388	**130**	Fluorotoluenes
2389	**128**	Furan
2390	**129**	2-Iodobutane
2391	**129**	Iodomethylpropanes
2392	**129**	Iodopropanes
2393	**129**	Isobutyl formate
2394	**129**	Isobutyl propionate
2395	**132**	Isobutyryl chloride
2396	**131P**	Methacrylaldehyde, stabilized
2397	**127**	3-Methylbutan-2-one
2398	**127**	Methyl tert-butyl ether
2399	**132**	1-Methylpiperidine
2400	**130**	Methyl isovalerate
2401	**132**	Piperidine
2402	**130**	Propanethiols
2403	**129P**	Isopropenyl acetate
2404	**131**	Propionitrile
2405	**129**	Isopropyl butyrate
2406	**127**	Isopropyl isobutyrate
2407	**155**	Isopropyl chloroformate
2409	**129**	Isopropyl propionate
2410	**129**	1,2,3,6-Tetrahydropyridine
2411	**131**	Butyronitrile
2412	**130**	Tetrahydrothiophene
2413	**128**	Tetrapropyl orthotitanate
2414	**130**	Thiophene
2416	**129**	Trimethyl borate
2417	**125**	Carbonyl fluoride
2417	**125**	Carbonyl fluoride, compressed
2418	**125**	Sulfur tetrafluoride
2418	**125**	Sulphur tetrafluoride
2419	**116**	Bromotrifluoroethylene
2420	**125**	Hexafluoroacetone
2421	**124**	Nitrogen trioxide
2422	**126**	Octafluorobut-2-ene
2422	**126**	Refrigerant gas R-1318
2424	**126**	Octafluoropropane
2424	**126**	Refrigerant gas R-218
2426	**140**	Ammonium nitrate, liquid (hot concentrated solution)
2427	**140**	Potassium chlorate, aqueous solution

ID No.	Guide No.	Name of Material
2428	**140**	Sodium chlorate, aqueous solution
2429	**140**	Calcium chlorate, aqueous solution
2430	**153**	Alkylphenols, solid, n.o.s. (including C2-C12 homologues)
2431	**153**	Anisidines
2432	**153**	N,N-Diethylaniline
2433	**152**	Chloronitrotoluenes, liquid
2434	**156**	Dibenzyldichlorosilane
2435	**156**	Ethylphenyldichlorosilane
2436	**129**	Thioacetic acid
2437	**156**	Methylphenyldichlorosilane
2438	**131**	Trimethylacetyl chloride
2439	**154**	Sodium hydrogendifluoride
2440	**154**	Stannic chloride, pentahydrate
2441	**135**	Titanium trichloride, pyrophoric
2441	**135**	Titanium trichloride mixture, pyrophoric
2442	**156**	Trichloroacetyl chloride
2443	**137**	Vanadium oxytrichloride
2444	**137**	Vanadium tetrachloride
2446	**153**	Nitrocresols, solid
2447	**136**	Phosphorus, white, molten
2447	**136**	White phosphorus, molten
2448	**133**	Molten sulfur
2448	**133**	Molten sulphur
2448	**133**	Sulfur, molten
2448	**133**	Sulphur, molten
2451	**122**	Nitrogen trifluoride
2451	**122**	Nitrogen trifluoride, compressed
2452	**116P**	Ethylacetylene, stabilized
2453	**115**	Ethyl fluoride
2453	**115**	Refrigerant gas R-161
2454	**115**	Methyl fluoride
2454	**115**	Refrigerant gas R-41
2455	**116**	Methyl nitrite
2456	**130P**	2-Chloropropene
2457	**128**	2,3-Dimethylbutane
2458	**130**	Hexadiene
2459	**128**	2-Methyl-1-butene
2460	**128**	2-Methyl-2-butene
2461	**128**	Methylpentadiene
2463	**138**	Aluminum hydride
2464	**141**	Beryllium nitrate
2465	**140**	Dichloroisocyanuric acid, dry
2465	**140**	Dichloroisocyanuric acid salts
2465	**140**	Sodium dichloroisocyanurate
2465	**140**	Sodium dichloro-s-triazinetrione
2466	**143**	Potassium superoxide
2468	**140**	Trichloroisocyanuric acid, dry
2469	**140**	Zinc bromate
2470	**152**	Phenylacetonitrile, liquid
2471	**154**	Osmium tetroxide
2473	**154**	Sodium arsanilate
2474	**157**	Thiophosgene
2475	**157**	Vanadium trichloride
2477	**131**	Methyl isothiocyanate
2478	**155**	Isocyanate solution, flammable, poisonous, n.o.s.
2478	**155**	Isocyanate solution, flammable, toxic, n.o.s.
2478	**155**	Isocyanates, flammable, poisonous, n.o.s.

ID No.	Guide No.	Name of Material
2478	**155**	Isocyanates, flammable, toxic, n.o.s.
2480	**155P**	Methyl isocyanate
2481	**155**	Ethyl isocyanate
2482	**155P**	n-Propyl isocyanate
2483	**155P**	Isopropyl isocyanate
2484	**155**	tert-Butyl isocyanate
2485	**155P**	n-Butyl isocyanate
2486	**155P**	Isobutyl isocyanate
2487	**155**	Phenyl isocyanate
2488	**155**	Cyclohexyl isocyanate
2490	**153**	Dichloroisopropyl ether
2491	**153**	Ethanolamine
2491	**153**	Ethanolamine, solution
2491	**153**	Monoethanolamine
2493	**132**	Hexamethyleneimine
2495	**144**	Iodine pentafluoride
2496	**156**	Propionic anhydride
2498	**129**	1,2,3,6-Tetrahydrobenzaldehyde
2501	**152**	Tris-(1-aziridinyl)phosphine oxide, solution
2502	**132**	Valeryl chloride
2503	**137**	Zirconium tetrachloride
2504	**159**	Acetylene tetrabromide
2504	**159**	Tetrabromoethane
2505	**154**	Ammonium fluoride
2506	**154**	Ammonium hydrogen sulfate
2506	**154**	Ammonium hydrogen sulphate
2507	**154**	Chloroplatinic acid, solid
2508	**156**	Molybdenum pentachloride
2509	**154**	Potassium hydrogen sulfate
2509	**154**	Potassium hydrogen sulphate
2511	**153**	2-Chloropropionic acid
2512	**152**	Aminophenols
2513	**156**	Bromoacetyl bromide
2514	**130**	Bromobenzene
2515	**159**	Bromoform
2516	**151**	Carbon tetrabromide
2517	**115**	1-Chloro-1,1-difluoroethane
2517	**115**	Difluorochloroethanes
2517	**115**	Refrigerant gas R-142b
2518	**153**	1,5,9-Cyclododecatriene
2520	**130P**	Cyclooctadienes
2521	**131P**	Diketene, stabilized
2522	**153P**	2-Dimethylaminoethyl methacrylate
2524	**129**	Ethyl orthoformate
2525	**156**	Ethyl oxalate
2526	**132**	Furfurylamine
2527	**129P**	Isobutyl acrylate, stabilized
2528	**130**	Isobutyl isobutyrate
2529	**132**	Isobutyric acid
2531	**153P**	Methacrylic acid, stabilized
2533	**156**	Methyl trichloroacetate
2534	**119**	Methylchlorosilane
2535	**132**	4-Methylmorpholine
2535	**132**	N-Methylmorpholine
2536	**127**	Methyltetrahydrofuran
2538	**133**	Nitronaphthalene
2541	**128**	Terpinolene
2542	**153**	Tributylamine
2545	**135**	Hafnium powder, dry
2546	**135**	Titanium powder, dry
2547	**143**	Sodium superoxide

ID No.	Guide No.	Name of Material
2548	**124**	Chlorine pentafluoride
2552	**151**	Hexafluoroacetone hydrate, liquid
2554	**130P**	Methylallyl chloride
2555	**113**	Nitrocellulose with water, not less than 25% water
2556	**113**	Nitrocellulose with alcohol, not less than 25% alcohol
2557	**133**	Nitrocellulose mixture, without pigment
2557	**133**	Nitrocellulose mixture, without plasticizer
2557	**133**	Nitrocellulose mixture, with pigment
2557	**133**	Nitrocellulose mixture, with plasticizer
2558	**131**	Epibromohydrin
2560	**129**	2-Methylpentan-2-ol
2561	**128**	3-Methyl-1-butene
2564	**153**	Trichloroacetic acid, solution
2565	**153**	Dicyclohexylamine
2567	**154**	Sodium pentachlorophenate
2570	**154**	Cadmium compound
2571	**156**	Alkylsulfuric acids
2571	**156**	Alkylsulphuric acids
2572	**153**	Phenylhydrazine
2573	**141**	Thallium chlorate
2574	**151**	Tricresyl phosphate
2576	**137**	Phosphorus oxybromide, molten
2577	**156**	Phenylacetyl chloride
2578	**157**	Phosphorus trioxide
2579	**153**	Piperazine
2580	**154**	Aluminum bromide, solution
2581	**154**	Aluminum chloride, solution
2582	**154**	Ferric chloride, solution
2583	**153**	Alkyl sulfonic acids, solid, with more than 5% free Sulfuric acid
2583	**153**	Alkyl sulphonic acids, solid, with more than 5% free Sulphuric acid
2583	**153**	Aryl sulfonic acids, solid, with more than 5% free Sulfuric acid
2583	**153**	Aryl sulphonic acids, solid, with more than 5% free Sulphuric acid
2584	**153**	Alkyl sulfonic acids, liquid, with more than 5% free Sulfuric acid
2584	**153**	Alkyl sulphonic acids, liquid, with more than 5% free Sulphuric acid
2584	**153**	Aryl sulfonic acids, liquid, with more than 5% free Sulfuric acid
2584	**153**	Aryl sulphonic acids, liquid, with more than 5% free Sulphuric acid
2585	**153**	Alkyl sulfonic acids, solid, with not more than 5% free Sulfuric acid
2585	**153**	Alkyl sulphonic acids, solid, with not more than 5% free Sulphuric acid
2585	**153**	Aryl sulfonic acids, solid, with not more than 5% free Sulfuric acid
2585	**153**	Aryl sulphonic acids, solid, with not more than 5% free Sulphuric acid
2586	**153**	Alkyl sulfonic acids, liquid, with not more than 5% free Sulfuric acid
2586	**153**	Alkyl sulphonic acids, liquid, with not more than 5% free Sulphuric acid

ID No.	Guide No.	Name of Material
2586	**153**	Aryl sulfonic acids, liquid, with not more than 5% free Sulfuric acid
2586	**153**	Aryl sulphonic acids, liquid, with not more than 5% free Sulphuric acid
2587	**153**	Benzoquinone
2588	**151**	Pesticide, solid, poisonous, n.o.s.
2588	**151**	Pesticide, solid, toxic, n.o.s.
2589	**155**	Vinyl chloroacetate
2590	**171**	Asbestos, chrysotile
2590	**171**	Asbestos, white
2590	**171**	White asbestos
2591	**120**	Xenon, refrigerated liquid (cryogenic liquid)
2599	**126**	Chlorotrifluoromethane and Trifluoromethane azeotropic mixture with approximately 60% Chlorotrifluoromethane
2599	**126**	Refrigerant gas R-503
2599	**126**	Trifluoromethane and Chlorotrifluoromethane azeotropic mixture with approximately 60% Chlorotrifluoromethane
2601	**115**	Cyclobutane
2602	**126**	Dichlorodifluoromethane and Difluoroethane azeotropic mixture with approximately 74% Dichlorodifluoromethane
2602	**126**	Difluoroethane and Dichlorodifluoromethane azeotropic mixture with approximately 74% Dichlorodifluoromethane
2602	**126**	Refrigerant gas R-500
2603	**131**	Cycloheptatriene
2604	**132**	Boron trifluoride diethyl etherate
2605	**155**	Methoxymethyl isocyanate
2606	**155**	Methyl orthosilicate
2607	**129P**	Acrolein dimer, stabilized
2608	**129**	Nitropropanes
2609	**156**	Triallyl borate
2610	**132**	Triallylamine
2611	**131**	Propylene chlorohydrin
2612	**127**	Methyl propyl ether
2614	**129**	Methallyl alcohol
2615	**127**	Ethyl propyl ether
2616	**129**	Triisopropyl borate
2617	**129**	Methylcyclohexanols
2618	**130P**	Vinyltoluenes, stabilized
2619	**132**	Benzyldimethylamine
2620	**130**	Amyl butyrates
2621	**127**	Acetyl methyl carbinol
2622	**131P**	Glycidaldehyde
2623	**133**	Firelighters, solid, with flammable liquid
2624	**138**	Magnesium silicide
2626	**140**	Chloric acid, aqueous solution, with not more than 10% Chloric acid
2627	**140**	Nitrites, inorganic, n.o.s.
2628	**151**	Potassium fluoroacetate
2629	**151**	Sodium fluoroacetate
2630	**151**	Selenates
2630	**151**	Selenites
2642	**154**	Fluoroacetic acid
2643	**155**	Methyl bromoacetate
2644	**151**	Methyl iodide
2645	**153**	Phenacyl bromide

ID No.	Guide No.	Name of Material
2646	**151**	Hexachlorocyclopentadiene
2647	**153**	Malononitrile
2648	**154**	1,2-Dibromobutan-3-one
2649	**153**	1,3-Dichloroacetone
2650	**153**	1,1-Dichloro-1-nitroethane
2651	**153**	4,4'-Diaminodiphenylmethane
2653	**156**	Benzyl iodide
2655	**151**	Potassium fluorosilicate
2656	**154**	Quinoline
2657	**153**	Selenium disulfide
2657	**153**	Selenium disulphide
2659	**151**	Sodium chloroacetate
2660	**153**	Mononitrotoluidines
2660	**153**	Nitrotoluidines (mono)
2661	**153**	Hexachloroacetone
2664	**160**	Dibromomethane
2667	**152**	Butyltoluenes
2668	**131**	Chloroacetonitrile
2669	**152**	Chlorocresols, solution
2670	**157**	Cyanuric chloride
2671	**153**	Aminopyridines
2672	**154**	Ammonia, solution, with more than 10% but not more than 35% Ammonia
2672	**154**	Ammonium hydroxide
2672	**154**	Ammonium hydroxide, with more than 10% but not more than 35% Ammonia
2673	**151**	2-Amino-4-chlorophenol
2674	**154**	Sodium fluorosilicate
2676	**119**	Stibine
2677	**154**	Rubidium hydroxide, solution
2678	**154**	Rubidium hydroxide, solid
2679	**154**	Lithium hydroxide, solution
2680	**154**	Lithium hydroxide
2681	**154**	Caesium hydroxide, solution
2681	**154**	Cesium hydroxide, solution
2682	**157**	Caesium hydroxide
2682	**157**	Cesium hydroxide
2683	**132**	Ammonium sulfide, solution
2683	**132**	Ammonium sulphide, solution
2684	**132**	3-Diethylaminopropylamine
2685	**132**	N,N-Diethylethylenediamine
2686	**132**	2-Diethylaminoethanol
2687	**133**	Dicyclohexylammonium nitrite
2688	**159**	1-Bromo-3-chloropropane
2689	**153**	Glycerol alpha-monochlorohydrin
2690	**152**	N,n-Butylimidazole
2691	**137**	Phosphorus pentabromide
2692	**157**	Boron tribromide
2693	**154**	Bisulfites, aqueous solution, n.o.s.
2693	**154**	Bisulphites, aqueous solution, n.o.s.
2698	**156**	Tetrahydrophthalic anhydrides
2699	**154**	Trifluoroacetic acid
2705	**153P**	1-Pentol
2707	**127**	Dimethyldioxanes
2709	**128**	Butylbenzenes
2710	**128**	Dipropyl ketone
2713	**153**	Acridine
2714	**133**	Zinc resinate
2715	**133**	Aluminum resinate
2716	**153**	1,4-Butynediol

ID No.	Guide No.	Name of Material
2717	**133**	Camphor, synthetic
2719	**141**	Barium bromate
2720	**141**	Chromium nitrate
2721	**140**	Copper chlorate
2722	**140**	Lithium nitrate
2723	**140**	Magnesium chlorate
2724	**140**	Manganese nitrate
2725	**140**	Nickel nitrate
2726	**140**	Nickel nitrite
2727	**141**	Thallium nitrate
2728	**140**	Zirconium nitrate
2729	**152**	Hexachlorobenzene
2730	**152**	Nitroanisoles, liquid
2732	**152**	Nitrobromobenzenes, liquid
2733	**132**	Amines, flammable, corrosive, n.o.s.
2733	**132**	Polyamines, flammable, corrosive, n.o.s.
2734	**132**	Amines, liquid, corrosive, flammable, n.o.s.
2734	**132**	Polyamines, liquid, corrosive, flammable, n.o.s.
2735	**153**	Amines, liquid, corrosive, n.o.s.
2735	**153**	Polyamines, liquid, corrosive, n.o.s.
2738	**153**	N-Butylaniline
2739	**156**	Butyric anhydride
2740	**155**	n-Propyl chloroformate
2741	**141**	Barium hypochlorite, with more than 22% available Chlorine
2742	**155**	sec-Butyl chloroformate
2742	**155**	Chloroformates, poisonous, corrosive, flammable, n.o.s.
2742	**155**	Chloroformates, toxic, corrosive, flammable, n.o.s.
2742	**155**	Isobutyl chloroformate
2743	**155**	n-Butyl chloroformate
2744	**155**	Cyclobutyl chloroformate
2745	**157**	Chloromethyl chloroformate
2746	**156**	Phenyl chloroformate
2747	**156**	tert-Butylcyclohexyl chloroformate
2748	**156**	2-Ethylhexyl chloroformate
2749	**130**	Tetramethylsilane
2750	**153**	1,3-Dichloropropanol-2
2751	**155**	Diethylthiophosphoryl chloride
2752	**127**	1,2-Epoxy-3-ethoxypropane
2753	**153**	N-Ethylbenzyltoluidines, liquid
2754	**153**	N-Ethyltoluidines
2757	**151**	Carbamate pesticide, solid, poisonous
2757	**151**	Carbamate pesticide, solid, toxic
2758	**131**	Carbamate pesticide, liquid, flammable, poisonous
2758	**131**	Carbamate pesticide, liquid, flammable, toxic
2759	**151**	Arsenical pesticide, solid, poisonous
2759	**151**	Arsenical pesticide, solid, toxic
2760	**131**	Arsenical pesticide, liquid, flammable, poisonous
2760	**131**	Arsenical pesticide, liquid, flammable, toxic
2761	**151**	Organochlorine pesticide, solid, poisonous
2761	**151**	Organochlorine pesticide, solid, toxic

ID No.	Guide No.	Name of Material
2762	**131**	Organochlorine pesticide, liquid, flammable, poisonous
2762	**131**	Organochlorine pesticide, liquid, flammable, toxic
2763	**151**	Triazine pesticide, solid, poisonous
2763	**151**	Triazine pesticide, solid, toxic
2764	**131**	Triazine pesticide, liquid, flammable, poisonous
2764	**131**	Triazine pesticide, liquid, flammable, toxic
2771	**151**	Thiocarbamate pesticide, solid, poisonous
2771	**151**	Thiocarbamate pesticide, solid, toxic
2772	**131**	Thiocarbamate pesticide, liquid, flammable, poisonous
2772	**131**	Thiocarbamate pesticide, liquid, flammable, toxic
2775	**151**	Copper based pesticide, solid, poisonous
2775	**151**	Copper based pesticide, solid, toxic
2776	**131**	Copper based pesticide, liquid, flammable, poisonous
2776	**131**	Copper based pesticide, liquid, flammable, toxic
2777	**151**	Mercury based pesticide, solid, poisonous
2777	**151**	Mercury based pesticide, solid, toxic
2778	**131**	Mercury based pesticide, liquid, flammable, poisonous
2778	**131**	Mercury based pesticide, liquid, flammable, toxic
2779	**153**	Substituted nitrophenol pesticide, solid, poisonous
2779	**153**	Substituted nitrophenol pesticide, solid, toxic

ID No.	Guide No.	Name of Material
2780	**131**	Substituted nitrophenol pesticide, liquid, flammable, poisonous
2780	**131**	Substituted nitrophenol pesticide, liquid, flammable, toxic
2781	**151**	Bipyridilium pesticide, solid, poisonous
2781	**151**	Bipyridilium pesticide, solid, toxic
2782	**131**	Bipyridilium pesticide, liquid, flammable, poisonous
2782	**131**	Bipyridilium pesticide, liquid, flammable, toxic
2783	**152**	Organophosphorus pesticide, solid, poisonous
2783	**152**	Organophosphorus pesticide, solid, toxic
2784	**131**	Organophosphorus pesticide, liquid, flammable, poisonous
2784	**131**	Organophosphorus pesticide, liquid, flammable, toxic
2785	**152**	4-Thiapentanal
2786	**153**	Organotin pesticide, solid, poisonous
2786	**153**	Organotin pesticide, solid, toxic
2787	**131**	Organotin pesticide, liquid, flammable, poisonous
2787	**131**	Organotin pesticide, liquid, flammable, toxic
2788	**153**	Organotin compound, liquid, n.o.s.
2789	**132**	Acetic acid, glacial
2789	**132**	Acetic acid, solution, more than 80% acid
2790	**153**	Acetic acid, solution, more than 10% but not more than 80% acid

ID No.	Guide No.	Name of Material
2793	**170**	Ferrous metal borings, shavings, turnings or cuttings
2794	**154**	Batteries, wet, filled with acid
2795	**154**	Batteries, wet, filled with alkali
2796	**157**	Battery fluid, acid
2796	**157**	Sulfuric acid, with not more than 51% acid
2796	**157**	Sulphuric acid, with not more than 51% acid
2797	**154**	Battery fluid, alkali
2798	**137**	Benzene phosphorus dichloride
2798	**137**	Phenylphosphorus dichloride
2799	**137**	Benzene phosphorus thiodichloride
2799	**137**	Phenylphosphorus thiodichloride
2800	**154**	Batteries, wet, non-spillable
2801	**154**	Dye, liquid, corrosive, n.o.s.
2801	**154**	Dye intermediate, liquid, corrosive, n.o.s.
2802	**154**	Copper chloride
2803	**172**	Gallium
2805	**138**	Lithium hydride, fused solid
2806	**139**	Lithium nitride
2807	**171**	Magnetized material
2809	**172**	Mercury
2810	**153**	Compounds, tree or weed killing, liquid (toxic)
2810	**153**	Poisonous liquid, organic, n.o.s.
2810	**153**	Toxic liquid, organic, n.o.s.
2811	**154**	Poisonous solid, organic, n.o.s.
2811	**154**	Toxic solid, organic, n.o.s.
2812	**154**	Sodium aluminate, solid
2813	**138**	Water-reactive solid, n.o.s.
2814	**158**	Infectious substance, affecting humans
2815	**153**	N-Aminoethylpiperazine
2817	**154**	Ammonium bifluoride, solution
2817	**154**	Ammonium hydrogendifluoride, solution
2818	**154**	Ammonium polysulfide, solution
2818	**154**	Ammonium polysulphide, solution
2819	**153**	Amyl acid phosphate
2820	**153**	Butyric acid
2821	**153**	Phenol solution
2822	**153**	2-Chloropyridine
2823	**153**	Crotonic acid, solid
2826	**155**	Ethyl chlorothioformate
2829	**153**	Caproic acid
2829	**153**	Hexanoic acid
2830	**139**	Lithium ferrosilicon
2831	**160**	1,1,1-Trichloroethane
2834	**154**	Phosphorous acid
2835	**138**	Sodium aluminum hydride
2837	**154**	Bisulfates, aqueous solution
2837	**154**	Bisulphates, aqueous solution
2837	**154**	Sodium bisulfate, solution
2837	**154**	Sodium bisulphate, solution
2838	**129P**	Vinyl butyrate, stabilized
2839	**153**	Aldol
2840	**129**	Butyraldoxime
2841	**131**	Di-n-amylamine
2842	**129**	Nitroethane
2844	**138**	Calcium manganese silicon
2845	**135**	Ethyl phosphonous dichloride, anhydrous

ID No.	Guide No.	Name of Material
2845	**135**	Methyl phosphonous dichloride
2845	**135**	Pyrophoric liquid, organic, n.o.s.
2846	**135**	Pyrophoric solid, organic, n.o.s.
2849	**153**	3-Chloropropanol-1
2850	**128**	Propylene tetramer
2851	**157**	Boron trifluoride, dihydrate
2852	**113**	Dipicryl sulfide, wetted with not less than 10% water
2852	**113**	Dipicryl sulphide, wetted with not less than 10% water
2853	**151**	Magnesium fluorosilicate
2854	**151**	Ammonium fluorosilicate
2854	**151**	Ammonium silicofluoride
2855	**151**	Zinc fluorosilicate
2855	**151**	Zinc silicofluoride
2856	**151**	Fluorosilicates, n.o.s.
2857	**126**	Refrigerating machines, containing Ammonia solutions (UN2672)
2857	**126**	Refrigerating machines, containing non-flammable, non-poisonous gases
2857	**126**	Refrigerating machines, containing non-flammable, non-toxic gases
2858	**170**	Zirconium, dry, coiled wire, finished metal sheets or strip
2859	**154**	Ammonium metavanadate
2861	**151**	Ammonium polyvanadate
2862	**151**	Vanadium pentoxide
2863	**154**	Sodium ammonium vanadate
2864	**151**	Potassium metavanadate
2865	**154**	Hydroxylamine sulfate
2865	**154**	Hydroxylamine sulphate

ID No.	Guide No.	Name of Material
2869	**157**	Titanium trichloride mixture
2870	**135**	Aluminum borohydride
2870	**135**	Aluminum borohydride in devices
2871	**170**	Antimony powder
2872	**159**	Dibromochloropropanes
2873	**153**	Dibutylaminoethanol
2874	**153**	Furfuryl alcohol
2875	**151**	Hexachlorophene
2876	**153**	Resorcinol
2878	**170**	Titanium sponge granules
2878	**170**	Titanium sponge powders
2879	**157**	Selenium oxychloride
2880	**140**	Calcium hypochlorite, hydrated, with not less than 5.5% but not more than 16% water
2880	**140**	Calcium hypochlorite, hydrated mixture, with not less than 5.5% but not more than 16% water
2881	**135**	Metal catalyst, dry
2881	**135**	Nickel catalyst, dry
2900	**158**	Infectious substance, affecting animals only
2901	**124**	Bromine chloride
2902	**151**	Pesticide, liquid, poisonous, n.o.s.
2902	**151**	Pesticide, liquid, toxic, n.o.s.
2903	**131**	Pesticide, liquid, poisonous, flammable, n.o.s.
2903	**131**	Pesticide, liquid, toxic, flammable, n.o.s.
2904	**154**	Chlorophenolates, liquid
2904	**154**	Phenolates, liquid
2905	**154**	Chlorophenolates, solid

ID No.	Guide No.	Name of Material
2905	**154**	Phenolates, solid
2907	**133**	Isosorbide dinitrate mixture
2908	**161**	Radioactive material, excepted package, empty packaging
2909	**161**	Radioactive material, excepted package, articles manufactured from depleted Uranium
2909	**161**	Radioactive material, excepted package, articles manufactured from natural Thorium
2909	**161**	Radioactive material, excepted package, articles manufactured from natural Uranium
2910	**161**	Radioactive material, excepted package, limited quantity of material
2911	**161**	Radioactive material, excepted package, articles
2911	**161**	Radioactive material, excepted package, instruments
2912	**162**	Radioactive material, low specific activity (LSA-I), non fissile or fissile-excepted
2913	**162**	Radioactive material, surface contaminated objects (SCO-I), non fissile or fissile-excepted
2913	**162**	Radioactive material, surface contaminated objects (SCO-II), non fissile or fissile-excepted
2915	**163**	Radioactive material, Type A package, non-special form, non fissile or fissile-excepted
2916	**163**	Radioactive material, Type B(U) package, non fissile or fissile-excepted
2917	**163**	Radioactive material, Type B(M) package, non fissile or fissile-excepted
2919	**163**	Radioactive material, transported under special arrangement, non fissile or fissile-excepted
2920	**132**	Corrosive liquid, flammable, n.o.s.
2921	**134**	Corrosive solid, flammable, n.o.s.
2922	**154**	Corrosive liquid, poisonous, n.o.s.
2922	**154**	Corrosive liquid, toxic, n.o.s.
2923	**154**	Corrosive solid, poisonous, n.o.s.
2923	**154**	Corrosive solid, toxic, n.o.s.
2924	**132**	Flammable liquid, corrosive, n.o.s
2925	**134**	Flammable solid, corrosive, organic, n.o.s.
2926	**134**	Flammable solid, poisonous, organic, n.o.s.
2926	**134**	Flammable solid, toxic, organic, n.o.s.
2927	**154**	Ethyl phosphonothioic dichloride, anhydrous
2927	**154**	Ethyl phosphorodichloridate
2927	**154**	Poisonous liquid, corrosive, organic, n.o.s.
2927	**154**	Toxic liquid, corrosive, organic, n.o.s.
2928	**154**	Poisonous solid, corrosive, organic, n.o.s.
2928	**154**	Toxic solid, corrosive, organic, n.o.s.
2929	**131**	Poisonous liquid, flammable, organic, n.o.s.
2929	**131**	Toxic liquid, flammable, organic, n.o.s.
2930	**134**	Poisonous solid, flammable, organic, n.o.s.

ID No.	Guide No.	Name of Material
2930	**134**	Toxic solid, flammable, organic, n.o.s.
2931	**151**	Vanadyl sulfate
2931	**151**	Vanadyl sulphate
2933	**129**	Methyl 2-chloropropionate
2934	**129**	Isopropyl 2-chloropropionate
2935	**129**	Ethyl 2-chloropropionate
2936	**153**	Thiolactic acid
2937	**153**	alpha-Methylbenzyl alcohol, liquid
2937	**153**	Methylbenzyl (alpha) alcohol, liquid
2940	**135**	Cyclooctadiene phosphines
2940	**135**	9-Phosphabicyclononanes
2941	**153**	Fluoroanilines
2942	**153**	2-Trifluoromethylaniline
2943	**129**	Tetrahydrofurfurylamine
2945	**132**	N-Methylbutylamine
2946	**153**	2-Amino-5-diethylaminopentane
2947	**155**	Isopropyl chloroacetate
2948	**153**	3-Trifluoromethylaniline
2949	**154**	Sodium hydrosulfide, hydrated, with not less than 25% water of crystallization
2949	**154**	Sodium hydrosulfide, with not less than 25% water of crystallization
2949	**154**	Sodium hydrosulphide, hydrated, with not less than 25% water of crystallization
2949	**154**	Sodium hydrosulphide, with not less than 25% water of crystallization
2950	**138**	Magnesium granules, coated
2956	**149**	5-tert-Butyl-2,4,6-trinitro-m-xylene
2956	**149**	Musk xylene
2965	**139**	Boron trifluoride dimethyl etherate
2966	**153**	Thioglycol
2967	**154**	Sulfamic acid
2967	**154**	Sulphamic acid
2968	**135**	Maneb, stabilized
2968	**135**	Maneb preparation, stabilized
2969	**171**	Castor beans, meal, pomace or flake
2977	**166**	Radioactive material, Uranium hexafluoride, fissile
2977	**166**	Uranium hexafluoride, radioactive material, fissile
2978	**166**	Radioactive material, Uranium hexafluoride, non fissile or fissile-excepted
2978	**166**	Uranium hexafluoride, radioactive material, non fissile or fissile-excepted
2983	**131P**	Ethylene oxide and Propylene oxide mixture, with not more than 30% Ethylene oxide
2983	**131P**	Propylene oxide and Ethylene oxide mixture, with not more than 30% Ethylene oxide
2984	**140**	Hydrogen peroxide, aqueous solution, with not less than 8% but less than 20% Hydrogen peroxide
2985	**155**	Chlorosilanes, flammable, corrosive, n.o.s.
2986	**155**	Chlorosilanes, corrosive, flammable, n.o.s.
2987	**156**	Chlorosilanes, corrosive, n.o.s.
2988	**139**	Chlorosilanes, water-reactive, flammable, corrosive, n.o.s.
2989	**133**	Lead phosphite, dibasic

ID No.	Guide No.	Name of Material
2990	**171**	Life-saving appliances, self-inflating
2991	**131**	Carbamate pesticide, liquid, poisonous, flammable
2991	**131**	Carbamate pesticide, liquid, toxic, flammable
2992	**151**	Carbamate pesticide, liquid, poisonous
2992	**151**	Carbamate pesticide, liquid, toxic
2993	**131**	Arsenical pesticide, liquid, poisonous, flammable
2993	**131**	Arsenical pesticide, liquid, toxic, flammable
2994	**151**	Arsenical pesticide, liquid, poisonous
2994	**151**	Arsenical pesticide, liquid, toxic
2995	**131**	Organochlorine pesticide, liquid, poisonous, flammable
2995	**131**	Organochlorine pesticide, liquid, toxic, flammable
2996	**151**	Organochlorine pesticide, liquid, poisonous
2996	**151**	Organochlorine pesticide, liquid, toxic
2997	**131**	Triazine pesticide, liquid, poisonous, flammable
2997	**131**	Triazine pesticide, liquid, toxic, flammable
2998	**151**	Triazine pesticide, liquid, poisonous
2998	**151**	Triazine pesticide, liquid, toxic
3002	**151**	Phenyl urea pesticide, liquid, poisonous
3002	**151**	Phenyl urea pesticide, liquid, toxic
3005	**131**	Thiocarbamate pesticide, liquid, poisonous, flammable
3005	**131**	Thiocarbamate pesticide, liquid, toxic, flammable
3006	**151**	Thiocarbamate pesticide, liquid, poisonous
3006	**151**	Thiocarbamate pesticide, liquid, toxic
3009	**131**	Copper based pesticide, liquid, poisonous, flammable
3009	**131**	Copper based pesticide, liquid, toxic, flammable
3010	**151**	Copper based pesticide, liquid, poisonous
3010	**151**	Copper based pesticide, liquid, toxic
3011	**131**	Mercury based pesticide, liquid, poisonous, flammable
3011	**131**	Mercury based pesticide, liquid, toxic, flammable
3012	**151**	Mercury based pesticide, liquid, poisonous
3012	**151**	Mercury based pesticide, liquid, toxic
3013	**131**	Substituted nitrophenol pesticide, liquid, poisonous, flammable
3013	**131**	Substituted nitrophenol pesticide, liquid, toxic, flammable
3014	**153**	Substituted nitrophenol pesticide, liquid, poisonous
3014	**153**	Substituted nitrophenol pesticide, liquid, toxic
3015	**131**	Bipyridilium pesticide, liquid, poisonous, flammable
3015	**131**	Bipyridilium pesticide, liquid, toxic, flammable
3016	**151**	Bipyridilium pesticide, liquid, poisonous
3016	**151**	Bipyridilium pesticide, liquid, toxic

ID No.	Guide No.	Name of Material
3017	**131**	Organophosphorus pesticide, liquid, poisonous, flammable
3017	**131**	Organophosphorus pesticide, liquid, toxic, flammable
3018	**152**	Organophosphorus pesticide, liquid, poisonous
3018	**152**	Organophosphorus pesticide, liquid, toxic
3019	**131**	Organotin pesticide, liquid, poisonous, flammable
3019	**131**	Organotin pesticide, liquid, toxic, flammable
3020	**153**	Organotin pesticide, liquid, poisonous
3020	**153**	Organotin pesticide, liquid, toxic
3021	**131**	Pesticide, liquid, flammable, poisonous, n.o.s.
3021	**131**	Pesticide, liquid, flammable, toxic, n.o.s.
3022	**127P**	1,2-Butylene oxide, stabilized
3023	**131**	2-Methyl-2-heptanethiol
3024	**131**	Coumarin derivative pesticide, liquid, flammable, poisonous
3024	**131**	Coumarin derivative pesticide, liquid, flammable, toxic
3025	**131**	Coumarin derivative pesticide, liquid, poisonous, flammable
3025	**131**	Coumarin derivative pesticide, liquid, toxic, flammable
3026	**151**	Coumarin derivative pesticide, liquid, poisonous
3026	**151**	Coumarin derivative pesticide, liquid, toxic
3027	**151**	Coumarin derivative pesticide, solid, poisonous
3027	**151**	Coumarin derivative pesticide, solid, toxic
3028	**154**	Batteries, dry, containing Potassium hydroxide solid
3048	**157**	Aluminum phosphide pesticide
3051	**135**	Aluminum alkyls
3053	**135**	Magnesium alkyls
3054	**129**	Cyclohexanethiol
3054	**129**	Cyclohexyl mercaptan
3055	**154**	2-(2-Aminoethoxy)ethanol
3056	**129**	n-Heptaldehyde
3057	**125**	Trifluoroacetyl chloride
3064	**127**	Nitroglycerin, solution in alcohol, with more than 1% but not more than 5% Nitroglycerin
3065	**127**	Alcoholic beverages
3066	**153**	Paint (corrosive)
3066	**153**	Paint related material (corrosive)
3070	**126**	Dichlorodifluoromethane and Ethylene oxide mixture, with not more than 12.5% Ethylene oxide
3070	**126**	Ethylene oxide and Dichlorodifluoromethane mixture, with not more than 12.5% Ethylene oxide
3071	**131**	Mercaptan mixture, liquid, poisonous, flammable, n.o.s.
3071	**131**	Mercaptan mixture, liquid, toxic, flammable, n.o.s.
3071	**131**	Mercaptans, liquid, poisonous, flammable, n.o.s.
3071	**131**	Mercaptans, liquid, toxic, flammable, n.o.s.
3072	**171**	Life-saving appliances, not self-inflating
3073	**131P**	Vinylpyridines, stabilized
3076	**138**	Aluminum alkyl hydrides
3077	**171**	Environmentally hazardous substance, solid, n.o.s.

ID No.	Guide No.	Name of Material
3077	**171**	Hazardous waste, solid, n.o.s.
3077	**171**	Other regulated substances, solid, n.o.s.
3078	**138**	Cerium, turnings or gritty powder
3079	**131P**	Methacrylonitrile, stabilized
3080	**155**	Isocyanate solution, poisonous, flammable, n.o.s.
3080	**155**	Isocyanate solution, toxic, flammable, n.o.s.
3080	**155**	Isocyanates, poisonous, flammable, n.o.s.
3080	**155**	Isocyanates, toxic, flammable, n.o.s.
3082	**171**	Environmentally hazardous substance, liquid, n.o.s.
3082	**171**	Hazardous waste, liquid, n.o.s.
3082	**171**	Other regulated substances, liquid, n.o.s.
3083	**124**	Perchloryl fluoride
3084	**157**	Corrosive solid, oxidizing, n.o.s.
3085	**140**	Oxidizing solid, corrosive, n.o.s.
3086	**141**	Poisonous solid, oxidizing, n.o.s.
3086	**141**	Toxic solid, oxidizing, n.o.s.
3087	**141**	Oxidizing solid, poisonous, n.o.s.
3087	**141**	Oxidizing solid, toxic, n.o.s.
3088	**135**	Self-heating solid, organic, n.o.s.
3089	**170**	Metal powder, flammable, n.o.s.
3090	**138**	Lithium batteries
3090	**138**	Lithium metal batteries (including lithium alloy batteries)
3091	**138**	Lithium batteries contained in equipment
3091	**138**	Lithium batteries packed with equipment
3091	**138**	Lithium metal batteries contained in equipment (including lithium alloy batteries)
3091	**138**	Lithium metal batteries packed with equipment (including lithium alloy batteries)
3092	**129**	1-Methoxy-2-propanol
3093	**157**	Corrosive liquid, oxidizing, n.o.s.
3094	**138**	Corrosive liquid, water-reactive, n.o.s.
3095	**136**	Corrosive solid, self-heating, n.o.s.
3096	**138**	Corrosive solid, water-reactive, n.o.s.
3097	**140**	Flammable solid, oxidizing, n.o.s.
3098	**140**	Oxidizing liquid, corrosive, n.o.s.
3099	**142**	Oxidizing liquid, poisonous, n.o.s.
3099	**142**	Oxidizing liquid, toxic, n.o.s.
3100	**135**	Oxidizing solid, self-heating, n.o.s.
3101	**146**	Organic peroxide type B, liquid
3102	**146**	Organic peroxide type B, solid
3103	**146**	Organic peroxide type C, liquid
3104	**146**	Organic peroxide type C, solid
3105	**145**	Organic peroxide type D, liquid
3106	**145**	Organic peroxide type D, solid
3107	**145**	Organic peroxide type E, liquid
3108	**145**	Organic peroxide type E, solid
3109	**145**	Organic peroxide type F, liquid
3110	**145**	Organic peroxide type F, solid

ID No.	Guide No.	Name of Material
3111	**148**	Organic peroxide type B, liquid, temperature controlled
3112	**148**	Organic peroxide type B, solid, temperature controlled
3113	**148**	Organic peroxide type C, liquid, temperature controlled
3114	**148**	Organic peroxide type C, solid, temperature controlled
3115	**148**	Organic peroxide type D, liquid, temperature controlled
3116	**148**	Organic peroxide type D, solid, temperature controlled
3117	**148**	Organic peroxide type E, liquid, temperature controlled
3118	**148**	Organic peroxide type E, solid, temperature controlled
3119	**148**	Organic peroxide type F, liquid, temperature controlled
3120	**148**	Organic peroxide type F, solid, temperature controlled
3121	**144**	Oxidizing solid, water-reactive, n.o.s.
3122	**142**	Poisonous liquid, oxidizing, n.o.s.
3122	**142**	Toxic liquid, oxidizing, n.o.s.
3123	**139**	Poisonous liquid, water-reactive, n.o.s.
3123	**139**	Toxic liquid, water-reactive, n.o.s.
3124	**136**	Poisonous solid, self-heating, n.o.s.
3124	**136**	Toxic solid, self-heating, n.o.s.
3125	**139**	Poisonous solid, water-reactive, n.o.s.
3125	**139**	Toxic solid, water-reactive, n.o.s.
3126	**136**	Self-heating solid, corrosive, organic, n.o.s.
3127	**135**	Self-heating solid, oxidizing, n.o.s.
3128	**136**	Self-heating solid, poisonous, organic, n.o.s.
3128	**136**	Self-heating solid, toxic, organic, n.o.s.
3129	**138**	Water-reactive liquid, corrosive, n.o.s.
3130	**139**	Water-reactive liquid, poisonous, n.o.s.
3130	**139**	Water-reactive liquid, toxic, n.o.s.
3131	**138**	Water-reactive solid, corrosive, n.o.s.
3132	**138**	Water-reactive solid, flammable, n.o.s.
3133	**138**	Water-reactive solid, oxidizing, n.o.s.
3134	**139**	Water-reactive solid, poisonous, n.o.s.
3134	**139**	Water-reactive solid, toxic, n.o.s.
3135	**138**	Water-reactive solid, self-heating, n.o.s.
3136	**120**	Trifluoromethane, refrigerated liquid
3137	**140**	Oxidizing solid, flammable, n.o.s.
3138	**115**	Acetylene, Ethylene and Propylene in mixture, refrigerated liquid containing at least 71.5% Ethylene with not more than 22.5% Acetylene and not more than 6% Propylene
3138	**115**	Ethylene, Acetylene and Propylene in mixture, refrigerated liquid containing at least 71.5% Ethylene with not more than 22.5% Acetylene and not more than 6% Propylene

ID No.	Guide No.	Name of Material
3138	**115**	Propylene, Ethylene and Acetylene in mixture, refrigerated liquid containing at least 71.5% Ethylene with not more than 22.5% Acetylene and not more than 6% Propylene
3139	**140**	Oxidizing liquid, n.o.s.
3140	**151**	Alkaloids, liquid, n.o.s. (poisonous)
3140	**151**	Alkaloid salts, liquid, n.o.s. (poisonous)
3141	**157**	Antimony compound, inorganic, liquid, n.o.s.
3142	**151**	Disinfectant, liquid, poisonous, n.o.s.
3142	**151**	Disinfectant, liquid, toxic, n.o.s.
3143	**151**	Dye, solid, poisonous, n.o.s.
3143	**151**	Dye, solid, toxic, n.o.s.
3143	**151**	Dye intermediate, solid, poisonous, n.o.s.
3143	**151**	Dye intermediate, solid, toxic, n.o.s.
3144	**151**	Nicotine compound, liquid, n.o.s.
3144	**151**	Nicotine preparation, liquid, n.o.s.
3145	**153**	Alkylphenols, liquid, n.o.s. (including C2-C12 homologues)
3146	**153**	Organotin compound, solid, n.o.s.
3147	**154**	Dye, solid, corrosive, n.o.s.
3147	**154**	Dye intermediate, solid, corrosive, n.o.s.
3148	**138**	Water-reactive liquid, n.o.s.
3149	**140**	Hydrogen peroxide and Peroxyacetic acid mixture, with acid(s), water and not more than 5% Peroxyacetic acid, stabilized
3149	**140**	Peroxyacetic acid and hydrogen peroxide mixture, with acid(s), water and not more than 5% Peroxyacetic acid, stabilized
3150	**115**	Devices, small, hydrocarbon gas powered, with release device
3150	**115**	Hydrocarbon gas refills for small devices, with release device
3151	**171**	Halogenated monomethyldiphenylmethanes, liquid
3151	**171**	Polyhalogenated biphenyls, liquid
3151	**171**	Polyhalogenated terphenyls, liquid
3152	**171**	Halogenated monomethyldiphenylmethanes, solid
3152	**171**	Polyhalogenated biphenyls, solid
3152	**171**	Polyhalogenated terphenyls, solid
3153	**115**	Perfluoro(methyl vinyl ether)
3154	**115**	Perfluoro(ethyl vinyl ether)
3155	**154**	Pentachlorophenol
3156	**122**	Compressed gas, oxidizing, n.o.s.
3157	**122**	Liquefied gas, oxidizing, n.o.s.
3158	**120**	Gas, refrigerated liquid, n.o.s.
3159	**126**	Refrigerant gas R-134a
3159	**126**	1,1,1,2-Tetrafluoroethane
3160	**119**	Liquefied gas, poisonous, flammable, n.o.s.

ID No.	Guide No.	Name of Material
3160	**119**	Liquefied gas, poisonous, flammable, n.o.s. (Inhalation Hazard Zone A)
3160	**119**	Liquefied gas, poisonous, flammable, n.o.s. (Inhalation Hazard Zone B)
3160	**119**	Liquefied gas, poisonous, flammable, n.o.s. (Inhalation Hazard Zone C)
3160	**119**	Liquefied gas, poisonous, flammable, n.o.s. (Inhalation Hazard Zone D)
3160	**119**	Liquefied gas, toxic, flammable, n.o.s.
3160	**119**	Liquefied gas, toxic, flammable, n.o.s. (Inhalation Hazard Zone A)
3160	**119**	Liquefied gas, toxic, flammable, n.o.s. (Inhalation Hazard Zone B)
3160	**119**	Liquefied gas, toxic, flammable, n.o.s. (Inhalation Hazard Zone C)
3160	**119**	Liquefied gas, toxic, flammable, n.o.s. (Inhalation Hazard Zone D)
3161	**115**	Liquefied gas, flammable, n.o.s.
3162	**123**	Liquefied gas, poisonous, n.o.s.
3162	**123**	Liquefied gas, poisonous, n.o.s. (Inhalation Hazard Zone A)
3162	**123**	Liquefied gas, poisonous, n.o.s. (Inhalation Hazard Zone B)
3162	**123**	Liquefied gas, poisonous, n.o.s. (Inhalation Hazard Zone C)
3162	**123**	Liquefied gas, poisonous, n.o.s. (Inhalation Hazard Zone D)
3162	**123**	Liquefied gas, toxic, n.o.s.
3162	**123**	Liquefied gas, toxic, n.o.s. (Inhalation Hazard Zone A)
3162	**123**	Liquefied gas, toxic, n.o.s. (Inhalation Hazard Zone B)
3162	**123**	Liquefied gas, toxic, n.o.s. (Inhalation Hazard Zone C)
3162	**123**	Liquefied gas, toxic, n.o.s. (Inhalation Hazard Zone D)
3163	**126**	Liquefied gas, n.o.s.
3164	**126**	Articles, pressurized, hydraulic (containing non-flammable gas)
3164	**126**	Articles, pressurized, pneumatic (containing non-flammable gas)
3165	**131**	Aircraft hydraulic power unit fuel tank
3166	**115**	Engine, fuel cell, flammable gas powered
3166	**128**	Engine, fuel cell, flammable liquid powered
3166	**128**	Engine, internal combustion
3166	**115**	Engines, internal combustion, flammable gas powered
3166	**128**	Engines, internal combustion, flammable liquid powered
3166	**115**	Vehicle, flammable gas powered
3166	**128**	Vehicle, flammable liquid powered
3166	**115**	Vehicle, fuel cell, flammable gas powered
3166	**128**	Vehicle, fuel cell, flammable liquid powered
3167	**115**	Gas sample, non-pressurized, flammable, n.o.s., not refrigerated liquid
3168	**119**	Gas sample, non-pressurized, poisonous, flammable, n.o.s., not refrigerated liquid
3168	**119**	Gas sample, non-pressurized, toxic, flammable, n.o.s., not refrigerated liquid

ID No.	Guide No.	Name of Material
3169	**123**	Gas sample, non-pressurized, poisonous, n.o.s., not refrigerated liquid
3169	**123**	Gas sample, non-pressurized, toxic, n.o.s., not refrigerated liquid
3170	**138**	Aluminum dross
3170	**138**	Aluminum remelting by-products
3170	**138**	Aluminum smelting by-products
3171	**154**	Battery-powered equipment (wet battery)
3171	**147**	Battery-powered equipment (with lithium ion batteries)
3171	**138**	Battery-powered equipment (with lithium metal batteries)
3171	**138**	Battery-powered equipment (with sodium batteries)
3171	**154**	Battery-powered vehicle (wet battery)
3171	**147**	Battery-powered vehicle (with lithium ion batteries)
3171	**138**	Battery-powered vehicle (with sodium batteries)
3171	**154**	Wheelchair, electric, with batteries
3172	**153**	Toxins, extracted from living sources, liquid, n.o.s.
3174	**135**	Titanium disulfide
3174	**135**	Titanium disulphide
3175	**133**	Solids containing flammable liquid, n.o.s.
3176	**133**	Flammable solid, organic, molten, n.o.s.
3178	**133**	Flammable solid, inorganic, n.o.s.
3178	**133**	Smokeless powder for small arms
3179	**134**	Flammable solid, poisonous, inorganic, n.o.s.
3179	**134**	Flammable solid, toxic, inorganic, n.o.s.
3180	**134**	Flammable solid, corrosive, inorganic, n.o.s.
3181	**133**	Metal salts of organic compounds, flammable, n.o.s.
3182	**170**	Metal hydrides, flammable, n.o.s.
3183	**135**	Self-heating liquid, organic, n.o.s.
3184	**136**	Self-heating liquid, poisonous, organic, n.o.s.
3184	**136**	Self-heating liquid, toxic, organic, n.o.s.
3185	**136**	Self-heating liquid, corrosive, organic, n.o.s.
3186	**135**	Self-heating liquid, inorganic, n.o.s.
3187	**136**	Self-heating liquid, poisonous, inorganic, n.o.s.
3187	**136**	Self-heating liquid, toxic, inorganic, n.o.s.
3188	**136**	Self-heating liquid, corrosive, inorganic, n.o.s.
3189	**135**	Metal powder, self-heating, n.o.s.
3190	**135**	Self-heating solid, inorganic, n.o.s.
3191	**136**	Self-heating solid, poisonous, inorganic, n.o.s.
3191	**136**	Self-heating solid, toxic, inorganic, n.o.s.
3192	**136**	Self-heating solid, corrosive, inorganic, n.o.s.
3194	**135**	Pyrophoric liquid, inorganic, n.o.s.
3200	**135**	Pyrophoric solid, inorganic, n.o.s.

ID No.	Guide No.	Name of Material
3205	**135**	Alkaline earth metal alcoholates, n.o.s.
3206	**136**	Alkali metal alcoholates, self-heating, corrosive, n.o.s.
3208	**138**	Metallic substance, water-reactive, n.o.s.
3209	**138**	Metallic substance, water-reactive, self-heating, n.o.s.
3210	**140**	Chlorates, inorganic, aqueous solution, n.o.s.
3211	**140**	Perchlorates, inorganic, aqueous solution, n.o.s.
3212	**140**	Hypochlorites, inorganic, n.o.s.
3213	**140**	Bromates, inorganic, aqueous solution, n.o.s.
3214	**140**	Permanganates, inorganic, aqueous solution, n.o.s.
3215	**140**	Persulfates, inorganic, n.o.s.
3215	**140**	Persulphates, inorganic, n.o.s.
3216	**140**	Persulfates, inorganic, aqueous solution, n.o.s.
3216	**140**	Persulphates, inorganic, aqueous solution, n.o.s.
3218	**140**	Nitrates, inorganic, aqueous solution, n.o.s.
3219	**140**	Nitrites, inorganic, aqueous solution, n.o.s.
3220	**126**	Pentafluoroethane
3220	**126**	Refrigerant gas R-125
3221	**149**	Self-reactive liquid type B
3222	**149**	Self-reactive solid type B
3223	**149**	Self-reactive liquid type C
3224	**149**	Self-reactive solid type C
3225	**149**	Self-reactive liquid type D
3226	**149**	Self-reactive solid type D
3227	**149**	Self-reactive liquid type E
3228	**149**	Self-reactive solid type E
3229	**149**	Self-reactive liquid type F
3230	**149**	Self-reactive solid type F
3231	**150**	Self-reactive liquid type B, temperature controlled
3232	**150**	Self-reactive solid type B, temperature controlled
3233	**150**	Self-reactive liquid type C, temperature controlled
3234	**150**	Self-reactive solid type C, temperature controlled
3235	**150**	Self-reactive liquid type D, temperature controlled
3236	**150**	Self-reactive solid type D, temperature controlled
3237	**150**	Self-reactive liquid type E, temperature controlled
3238	**150**	Self-reactive solid type E, temperature controlled
3239	**150**	Self-reactive liquid type F, temperature controlled
3240	**150**	Self-reactive solid type F, temperature controlled
3241	**133**	2-Bromo-2-nitropropane-1, 3-diol
3242	**149**	Azodicarbonamide
3243	**151**	Solids containing poisonous liquid, n.o.s.
3243	**151**	Solids containing toxic liquid, n.o.s.
3244	**154**	Solids containing corrosive liquid, n.o.s.
3245	**171**	Genetically modified micro-organisms
3245	**171**	Genetically modified organisms
3246	**156**	Methanesulfonyl chloride
3246	**156**	Methanesulphonyl chloride

ID No.	Guide No.	Name of Material
3247	**140**	Sodium peroxoborate, anhydrous
3248	**131**	Medicine, liquid, flammable, poisonous, n.o.s.
3248	**131**	Medicine, liquid, flammable, toxic, n.o.s.
3249	**151**	Medicine, solid, poisonous, n.o.s.
3249	**151**	Medicine, solid, toxic, n.o.s.
3250	**153**	Chloroacetic acid, molten
3251	**133**	Isosorbide-5-mononitrate
3252	**115**	Difluoromethane
3252	**115**	Refrigerant gas R-32
3253	**154**	Disodium trioxosilicate
3254	**135**	Tributylphosphane
3255	**135**	tert-Butyl hypochlorite
3256	**128**	Elevated temperature liquid, flammable, n.o.s., with flash point above 37.8°C (100°F), at or above its flash point
3256	**128**	Elevated temperature liquid, flammable, n.o.s., with flash point above 60°C (140°F), at or above its flash point
3257	**171**	Elevated temperature liquid, n.o.s., at or above 100°C (212°F), and below its flash point
3258	**171**	Elevated temperature solid, n.o.s., at or above 240°C (464°F)
3259	**154**	Amines, solid, corrosive, n.o.s.
3259	**154**	Polyamines, solid, corrosive, n.o.s.
3260	**154**	Corrosive solid, acidic, inorganic, n.o.s.
3261	**154**	Corrosive solid, acidic, organic, n.o.s.
3262	**154**	Corrosive solid, basic, inorganic, n.o.s.
3263	**154**	Corrosive solid, basic, organic, n.o.s.
3264	**154**	Corrosive liquid, acidic, inorganic, n.o.s.
3265	**153**	Corrosive liquid, acidic, organic, n.o.s.
3266	**154**	Corrosive liquid, basic, inorganic, n.o.s.
3267	**153**	Corrosive liquid, basic, organic, n.o.s.
3268	**171**	Air bag inflators
3268	**171**	Air bag modules
3268	**171**	Safety devices
3268	**171**	Seat-belt pre-tensioners
3269	**128**	Polyester resin kit, liquid base material
3270	**133**	Nitrocellulose membrane filters
3271	**127**	Ethers, n.o.s.
3272	**127**	Esters, n.o.s.
3273	**131**	Nitriles, flammable, poisonous, n.o.s.
3273	**131**	Nitriles, flammable, toxic, n.o.s.
3274	**132**	Alcoholates solution, n.o.s., in alcohol
3275	**131**	Nitriles, poisonous, flammable, n.o.s.
3275	**131**	Nitriles, toxic, flammable, n.o.s.
3276	**151**	Nitriles, liquid, poisonous, n.o.s.
3276	**151**	Nitriles, liquid, toxic, n.o.s.
3276	**151**	Nitriles, poisonous, liquid, n.o.s.
3276	**151**	Nitriles, toxic, liquid, n.o.s.
3277	**154**	Chloroformates, poisonous, corrosive, n.o.s.

ID No.	Guide No.	Name of Material
3277	**154**	Chloroformates, toxic, corrosive, n.o.s.
3278	**151**	Organophosphorus compound, liquid, poisonous, n.o.s.
3278	**151**	Organophosphorus compound, liquid, toxic, n.o.s.
3278	**151**	Organophosphorus compound, poisonous, liquid, n.o.s.
3278	**151**	Organophosphorus compound, toxic, liquid, n.o.s.
3279	**131**	Organophosphorus compound, poisonous, flammable, n.o.s.
3279	**131**	Organophosphorus compound, toxic, flammable, n.o.s.
3280	**151**	Organoarsenic compound, liquid, n.o.s.
3281	**151**	Metal carbonyls, liquid, n.o.s.
3282	**151**	Organometallic compound, liquid, poisonous, n.o.s.
3282	**151**	Organometallic compound, liquid, toxic, n.o.s.
3282	**151**	Organometallic compound, poisonous, liquid, n.o.s.
3282	**151**	Organometallic compound, toxic, liquid, n.o.s.
3283	**151**	Selenium compound, solid, n.o.s.
3284	**151**	Tellurium compound, n.o.s.
3285	**151**	Vanadium compound, n.o.s.
3286	**131**	Flammable liquid, poisonous, corrosive, n.o.s.
3286	**131**	Flammable liquid, toxic, corrosive, n.o.s.
3287	**151**	Poisonous liquid, inorganic, n.o.s.
3287	**151**	Toxic liquid, inorganic, n.o.s.
3288	**151**	Poisonous solid, inorganic, n.o.s.
3288	**151**	Toxic solid, inorganic, n.o.s.
3289	**154**	Poisonous liquid, corrosive, inorganic, n.o.s.
3289	**154**	Toxic liquid, corrosive, inorganic, n.o.s.
3290	**154**	Poisonous solid, corrosive, inorganic, n.o.s.
3290	**154**	Toxic solid, corrosive, inorganic, n.o.s.
3291	**158**	(Bio)Medical waste, n.o.s.
3291	**158**	Clinical waste, unspecified, n.o.s.
3291	**158**	Medical waste, n.o.s.
3291	**158**	Regulated medical waste, n.o.s.
3292	**138**	Batteries, containing Sodium
3292	**138**	Cells, containing Sodium
3292	**138**	Sodium, batteries containing
3293	**152**	Hydrazine, aqueous solution, with not more than 37% Hydrazine
3294	**131**	Hydrogen cyanide, solution in alcohol, with not more than 45% Hydrogen cyanide
3295	**128**	Hydrocarbons, liquid, n.o.s.
3296	**126**	Heptafluoropropane
3296	**126**	Refrigerant gas R-227
3297	**126**	Chlorotetrafluoroethane and Ethylene oxide mixture, with not more than 8.8% Ethylene oxide
3297	**126**	Ethylene oxide and Chlorotetrafluoroethane mixture, with not more than 8.8% Ethylene oxide
3298	**126**	Ethylene oxide and Pentafluoroethane mixture, with not more than 7.9% Ethylene oxide

ID No.	Guide No.	Name of Material
3298	**126**	Pentafluoroethane and Ethylene oxide mixture, with not more than 7.9% Ethylene oxide
3299	**126**	Ethylene oxide and Tetrafluoroethane mixture, with not more than 5.6% Ethylene oxide
3299	**126**	Tetrafluoroethane and Ethylene oxide mixture, with not more than 5.6% Ethylene oxide
3300	**119P**	Carbon dioxide and Ethylene oxide mixture, with more than 87% Ethylene oxide
3300	**119P**	Ethylene oxide and Carbon dioxide mixture, with more than 87% Ethylene oxide
3301	**136**	Corrosive liquid, self-heating, n.o.s.
3302	**152**	2-Dimethylaminoethyl acrylate
3303	**124**	Compressed gas, poisonous, oxidizing, n.o.s.
3303	**124**	Compressed gas, poisonous, oxidizing, n.o.s. (Inhalation Hazard Zone A)
3303	**124**	Compressed gas, poisonous, oxidizing, n.o.s. (Inhalation Hazard Zone B)
3303	**124**	Compressed gas, poisonous, oxidizing, n.o.s. (Inhalation Hazard Zone C)
3303	**124**	Compressed gas, poisonous, oxidizing, n.o.s. (Inhalation Hazard Zone D)
3303	**124**	Compressed gas, toxic, oxidizing, n.o.s.
3303	**124**	Compressed gas, toxic, oxidizing, n.o.s. (Inhalation Hazard Zone A)
3303	**124**	Compressed gas, toxic, oxidizing, n.o.s. (Inhalation Hazard Zone B)
3303	**124**	Compressed gas, toxic, oxidizing, n.o.s. (Inhalation Hazard Zone C)
3303	**124**	Compressed gas, toxic, oxidizing, n.o.s. (Inhalation Hazard Zone D)
3304	**125**	Compressed gas, poisonous, corrosive, n.o.s.
3304	**125**	Compressed gas, poisonous, corrosive, n.o.s. (Inhalation Hazard Zone A)
3304	**125**	Compressed gas, poisonous, corrosive, n.o.s. (Inhalation Hazard Zone B)
3304	**125**	Compressed gas, poisonous, corrosive, n.o.s. (Inhalation Hazard Zone C)
3304	**125**	Compressed gas, poisonous, corrosive, n.o.s. (Inhalation Hazard Zone D)
3304	**125**	Compressed gas, toxic, corrosive, n.o.s.
3304	**125**	Compressed gas, toxic, corrosive, n.o.s. (Inhalation Hazard Zone A)
3304	**125**	Compressed gas, toxic, corrosive, n.o.s. (Inhalation Hazard Zone B)
3304	**125**	Compressed gas, toxic, corrosive, n.o.s. (Inhalation Hazard Zone C)
3304	**125**	Compressed gas, toxic, corrosive, n.o.s. (Inhalation Hazard Zone D)
3305	**119**	Compressed gas, poisonous, flammable, corrosive, n.o.s.
3305	**119**	Compressed gas, poisonous, flammable, corrosive, n.o.s. (Inhalation Hazard Zone A)
3305	**119**	Compressed gas, poisonous, flammable, corrosive, n.o.s. (Inhalation Hazard Zone B)

ID No.	Guide No.	Name of Material
3305	**119**	Compressed gas, poisonous, flammable, corrosive, n.o.s. (Inhalation Hazard Zone C)
3305	**119**	Compressed gas, poisonous, flammable, corrosive, n.o.s. (Inhalation Hazard Zone D)
3305	**119**	Compressed gas, toxic, flammable, corrosive, n.o.s.
3305	**119**	Compressed gas, toxic, flammable, corrosive, n.o.s. (Inhalation Hazard Zone A)
3305	**119**	Compressed gas, toxic, flammable, corrosive, n.o.s. (Inhalation Hazard Zone B)
3305	**119**	Compressed gas, toxic, flammable, corrosive, n.o.s. (Inhalation Hazard Zone C)
3305	**119**	Compressed gas, toxic, flammable, corrosive, n.o.s. (Inhalation Hazard Zone D)
3306	**124**	Compressed gas, poisonous, oxidizing, corrosive, n.o.s.
3306	**124**	Compressed gas, poisonous, oxidizing, corrosive, n.o.s. (Inhalation Hazard Zone A)
3306	**124**	Compressed gas, poisonous, oxidizing, corrosive, n.o.s. (Inhalation Hazard Zone B)
3306	**124**	Compressed gas, poisonous, oxidizing, corrosive, n.o.s. (Inhalation Hazard Zone C)
3306	**124**	Compressed gas, poisonous, oxidizing, corrosive, n.o.s. (Inhalation Hazard Zone D)
3306	**124**	Compressed gas, toxic, oxidizing, corrosive, n.o.s.
3306	**124**	Compressed gas, toxic, oxidizing, corrosive, n.o.s. (Inhalation Hazard Zone A)
3306	**124**	Compressed gas, toxic, oxidizing, corrosive, n.o.s. (Inhalation Hazard Zone B)

ID No.	Guide No.	Name of Material
3306	**124**	Compressed gas, toxic, oxidizing, corrosive, n.o.s. (Inhalation Hazard Zone C)
3306	**124**	Compressed gas, toxic, oxidizing, corrosive, n.o.s. (Inhalation Hazard Zone D)
3307	**124**	Liquefied gas, poisonous, oxidizing, n.o.s.
3307	**124**	Liquefied gas, poisonous, oxidizing, n.o.s. (Inhalation Hazard Zone A)
3307	**124**	Liquefied gas, poisonous, oxidizing, n.o.s. (Inhalation Hazard Zone B)
3307	**124**	Liquefied gas, poisonous, oxidizing, n.o.s. (Inhalation Hazard Zone C)
3307	**124**	Liquefied gas, poisonous, oxidizing, n.o.s. (Inhalation Hazard Zone D)
3307	**124**	Liquefied gas, toxic, oxidizing, n.o.s.
3307	**124**	Liquefied gas, toxic, oxidizing, n.o.s. (Inhalation Hazard Zone A)
3307	**124**	Liquefied gas, toxic, oxidizing, n.o.s. (Inhalation Hazard Zone B)
3307	**124**	Liquefied gas, toxic, oxidizing, n.o.s. (Inhalation Hazard Zone C)
3307	**124**	Liquefied gas, toxic, oxidizing, n.o.s. (Inhalation Hazard Zone D)
3308	**125**	Liquefied gas, poisonous, corrosive, n.o.s.
3308	**125**	Liquefied gas, poisonous, corrosive, n.o.s. (Inhalation Hazard Zone A)
3308	**125**	Liquefied gas, poisonous, corrosive, n.o.s. (Inhalation Hazard Zone B)

ID No.	Guide No.	Name of Material
3308	**125**	Liquefied gas, poisonous, corrosive, n.o.s. (Inhalation Hazard Zone C)
3308	**125**	Liquefied gas, poisonous, corrosive, n.o.s. (Inhalation Hazard Zone D)
3308	**125**	Liquefied gas, toxic, corrosive, n.o.s.
3308	**125**	Liquefied gas, toxic, corrosive, n.o.s. (Inhalation Hazard Zone A)
3308	**125**	Liquefied gas, toxic, corrosive, n.o.s. (Inhalation Hazard Zone B)
3308	**125**	Liquefied gas, toxic, corrosive, n.o.s. (Inhalation Hazard Zone C)
3308	**125**	Liquefied gas, toxic, corrosive, n.o.s. (Inhalation Hazard Zone D)
3309	**119**	Liquefied gas, poisonous, flammable, corrosive, n.o.s.
3309	**119**	Liquefied gas, poisonous, flammable, corrosive, n.o.s. (Inhalation Hazard Zone A)
3309	**119**	Liquefied gas, poisonous, flammable, corrosive, n.o.s. (Inhalation Hazard Zone B)
3309	**119**	Liquefied gas, poisonous, flammable, corrosive, n.o.s. (Inhalation Hazard Zone C)
3309	**119**	Liquefied gas, poisonous, flammable, corrosive, n.o.s. (Inhalation Hazard Zone D)
3309	**119**	Liquefied gas, toxic, flammable, corrosive, n.o.s.
3309	**119**	Liquefied gas, toxic, flammable, corrosive, n.o.s. (Inhalation Hazard Zone A)
3309	**119**	Liquefied gas, toxic, flammable, corrosive, n.o.s. (Inhalation Hazard Zone B)
3309	**119**	Liquefied gas, toxic, flammable, corrosive, n.o.s. (Inhalation Hazard Zone C)
3309	**119**	Liquefied gas, toxic, flammable, corrosive, n.o.s. (Inhalation Hazard Zone D)
3310	**124**	Liquefied gas, poisonous, oxidizing, corrosive, n.o.s.
3310	**124**	Liquefied gas, poisonous, oxidizing, corrosive, n.o.s. (Inhalation Hazard Zone A)
3310	**124**	Liquefied gas, poisonous, oxidizing, corrosive, n.o.s. (Inhalation Hazard Zone B)
3310	**124**	Liquefied gas, poisonous, oxidizing, corrosive, n.o.s. (Inhalation Hazard Zone C)
3310	**124**	Liquefied gas, poisonous, oxidizing, corrosive, n.o.s. (Inhalation Hazard Zone D)
3310	**124**	Liquefied gas, toxic, oxidizing, corrosive, n.o.s.
3310	**124**	Liquefied gas, toxic, oxidizing, corrosive, n.o.s. (Inhalation Hazard Zone A)
3310	**124**	Liquefied gas, toxic, oxidizing, corrosive, n.o.s. (Inhalation Hazard Zone B)
3310	**124**	Liquefied gas, toxic, oxidizing, corrosive, n.o.s. (Inhalation Hazard Zone C)
3310	**124**	Liquefied gas, toxic, oxidizing, corrosive, n.o.s. (Inhalation Hazard Zone D)
3311	**122**	Gas, refrigerated liquid, oxidizing, n.o.s.
3312	**115**	Gas, refrigerated liquid, flammable, n.o.s.
3313	**135**	Organic pigments, self-heating
3314	**171**	Plastic molding compound
3314	**171**	Plastics moulding compound

ID No.	Guide No.	Name of Material
3315	**151**	Chemical sample, poisonous
3315	**151**	Chemical sample, toxic
3316	**171**	Chemical kit
3316	**171**	First aid kit
3317	**113**	2-Amino-4,6-dinitrophenol, wetted with not less than 20% water
3318	**125**	Ammonia solution, with more than 50% Ammonia
3319	**113**	Nitroglycerin mixture, desensitized, solid, n.o.s., with more than 2% but not more than 10% Nitroglycerin
3320	**157**	Sodium borohydride and Sodium hydroxide solution, with not more than 12% Sodium borohydride and not more than 40% Sodium hydroxide
3321	**162**	Radioactive material, low specific activity (LSA-II), non fissile or fissile-excepted
3322	**162**	Radioactive material, low specific activity (LSA-III), non fissile or fissile-excepted
3323	**163**	Radioactive material, Type C package, non fissile or fissile excepted
3324	**165**	Radioactive material, low specific activity (LSA-II), fissile
3325	**165**	Radioactive material, low specific activity (LSA-III), fissile
3326	**165**	Radioactive material, surface contaminated objects (SCO-I), fissile
3326	**165**	Radioactive material, surface contaminated objects (SCO-II), fissile
3327	**165**	Radioactive material, Type A package, fissile, non-special form
3328	**165**	Radioactive material, Type B(U) package, fissile
3329	**165**	Radioactive material, Type B(M) package, fissile
3330	**165**	Radioactive material, Type C package, fissile
3331	**165**	Radioactive material, transported under special arrangement, fissile
3332	**164**	Radioactive material, Type A package, special form, non fissile or fissile-excepted
3333	**165**	Radioactive material, Type A package, special form, fissile
3334	**171**	Aviation regulated liquid, n.o.s.
3334	**171**	Self-defense spray, non-pressurized
3335	**171**	Aviation regulated solid, n.o.s.
3336	**130**	Mercaptan mixture, liquid, flammable, n.o.s.
3336	**130**	Mercaptans, liquid, flammable, n.o.s.
3337	**126**	Refrigerant gas R-404A
3338	**126**	Refrigerant gas R-407A
3339	**126**	Refrigerant gas R-407B
3340	**126**	Refrigerant gas R-407C
3341	**135**	Thiourea dioxide
3342	**135**	Xanthates
3343	**113**	Nitroglycerin mixture, desensitized, liquid, flammable, n.o.s., with not more than 30% Nitroglycerin
3344	**113**	Pentaerythrite tetranitrate mixture, desensitized, solid, n.o.s., with more than 10% but not more than 20% PETN

ID No.	Guide No.	Name of Material
3344	**113**	Pentaerythritol tetranitrate mixture, desensitized, solid, n.o.s., with more than 10% but not more than 20% PETN
3344	**113**	PETN mixture, desensitized, solid, n.o.s., with more than 10% but not more than 20% PETN
3345	**153**	Phenoxyacetic acid derivative pesticide, solid, poisonous
3345	**153**	Phenoxyacetic acid derivative pesticide, solid, toxic
3346	**131**	Phenoxyacetic acid derivative pesticide, liquid, flammable, poisonous
3346	**131**	Phenoxyacetic acid derivative pesticide, liquid, flammable, toxic
3347	**131**	Phenoxyacetic acid derivative pesticide, liquid, poisonous, flammable
3347	**131**	Phenoxyacetic acid derivative pesticide, liquid, toxic, flammable
3348	**153**	Phenoxyacetic acid derivative pesticide, liquid, poisonous
3348	**153**	Phenoxyacetic acid derivative pesticide, liquid, toxic
3349	**151**	Pyrethroid pesticide, solid, poisonous
3349	**151**	Pyrethroid pesticide, solid, toxic
3350	**131**	Pyrethroid pesticide, liquid, flammable, poisonous
3350	**131**	Pyrethroid pesticide, liquid, flammable, toxic
3351	**131**	Pyrethroid pesticide, liquid, poisonous, flammable
3351	**131**	Pyrethroid pesticide, liquid, toxic, flammable
3352	**151**	Pyrethroid pesticide, liquid, poisonous
3352	**151**	Pyrethroid pesticide, liquid, toxic
3354	**115**	Insecticide gas, flammable, n.o.s.
3355	**119**	Insecticide gas, poisonous, flammable, n.o.s.
3355	**119**	Insecticide gas, poisonous, flammable, n.o.s. (Inhalation Hazard Zone A)
3355	**119**	Insecticide gas, poisonous, flammable, n.o.s. (Inhalation Hazard Zone B)
3355	**119**	Insecticide gas, poisonous, flammable, n.o.s. (Inhalation Hazard Zone C)
3355	**119**	Insecticide gas, poisonous, flammable, n.o.s. (Inhalation Hazard Zone D)
3355	**119**	Insecticide gas, toxic, flammable, n.o.s.
3355	**119**	Insecticide gas, toxic, flammable, n.o.s. (Inhalation Hazard Zone A)
3355	**119**	Insecticide gas, toxic, flammable, n.o.s. (Inhalation Hazard Zone B)
3355	**119**	Insecticide gas, toxic, flammable, n.o.s. (Inhalation Hazard Zone C)
3355	**119**	Insecticide gas, toxic, flammable, n.o.s. (Inhalation Hazard Zone D)
3356	**140**	Oxygen generator, chemical
3356	**140**	Oxygen generator, chemical, spent
3357	**113**	Nitroglycerin mixture, desensitized, liquid, n.o.s., with not more than 30% Nitroglycerin
3358	**115**	Refrigerating machines, containing flammable, non-poisonous, liquefied gas

ID No.	Guide No.	Name of Material
3358	**115**	Refrigerating machines, containing flammable, non-toxic, liquefied gas
3359	**171**	Fumigated cargo transport unit
3360	**133**	Fibers, vegetable, dry
3360	**133**	Fibres, vegetable, dry
3361	**156**	Chlorosilanes, poisonous, corrosive, n.o.s.
3361	**156**	Chlorosilanes, toxic, corrosive, n.o.s.
3362	**155**	Chlorosilanes, poisonous, corrosive, flammable, n.o.s.
3362	**155**	Chlorosilanes, toxic, corrosive, flammable, n.o.s.
3363	**171**	Dangerous goods in apparatus
3363	**171**	Dangerous goods in articles
3363	**171**	Dangerous goods in machinery
3364	**113**	Picric acid, wetted with not less than 10% water
3364	**113**	Trinitrophenol, wetted with not less than 10% water
3365	**113**	Picryl chloride, wetted with not less than 10% water
3365	**113**	Trinitrochlorobenzene, wetted with not less than 10% water
3366	**113**	TNT, wetted with not less than 10% water
3366	**113**	Trinitrotoluene, wetted with not less than 10% water
3367	**113**	Trinitrobenzene, wetted with not less than 10% water
3368	**113**	Trinitrobenzoic acid, wetted with not less than 10% water
3369	**113**	Sodium dinitro-o-cresolate, wetted with not less than 10% water
3370	**113**	Urea nitrate, wetted with not less than 10% water
3371	**129**	2-Methylbutanal

ID No.	Guide No.	Name of Material
3373	**158**	Biological substance, category B
3374	**116**	Acetylene, solvent free
3375	**140**	Ammonium nitrate emulsion
3375	**140**	Ammonium nitrate gel
3375	**140**	Ammonium nitrate suspension
3376	**113**	4-Nitrophenylhydrazine, with not less than 30% water
3377	**140**	Sodium perborate monohydrate
3378	**140**	Sodium carbonate peroxyhydrate
3379	**113**	Desensitized explosive, liquid, n.o.s.
3380	**113**	Desensitized explosive, solid, n.o.s.
3381	**151**	Poisonous by inhalation liquid, n.o.s. (Inhalation Hazard Zone A)
3381	**151**	Toxic by inhalation liquid, n.o.s. (Inhalation Hazard Zone A)
3382	**151**	Poisonous by inhalation liquid, n.o.s. (Inhalation Hazard Zone B)
3382	**151**	Toxic by inhalation liquid, n.o.s. (Inhalation Hazard Zone B)
3383	**131**	Poisonous by inhalation liquid, flammable, n.o.s. (Inhalation Hazard Zone A)
3383	**131**	Toxic by inhalation liquid, flammable, n.o.s. (Inhalation Hazard Zone A)
3384	**131**	Poisonous by inhalation liquid, flammable, n.o.s. (Inhalation Hazard Zone B)
3384	**131**	Toxic by inhalation liquid, flammable, n.o.s. (Inhalation Hazard Zone B)
3385	**139**	Poisonous by inhalation liquid, water-reactive, n.o.s. (Inhalation Hazard Zone A)

ID No.	Guide No.	Name of Material
3385	**139**	Toxic by inhalation liquid, water-reactive, n.o.s. (Inhalation Hazard Zone A)
3386	**139**	Poisonous by inhalation liquid, water-reactive, n.o.s. (Inhalation Hazard Zone B)
3386	**139**	Toxic by inhalation liquid, water-reactive, n.o.s. (Inhalation Hazard Zone B)
3387	**142**	Poisonous by inhalation liquid, oxidizing, n.o.s. (Inhalation Hazard Zone A)
3387	**142**	Toxic by inhalation liquid, oxidizing, n.o.s. (Inhalation Hazard Zone A)
3388	**142**	Poisonous by inhalation liquid, oxidizing, n.o.s. (Inhalation Hazard Zone B)
3388	**142**	Toxic by inhalation liquid, oxidizing, n.o.s. (Inhalation Hazard Zone B)
3389	**154**	Poisonous by inhalation liquid, corrosive, n.o.s. (Inhalation Hazard Zone A)
3389	**154**	Toxic by inhalation liquid, corrosive, n.o.s. (Inhalation Hazard Zone A)
3390	**154**	Poisonous by inhalation liquid, corrosive, n.o.s. (Inhalation Hazard Zone B)
3390	**154**	Toxic by inhalation liquid, corrosive, n.o.s. (Inhalation Hazard Zone B)
3391	**135**	Organometallic substance, solid, pyrophoric
3392	**135**	Organometallic substance, liquid, pyrophoric
3393	**135**	Organometallic substance, solid, pyrophoric, water-reactive
3394	**135**	Organometallic substance, liquid, pyrophoric, water-reactive

ID No.	Guide No.	Name of Material
3395	**135**	Organometallic substance, solid, water-reactive
3396	**138**	Organometallic substance, solid, water-reactive, flammable
3397	**138**	Organometallic substance, solid, water-reactive, self-heating
3398	**135**	Organometallic substance, liquid, water-reactive
3399	**138**	Organometallic substance, liquid, water-reactive, flammable
3400	**138**	Organometallic substance, solid, self-heating
3401	**138**	Alkali metal amalgam, solid
3402	**138**	Alkaline earth metal amalgam, solid
3403	**138**	Potassium, metal alloys, solid
3404	**138**	Potassium sodium alloys, solid
3404	**138**	Sodium potassium alloys, solid
3405	**141**	Barium chlorate, solution
3406	**141**	Barium perchlorate, solution
3407	**140**	Chlorate and Magnesium chloride mixture, solution
3407	**140**	Magnesium chloride and Chlorate mixture, solution
3408	**141**	Lead perchlorate, solution
3409	**152**	Chloronitrobenzenes, liquid
3410	**153**	4-Chloro-o-toluidine hydrochloride, solution
3411	**153**	beta-Naphthylamine, solution
3411	**153**	Naphthylamine (beta), solution
3412	**153**	Formic acid, with not less than 5% but less than 10% acid
3412	**153**	Formic acid, with not less than 10% but not more than 85% acid

ID No.	Guide No.	Name of Material
3413	**157**	Potassium cyanide, solution
3414	**157**	Sodium cyanide, solution
3415	**154**	Sodium fluoride, solution
3416	**153**	Chloroacetophenone, liquid
3417	**152**	Xylyl bromide, solid
3418	**151**	2,4-Toluenediamine, solution
3418	**151**	2,4-Toluylenediamine, solution
3419	**157**	Boron trifluoride acetic acid complex, solid
3420	**157**	Boron trifluoride propionic acid complex, solid
3421	**154**	Potassium hydrogen difluoride, solution
3422	**154**	Potassium fluoride, solution
3423	**153**	Tetramethylammonium hydroxide, solid
3424	**141**	Ammonium dinitro-o-cresolate, solution
3425	**156**	Bromoacetic acid, solid
3426	**153P**	Acrylamide, solution
3427	**153**	Chlorobenzyl chlorides, solid
3428	**156**	3-Chloro-4-methylphenyl isocyanate, solid
3429	**153**	Chlorotoluidines, liquid
3430	**153**	Xylenols, liquid
3431	**152**	Nitrobenzotrifluorides, solid
3432	**171**	Polychlorinated biphenyls, solid
3434	**153**	Nitrocresols, liquid
3436	**151**	Hexafluoroacetone hydrate, solid
3437	**152**	Chlorocresols, solid
3438	**153**	alpha-Methylbenzyl alcohol, solid
3438	**153**	Methylbenzyl (alpha) alcohol, solid
3439	**151**	Nitriles, poisonous, solid, n.o.s.
3439	**151**	Nitriles, solid, poisonous, n.o.s.
3439	**151**	Nitriles, solid, toxic, n.o.s.
3439	**151**	Nitriles, toxic, solid, n.o.s.
3440	**151**	Selenium compound, liquid, n.o.s.
3441	**153**	Chlorodinitrobenzenes, solid
3442	**153**	Dichloroanilines, solid
3443	**152**	Dinitrobenzenes, solid
3444	**151**	Nicotine hydrochloride, solid
3445	**151**	Nicotine sulfate, solid
3445	**151**	Nicotine sulphate, solid
3446	**152**	Nitrotoluenes, solid
3447	**152**	Nitroxylenes, solid
3448	**159**	Tear gas substance, solid, n.o.s.
3449	**159**	Bromobenzyl cyanides, solid
3450	**151**	Diphenylchloroarsine, solid
3451	**153**	Toluidines, solid
3452	**153**	Xylidines, solid
3453	**154**	Phosphoric acid, solid
3454	**152**	Dinitrotoluenes, solid
3455	**153**	Cresols, solid
3456	**157**	Nitrosylsulfuric acid, solid
3456	**157**	Nitrosylsulphuric acid, solid
3457	**152**	Chloronitrotoluenes, solid
3458	**152**	Nitroanisoles, solid
3459	**152**	Nitrobromobenzenes, solid
3460	**153**	N-Ethylbenzyltoluidines, solid
3462	**153**	Toxins, extracted from living sources, solid, n.o.s.
3463	**153**	Propionic acid, with not less than 90% acid

ID No.	Guide No.	Name of Material
3464	**151**	Organophosphorus compound, poisonous, solid, n.o.s.
3464	**151**	Organophosphorus compound, solid, poisonous, n.o.s.
3464	**151**	Organophosphorus compound, solid, toxic, n.o.s.
3464	**151**	Organophosphorus compound, toxic, solid, n.o.s.
3465	**151**	Organoarsenic compound, solid, n.o.s.
3466	**151**	Metal carbonyls, solid, n.o.s.
3467	**151**	Organometallic compound, poisonous, solid, n.o.s.
3467	**151**	Organometallic compound, solid, poisonous, n.o.s.
3467	**151**	Organometallic compound, solid, toxic, n.o.s.
3467	**151**	Organometallic compound, toxic, solid, n.o.s.
3468	**115**	Hydrogen in a metal hydride storage system
3468	**115**	Hydrogen in a metal hydride storage system contained in equipment
3468	**115**	Hydrogen in a metal hydride storage system packed with equipment
3469	**132**	Paint, flammable, corrosive
3469	**132**	Paint related material, flammable, corrosive
3470	**132**	Paint, corrosive, flammable
3470	**132**	Paint related material, corrosive, flammable
3471	**154**	Hydrogendifluorides, solution, n.o.s.
3472	**153**	Crotonic acid, liquid
3473	**128**	Fuel cell cartridges, containing flammable liquids

ID No.	Guide No.	Name of Material
3473	**128**	Fuel cell cartridges contained in equipment, containing flammable liquids
3473	**128**	Fuel cell cartridges packed with equipment, containing flammable liquids
3474	**113**	1-Hydroxybenzotriazole, anhydrous, wetted with not less than 20% water
3474	**113**	1-Hydroxybenzotriazole, monohydrate
3475	**127**	Ethanol and gasoline mixture, with more than 10% ethanol
3475	**127**	Ethanol and motor spirit mixture, with more than 10% ethanol
3475	**127**	Ethanol and petrol mixture, with more than 10% ethanol
3475	**127**	Gasoline and ethanol mixture, with more than 10% ethanol
3475	**127**	Motor spirit and ethanol mixture, with more than 10% ethanol
3475	**127**	Petrol and ethanol mixture, with more than 10% ethanol
3476	**138**	Fuel cell cartridges, containing water-reactive substances
3476	**138**	Fuel cell cartridges contained in equipment, containing water-reactive substances
3476	**138**	Fuel cell cartridges packed with equipment, containing water-reactive substances
3477	**153**	Fuel cell cartridges, containing corrosive substances
3477	**153**	Fuel cell cartridges contained in equipment, containing corrosive substances
3477	**153**	Fuel cell cartridges packed with equipment, containing corrosive substances

ID No.	Guide No.	Name of Material
3478	**115**	Fuel cell cartridges, containing liquefied flammable gas
3478	**115**	Fuel cell cartridges contained in equipment, containing liquefied flammable gas
3478	**115**	Fuel cell cartridges packed with equipment, containing liquefied flammable gas
3479	**115**	Fuel cell cartridges, containing hydrogen in metal hydride
3479	**115**	Fuel cell cartridges contained in equipment, containing hydrogen in metal hydride
3479	**115**	Fuel cell cartridges packed with equipment, containing hydrogen in metal hydride
3480	**147**	Lithium ion batteries (including lithium ion polymer batteries)
3481	**147**	Lithium ion batteries contained in equipment (including lithium ion polymer batteries)
3481	**147**	Lithium ion batteries packed with equipment (including lithium ion polymer batteries)
3482	**138**	Alkali metal dispersion, flammable
3482	**138**	Alkaline earth metal dispersion, flammable
3483	**131**	Motor fuel anti-knock mixture, flammable
3484	**132**	Hydrazine aqueous solution, flammable, with more than 37% hydrazine, by mass
3485	**140**	Calcium hypochlorite, dry, corrosive, with more than 39% available chlorine (8.8% available oxygen)
3485	**140**	Calcium hypochlorite mixture, dry, corrosive, with more than 39% available chlorine (8.8% available oxygen)
3486	**140**	Calcium hypochlorite mixture, dry, corrosive, with more than 10% but not more than 39% available chlorine
3487	**140**	Calcium hypochlorite, hydrated, corrosive, with not less than 5.5% but not more than 16% water
3487	**140**	Calcium hypochlorite, hydrated mixture, corrosive, with not less than 5.5% but not more than 16% water
3488	**131**	Poisonous by inhalation liquid, flammable, corrosive, n.o.s. (Inhalation Hazard Zone A)
3488	**131**	Toxic by inhalation liquid, flammable, corrosive, n.o.s. (Inhalation Hazard Zone A)
3489	**131**	Poisonous by inhalation liquid, flammable, corrosive, n.o.s. (Inhalation Hazard Zone B)
3489	**131**	Toxic by inhalation liquid, flammable, corrosive, n.o.s. (Inhalation Hazard Zone B)
3490	**155**	Poisonous by inhalation liquid, water-reactive, flammable, n.o.s. (Inhalation Hazard Zone A)
3490	**155**	Toxic by inhalation liquid, water-reactive, flammable, n.o.s. (Inhalation Hazard Zone A)
3491	**155**	Poisonous by inhalation liquid, water-reactive, flammable, n.o.s. (Inhalation Hazard Zone B)
3491	**155**	Toxic by inhalation liquid, water-reactive, flammable, n.o.s. (Inhalation Hazard Zone B)
3492	**131**	Poisonous by inhalation liquid, corrosive, flammable, n.o.s. (Inhalation Hazard Zone A)
3492	**131**	Toxic by inhalation liquid, corrosive, flammable, n.o.s. (Inhalation Hazard Zone A)

ID No.	Guide No.	Name of Material
3493	**131**	Poisonous by inhalation liquid, corrosive, flammable, n.o.s. (Inhalation Hazard Zone B)
3493	**131**	Toxic by inhalation liquid, corrosive, flammable, n.o.s. (Inhalation Hazard Zone B)
3494	**131**	Petroleum sour crude oil, flammable, poisonous
3494	**131**	Petroleum sour crude oil, flammable, toxic
3495	**154**	Iodine
3496	**171**	Batteries, nickel-metal hydride
3497	**133**	Krill meal
3498	**157**	Iodine monochloride, liquid
3499	**171**	Capacitor, electric double layer
3500	**126**	Chemical under pressure, n.o.s.
3501	**115**	Chemical under pressure, flammable, n.o.s.
3502	**123**	Chemical under pressure, poisonous, n.o.s.
3502	**123**	Chemical under pressure, toxic, n.o.s.
3503	**125**	Chemical under pressure, corrosive, n.o.s.
3504	**119**	Chemical under pressure, flammable, poisonous, n.o.s.
3504	**119**	Chemical under pressure, flammable, toxic, n.o.s.
3505	**118**	Chemical under pressure, flammable, corrosive, n.o.s.
3506	**172**	Mercury contained in manufactured articles
3507	**166**	Uranium hexafluoride, radioactive material, excepted package, less than 0.1 kg per package, non-fissile or fissile-excepted
3508	**171**	Capacitor, asymmetric
3509	**171**	Packagings discarded, empty, uncleaned
3510	**174**	Adsorbed gas, flammable, n.o.s.
3511	**174**	Adsorbed gas, n.o.s.
3512	**173**	Adsorbed gas, poisonous, n.o.s.
3512	**173**	Adsorbed gas, poisonous, n.o.s. (Inhalation hazard zone A)
3512	**173**	Adsorbed gas, poisonous, n.o.s. (Inhalation hazard zone B)
3512	**173**	Adsorbed gas, poisonous, n.o.s. (Inhalation hazard zone C)
3512	**173**	Adsorbed gas, poisonous, n.o.s. (Inhalation hazard zone D)
3512	**173**	Adsorbed gas, toxic, n.o.s.
3512	**173**	Adsorbed gas, toxic, n.o.s. (Inhalation hazard zone A)
3512	**173**	Adsorbed gas, toxic, n.o.s. (Inhalation hazard zone B)
3512	**173**	Adsorbed gas, toxic, n.o.s. (Inhalation hazard zone C)
3512	**173**	Adsorbed gas, toxic, n.o.s. (Inhalation hazard zone D)
3513	**174**	Adsorbed gas, oxidizing, n.o.s.
3514	**173**	Adsorbed gas, poisonous, flammable, n.o.s.
3514	**173**	Adsorbed gas, poisonous, flammable, n.o.s. (Inhalation hazard zone A)
3514	**173**	Adsorbed gas, poisonous, flammable, n.o.s. (Inhalation hazard zone B)
3514	**173**	Adsorbed gas, poisonous, flammable, n.o.s. (Inhalation hazard zone C)
3514	**173**	Adsorbed gas, poisonous, flammable, n.o.s. (Inhalation hazard zone D)
3514	**173**	Adsorbed gas, toxic, flammable, n.o.s.

ID No.	Guide No.	Name of Material
3514	**173**	Adsorbed gas, toxic, flammable, n.o.s. (Inhalation hazard zone A)
3514	**173**	Adsorbed gas, toxic, flammable, n.o.s. (Inhalation hazard zone B)
3514	**173**	Adsorbed gas, toxic, flammable, n.o.s. (Inhalation hazard zone C)
3514	**173**	Adsorbed gas, toxic, flammable, n.o.s. (Inhalation hazard zone D)
3515	**173**	Adsorbed gas, poisonous, oxidizing, n.o.s.
3515	**173**	Adsorbed gas, poisonous, oxidizing, n.o.s. (Inhalation hazard zone A)
3515	**173**	Adsorbed gas, poisonous, oxidizing, n.o.s. (Inhalation hazard zone B)
3515	**173**	Adsorbed gas, poisonous, oxidizing, n.o.s. (Inhalation hazard zone C)
3515	**173**	Adsorbed gas, poisonous, oxidizing, n.o.s. (Inhalation hazard zone D)
3515	**173**	Adsorbed gas, toxic, oxidizing, n.o.s.
3515	**173**	Adsorbed gas, toxic, oxidizing, n.o.s. (Inhalation hazard zone A)
3515	**173**	Adsorbed gas, toxic, oxidizing, n.o.s. (Inhalation hazard zone B)
3515	**173**	Adsorbed gas, toxic, oxidizing, n.o.s. (Inhalation hazard zone C)
3515	**173**	Adsorbed gas, toxic, oxidizing, n.o.s. (Inhalation hazard zone D)
3516	**173**	Adsorbed gas, poisonous, corrosive, n.o.s.
3516	**173**	Adsorbed gas, poisonous, corrosive, n.o.s. (Inhalation hazard zone A)
3516	**173**	Adsorbed gas, poisonous, corrosive, n.o.s. (Inhalation hazard zone B)
3516	**173**	Adsorbed gas, poisonous, corrosive, n.o.s. (Inhalation hazard zone C)
3516	**173**	Adsorbed gas, poisonous, corrosive, n.o.s. (Inhalation hazard zone D)
3516	**173**	Adsorbed gas, toxic, corrosive, n.o.s.
3516	**173**	Adsorbed gas, toxic, corrosive, n.o.s. (Inhalation hazard zone A)
3516	**173**	Adsorbed gas, toxic, corrosive, n.o.s. (Inhalation hazard zone B)
3516	**173**	Adsorbed gas, toxic, corrosive, n.o.s. (Inhalation hazard zone C)
3516	**173**	Adsorbed gas, toxic, corrosive, n.o.s. (Inhalation hazard zone D)
3517	**173**	Adsorbed gas, poisonous, flammable, corrosive, n.o.s.
3517	**173**	Adsorbed gas, poisonous, flammable, corrosive, n.o.s. (Inhalation hazard zone A)
3517	**173**	Adsorbed gas, poisonous, flammable, corrosive, n.o.s. (Inhalation hazard zone B)
3517	**173**	Adsorbed gas, poisonous, flammable, corrosive, n.o.s. (Inhalation hazard zone C)
3517	**173**	Adsorbed gas, poisonous, flammable, corrosive, n.o.s. (Inhalation hazard zone D)
3517	**173**	Adsorbed gas, toxic, flammable, corrosive, n.o.s.

ID No.	Guide No.	Name of Material
3517	**173**	Adsorbed gas, toxic, flammable, corrosive, n.o.s. (Inhalation hazard zone A)
3517	**173**	Adsorbed gas, toxic, flammable, corrosive, n.o.s. (Inhalation hazard zone B)
3517	**173**	Adsorbed gas, toxic, flammable, corrosive, n.o.s. (Inhalation hazard zone C)
3517	**173**	Adsorbed gas, toxic, flammable, corrosive, n.o.s. (Inhalation hazard zone D)
3518	**173**	Adsorbed gas, poisonous, oxidizing, corrosive, n.o.s.
3518	**173**	Adsorbed gas, poisonous, oxidizing, corrosive, n.o.s. (Inhalation hazard zone A)
3518	**173**	Adsorbed gas, poisonous, oxidizing, corrosive, n.o.s. (Inhalation hazard zone B)
3518	**173**	Adsorbed gas, poisonous, oxidizing, corrosive, n.o.s. (Inhalation hazard zone C)
3518	**173**	Adsorbed gas, poisonous, oxidizing, corrosive, n.o.s. (Inhalation hazard zone D)
3518	**173**	Adsorbed gas, toxic, oxidizing, corrosive, n.o.s.
3518	**173**	Adsorbed gas, toxic, oxidizing, corrosive, n.o.s. (Inhalation hazard zone A)
3518	**173**	Adsorbed gas, toxic, oxidizing, corrosive, n.o.s. (Inhalation hazard zone B)
3518	**173**	Adsorbed gas, toxic, oxidizing, corrosive, n.o.s. (Inhalation hazard zone C)
3518	**173**	Adsorbed gas, toxic, oxidizing, corrosive, n.o.s. (Inhalation hazard zone D)
3519	**173**	Boron trifluoride, adsorbed
3520	**173**	Chlorine, adsorbed

ID No.	Guide No.	Name of Material
3521	**173**	Silicon tetrafluoride, adsorbed
3522	**173**	Arsine, adsorbed
3523	**173**	Germane, adsorbed
3524	**173**	Phosphorus pentafluoride, adsorbed
3525	**173**	Phosphine, adsorbed
3526	**173**	Hydrogen selenide, adsorbed
3527	**128P**	Polyester resin kit, solid base material
3528	**128**	Engine, fuel cell, flammable liquid powered
3528	**128**	Engine, internal combustion, flammable liquid powered
3528	**128**	Machinery, fuel cell, flammable liquid powered
3528	**128**	Machinery, internal combustion, flammable liquid powered
3529	**115**	Engine, fuel cell, flammable gas powered
3529	**115**	Engine, internal combustion, flammable gas powered
3529	**115**	Machinery, fuel cell, flammable gas powered
3529	**115**	Machinery, internal combustion, flammable gas powered
3530	**171**	Engine, internal combustion
3530	**171**	Machinery, internal combustion
3531	**149P**	Polymerizing substance, solid, stabilized, n.o.s.
3532	**149P**	Polymerizing substance, liquid, stabilized, n.o.s.
3533	**150P**	Polymerizing substance, solid, temperature controlled, n.o.s.
3534	**150P**	Polymerizing substance, liquid, temperature controlled, n.o.s.
3535	**134**	Toxic solid, flammable, inorganic, n.o.s.

ID No.	Guide No.	Name of Material
3536	**147**	Lithium batteries installed in cargo transport unit (lithium ion batteries)
3536	**138**	Lithium batteries installed in cargo transport unit (lithium metal batteries)
3537	**115**	Articles containing flammable gas, n.o.s.
3538	**120**	Articles containing non-flammable, non-toxic gas, n.o.s.
3539	**123**	Articles containing toxic gas, n.o.s.
3540	**127**	Articles containing flammable liquid, n.o.s.
3541	**133**	Articles containing flammable solid, n.o.s.
3542	**135**	Articles containing a substance liable to spontaneous combustion, n.o.s.
3543	**138**	Articles containing a substance which emits flammable gas in contact with water, n.o.s.
3544	**140**	Articles containing oxidizing substance, n.o.s.
3545	**145**	Articles containing organic peroxide, n.o.s.
3546	**151**	Articles containing toxic substance, n.o.s.
3547	**154**	Articles containing corrosive substance, n.o.s.
3548	**171**	Articles containing miscellaneous dangerous goods, n.o.s.
3549	**158**	Medical waste, category A, affecting humans, solid
3549	**158**	Medical waste, category A, affecting animals only, solid
8000	**171**	Consumer commodity
9035	**123**	Gas identification set
9191	**143**	Chlorine dioxide, hydrate, frozen
9202	**168**	Carbon monoxide, refrigerated liquid (cryogenic liquid)
9206	**137**	Methyl phosphonic dichloride
9260	**169**	Aluminum, molten
9263	**156**	Chloropivaloyl chloride
9264	**151**	3,5-Dichloro-2,4,6-trifluoropyridine
9269	**132**	Trimethoxysilane

NOTES

INTRODUCTION TO BLUE PAGES

For entries highlighted in green follow these steps:

- **IF THERE IS NO FIRE**:
  - Go directly to **Table 1** (green-bordered pages)
  - Look up the ID number and name of material
  - Identify initial isolation and protective action distances
  - Also consult the appropriate Orange Guide

- **IF A FIRE IS INVOLVED**:
  - Use the appropriate Orange Guide for **EVACUATION** distances
  - Also protect in downwind direction according to Table 1 for residual material release

Note 1: If the name in **Table 1** is shown with **(when spilled in water)**, these materials produce large amounts of Toxic Inhalation Hazard (TIH) (PIH in the US) gases when spilled in water. Some Water Reactive materials are also TIH materials themselves (e.g., UN1746 (Bromine trifluoride), UN1836 (Thionyl chloride)). In these instances, two entries are provided in **Table 1** for land-based and water-based spills. If a water-reactive material only has one entry in Table 1 for **(when spilled in water)** and the product is NOT spilled in water, Table 1 and Table 2 do not apply. You will find safe distances in the appropriate orange-bordered guide.

Note 2: **Explosives** are not individually listed by their name because in an emergency situation, the response will be based only on the division of the explosive, not on the individual explosive.

For divisions 1.1, 1.2, 1.3 and 1.5, refer to GUIDE 112.

For divisions 1.4 and 1.6, refer to GUIDE 114.

Note 3: Chemical warfare agents do not have an assigned ID number because they are not commercially transported. In an emergency situation, the assigned orange guide will provide guidance for the initial response. Also consult "Criminal or Terrorist Use of Chemical, Biological and Radiological Agents", pp. 368 to 372.

Name of Material	Guide No.	ID No.
AC	**117**	—
Acetal	**127**	1088
Acetaldehyde	**129P**	1089
Acetaldehyde ammonia	**171**	1841
Acetaldehyde oxime	**129**	2332
Acetic acid, glacial	**132**	2789
Acetic acid, solution, more than 10% but not more than 80% acid	**153**	2790
Acetic acid, solution, more than 80% acid	**132**	2789
Acetic anhydride	**137**	1715
Acetone	**127**	1090
Acetone cyanohydrin, stabilized	**155**	1541
Acetone oils	**127**	1091
Acetonitrile	**127**	1648
Acetyl bromide	**156**	1716
Acetyl chloride	**155**	1717
Acetylene, dissolved	**116**	1001
Acetylene, Ethylene and Propylene in mixture, refrigerated liquid containing at least 71.5% Ethylene with not more than 22.5% Acetylene and not more than 6% Propylene	**115**	3138
Acetylene, solvent free	**116**	3374
Acetylene tetrabromide	**159**	2504
Acetyl iodide	**156**	1898
Acetyl methyl carbinol	**127**	2621
Acid, sludge	**153**	1906
Acid butyl phosphate	**153**	1718
Acridine	**153**	2713
Acrolein, stabilized	**131P**	1092
Acrolein dimer, stabilized	**129P**	2607
Acrylamide, solid	**153P**	2074
Acrylamide, solution	**153P**	3426
Acrylic acid, stabilized	**132P**	2218
Acrylonitrile, stabilized	**131P**	1093
Adamsite	**154**	—
Adhesives (flammable)	**128**	1133
Adiponitrile	**153**	2205
Adsorbed gas, flammable, n.o.s.	**174**	3510
Adsorbed gas, n.o.s.	**174**	3511
Adsorbed gas, oxidizing, n.o.s.	**174**	3513
Adsorbed gas, poisonous, corrosive, n.o.s.	**173**	3516
Adsorbed gas, poisonous, corrosive, n.o.s. (Inhalation hazard zone A)	**173**	3516
Adsorbed gas, poisonous, corrosive, n.o.s. (Inhalation hazard zone B)	**173**	3516
Adsorbed gas, poisonous, corrosive, n.o.s. (Inhalation hazard zone C)	**173**	3516
Adsorbed gas, poisonous, corrosive, n.o.s. (Inhalation hazard zone D)	**173**	3516
Adsorbed gas, poisonous, flammable, corrosive, n.o.s.	**173**	3517
Adsorbed gas, poisonous, flammable, corrosive, n.o.s. (Inhalation hazard zone A)	**173**	3517
Adsorbed gas, poisonous, flammable, corrosive, n.o.s. (Inhalation hazard zone B)	**173**	3517
Adsorbed gas, poisonous, flammable, corrosive, n.o.s. (Inhalation hazard zone C)	**173**	3517
Adsorbed gas, poisonous, flammable, corrosive, n.o.s. (Inhalation hazard zone D)	**173**	3517

Name of Material	Guide No.	ID No.
Adsorbed gas, poisonous, flammable, n.o.s.	**173**	3514
Adsorbed gas, poisonous, flammable, n.o.s. (Inhalation hazard zone A)	**173**	3514
Adsorbed gas, poisonous, flammable, n.o.s. (Inhalation hazard zone B)	**173**	3514
Adsorbed gas, poisonous, flammable, n.o.s. (Inhalation hazard zone C)	**173**	3514
Adsorbed gas, poisonous, flammable, n.o.s. (Inhalation hazard zone D)	**173**	3514
Adsorbed gas, poisonous, n.o.s.	**173**	3512
Adsorbed gas, poisonous, n.o.s. (Inhalation hazard zone A)	**173**	3512
Adsorbed gas, poisonous, n.o.s. (Inhalation hazard zone B)	**173**	3512
Adsorbed gas, poisonous, n.o.s. (Inhalation hazard zone C)	**173**	3512
Adsorbed gas, poisonous, n.o.s. (Inhalation hazard zone D)	**173**	3512
Adsorbed gas, poisonous, oxidizing, corrosive, n.o.s.	**173**	3518
Adsorbed gas, poisonous, oxidizing, corrosive, n.o.s. (Inhalation hazard zone A)	**173**	3518
Adsorbed gas, poisonous, oxidizing, corrosive, n.o.s. (Inhalation hazard zone B)	**173**	3518
Adsorbed gas, poisonous, oxidizing, corrosive, n.o.s. (Inhalation hazard zone C)	**173**	3518
Adsorbed gas, poisonous, oxidizing, corrosive, n.o.s. (Inhalation hazard zone D)	**173**	3518
Adsorbed gas, poisonous, oxidizing, n.o.s.	**173**	3515
Adsorbed gas, poisonous, oxidizing, n.o.s. (Inhalation hazard zone A)	**173**	3515
Adsorbed gas, poisonous, oxidizing, n.o.s. (Inhalation hazard zone B)	**173**	3515
Adsorbed gas, poisonous, oxidizing, n.o.s. (Inhalation hazard zone C)	**173**	3515
Adsorbed gas, poisonous, oxidizing, n.o.s. (Inhalation hazard zone D)	**173**	3515
Adsorbed gas, toxic, corrosive, n.o.s.	**173**	3516
Adsorbed gas, toxic, corrosive, n.o.s. (Inhalation hazard zone A)	**173**	3516
Adsorbed gas, toxic, corrosive, n.o.s. (Inhalation hazard zone B)	**173**	3516
Adsorbed gas, toxic, corrosive, n.o.s. (Inhalation hazard zone C)	**173**	3516
Adsorbed gas, toxic, corrosive, n.o.s. (Inhalation hazard zone D)	**173**	3516
Adsorbed gas, toxic, flammable, corrosive, n.o.s.	**173**	3517
Adsorbed gas, toxic, flammable, corrosive, n.o.s. (Inhalation hazard zone A)	**173**	3517
Adsorbed gas, toxic, flammable, corrosive, n.o.s. (Inhalation hazard zone B)	**173**	3517
Adsorbed gas, toxic, flammable, corrosive, n.o.s. (Inhalation hazard zone C)	**173**	3517
Adsorbed gas, toxic, flammable, corrosive, n.o.s. (Inhalation hazard zone D)	**173**	3517

Name of Material	Guide No.	ID No.
Adsorbed gas, toxic, flammable, n.o.s.	173	3514
Adsorbed gas, toxic, flammable, n.o.s. (Inhalation hazard zone A)	173	3514
Adsorbed gas, toxic, flammable, n.o.s. (Inhalation hazard zone B)	173	3514
Adsorbed gas, toxic, flammable, n.o.s. (Inhalation hazard zone C)	173	3514
Adsorbed gas, toxic, flammable, n.o.s. (Inhalation hazard zone D)	173	3514
Adsorbed gas, toxic, n.o.s.	173	3512
Adsorbed gas, toxic, n.o.s. (Inhalation hazard zone A)	173	3512
Adsorbed gas, toxic, n.o.s. (Inhalation hazard zone B)	173	3512
Adsorbed gas, toxic, n.o.s. (Inhalation hazard zone C)	173	3512
Adsorbed gas, toxic, n.o.s. (Inhalation hazard zone D)	173	3512
Adsorbed gas, toxic, oxidizing, corrosive, n.o.s.	173	3518
Adsorbed gas, toxic, oxidizing, corrosive, n.o.s. (Inhalation hazard zone A)	173	3518
Adsorbed gas, toxic, oxidizing, corrosive, n.o.s. (Inhalation hazard zone B)	173	3518
Adsorbed gas, toxic, oxidizing, corrosive, n.o.s. (Inhalation hazard zone C)	173	3518
Adsorbed gas, toxic, oxidizing, corrosive, n.o.s. (Inhalation hazard zone D)	173	3518
Adsorbed gas, toxic, oxidizing, n.o.s.	173	3515
Adsorbed gas, toxic, oxidizing, n.o.s. (Inhalation hazard zone A)	173	3515

Name of Material	Guide No.	ID No.
Adsorbed gas, toxic, oxidizing, n.o.s. (Inhalation hazard zone B)	173	3515
Adsorbed gas, toxic, oxidizing, n.o.s. (Inhalation hazard zone C)	173	3515
Adsorbed gas, toxic, oxidizing, n.o.s. (Inhalation hazard zone D)	173	3515
Aerosols	126	1950
Air, compressed	122	1002
Air, refrigerated liquid (cryogenic liquid)	122	1003
Air bag inflators	171	3268
Air bag modules	171	3268
Aircraft hydraulic power unit fuel tank	131	3165
Alcoholates solution, n.o.s., in alcohol	132	3274
Alcoholic beverages	127	3065
Alcohols, flammable, poisonous, n.o.s.	131	1986
Alcohols, flammable, toxic, n.o.s.	131	1986
Alcohols, n.o.s.	127	1987
Aldehydes, flammable, poisonous, n.o.s.	131P	1988
Aldehydes, flammable, toxic, n.o.s.	131P	1988
Aldehydes, n.o.s.	129P	1989
Aldol	153	2839
Alkali metal alcoholates, self-heating, corrosive, n.o.s.	136	3206
Alkali metal alloy, liquid, n.o.s.	138	1421
Alkali metal amalgam, liquid	138	1389
Alkali metal amalgam, solid	138	3401
Alkali metal amides	139	1390

Name of Material	Guide No.	ID No.
Alkali metal dispersion	**138**	1391
Alkali metal dispersion, flammable	**138**	3482
Alkaline earth metal alcoholates, n.o.s.	**135**	3205
Alkaline earth metal alloy, n.o.s.	**138**	1393
Alkaline earth metal amalgam, liquid	**138**	1392
Alkaline earth metal amalgam, solid	**138**	3402
Alkaline earth metal dispersion	**138**	1391
Alkaline earth metal dispersion, flammable	**138**	3482
Alkaloids, liquid, n.o.s. (poisonous)	**151**	3140
Alkaloids, solid, n.o.s. (poisonous)	**151**	1544
Alkaloid salts, liquid, n.o.s. (poisonous)	**151**	3140
Alkaloid salts, solid, n.o.s. (poisonous)	**151**	1544
Alkylphenols, liquid, n.o.s. (including C2-C12 homologues)	**153**	3145
Alkylphenols, solid, n.o.s. (including C2-C12 homologues)	**153**	2430
Alkyl sulfonic acids, liquid, with more than 5% free Sulfuric acid	**153**	2584
Alkyl sulfonic acids, liquid, with not more than 5% free Sulfuric acid	**153**	2586
Alkyl sulfonic acids, solid, with more than 5% free Sulfuric acid	**153**	2583
Alkyl sulfonic acids, solid, with not more than 5% free Sulfuric acid	**153**	2585
Alkylsulfuric acids	**156**	2571

Name of Material	Guide No.	ID No.
Alkyl sulphonic acids, liquid, with more than 5% free Sulphuric acid	**153**	2584
Alkyl sulphonic acids, liquid, with not more than 5% free Sulphuric acid	**153**	2586
Alkyl sulphonic acids, solid, with more than 5% free Sulphuric acid	**153**	2583
Alkyl sulphonic acids, solid, with not more than 5% free Sulphuric acid	**153**	2585
Alkylsulphuric acids	**156**	2571
Allyl acetate	**131**	2333
Allyl alcohol	**131**	1098
Allylamine	**131**	2334
Allyl bromide	**131P**	1099
Allyl chloride	**131P**	1100
Allyl chlorocarbonate	**155**	1722
Allyl chloroformate	**155**	1722
Allyl ethyl ether	**131**	2335
Allyl formate	**131**	2336
Allyl glycidyl ether	**129**	2219
Allyl iodide	**132**	1723
Allyl isothiocyanate, stabilized	**155**	1545
Allyltrichlorosilane, stabilized	**155**	1724
alpha-Methylbenzyl alcohol, liquid	**153**	2937
alpha-Methylbenzyl alcohol, solid	**153**	3438
alpha-Methylvaleraldehyde	**130**	2367
alpha-Naphthylamine	**153**	2077
alpha-Pinene	**128**	2368
Aluminum, molten	**169**	9260
Aluminum alkyl hydrides	**138**	3076
Aluminum alkyls	**135**	3051

Name of Material	Guide No.	ID No.
Aluminum borohydride	**135**	2870
Aluminum borohydride in devices	**135**	2870
Aluminum bromide, anhydrous	**137**	1725
Aluminum bromide, solution	**154**	2580
Aluminum carbide	**138**	1394
Aluminum chloride, anhydrous	**137**	1726
Aluminum chloride, solution	**154**	2581
Aluminum dross	**138**	3170
Aluminum ferrosilicon powder	**139**	1395
Aluminum hydride	**138**	2463
Aluminum nitrate	**140**	1438
Aluminum phosphide	**139**	1397
Aluminum phosphide pesticide	**157**	3048
Aluminum powder, coated	**170**	1309
Aluminum powder, pyrophoric	**135**	1383
Aluminum powder, uncoated	**138**	1396
Aluminum remelting by-products	**138**	3170
Aluminum resinate	**133**	2715
Aluminum silicon powder, uncoated	**138**	1398
Aluminum smelting by-products	**138**	3170
Amines, flammable, corrosive, n.o.s.	**132**	2733
Amines, liquid, corrosive, flammable, n.o.s.	**132**	2734
Amines, liquid, corrosive, n.o.s.	**153**	2735
Amines, solid, corrosive, n.o.s.	**154**	3259
2-Amino-4-chlorophenol	**151**	2673
2-Amino-5-diethylaminopentane	**153**	2946
2-Amino-4,6-dinitrophenol, wetted with not less than 20% water	**113**	3317
2-(2-Aminoethoxy)ethanol	**154**	3055
N-Aminoethylpiperazine	**153**	2815
Aminophenols	**152**	2512
Aminopyridines	**153**	2671
Ammonia, anhydrous	**125**	1005
Ammonia, solution, with more than 10% but not more than 35% Ammonia	**154**	2672
Ammonia, solution, with more than 35% but not more than 50% Ammonia	**125**	2073
Ammonia solution, with more than 50% Ammonia	**125**	3318
Ammonium arsenate	**151**	1546
Ammonium bifluoride, solid	**154**	1727
Ammonium bifluoride, solution	**154**	2817
Ammonium dichromate	**141**	1439
Ammonium dinitro-o-cresolate, solid	**141**	1843
Ammonium dinitro-o-cresolate, solution	**141**	3424
Ammonium fluoride	**154**	2505
Ammonium fluorosilicate	**151**	2854
Ammonium hydrogendifluoride, solid	**154**	1727
Ammonium hydrogendifluoride, solution	**154**	2817
Ammonium hydrogen sulfate	**154**	2506
Ammonium hydrogen sulphate	**154**	2506
Ammonium hydroxide	**154**	2672
Ammonium hydroxide, with more than 10% but not more than 35% Ammonia	**154**	2672
Ammonium metavanadate	**154**	2859
Ammonium nitrate, liquid (hot concentrated solution)	**140**	2426

Name of Material	Guide No.	ID No.
Ammonium nitrate, with not more than 0.2% combustible substances	**140**	1942
Ammonium nitrate based fertilizer	**140**	2067
Ammonium nitrate based fertilizer	**140**	2071
Ammonium nitrate emulsion	**140**	3375
Ammonium nitrate-fuel oil mixtures	**112**	——
Ammonium nitrate gel	**140**	3375
Ammonium nitrate suspension	**140**	3375
Ammonium perchlorate	**143**	1442
Ammonium persulfate	**140**	1444
Ammonium persulphate	**140**	1444
Ammonium picrate, wetted with not less than 10% water	**113**	1310
Ammonium polysulfide, solution	**154**	2818
Ammonium polysulphide, solution	**154**	2818
Ammonium polyvanadate	**151**	2861
Ammonium silicofluoride	**151**	2854
Ammonium sulfide, solution	**132**	2683
Ammonium sulphide, solution	**132**	2683
Ammunition, poisonous, non-explosive	**151**	2016
Ammunition, tear-producing, non-explosive	**159**	2017
Ammunition, toxic, non-explosive	**151**	2016
Amyl acetates	**129**	1104
Amyl acid phosphate	**153**	2819
Amylamine	**132**	1106
Amyl butyrates	**130**	2620
Amyl chloride	**129**	1107
n-Amylene	**128**	1108
Amyl formates	**129**	1109
Amyl mercaptan	**130**	1111
n-Amyl methyl ketone	**127**	1110
Amyl nitrate	**128**	1112
Amyl nitrite	**129**	1113
Amyltrichlorosilane	**155**	1728
Anhydrous ammonia	**125**	1005
Aniline	**153**	1547
Aniline hydrochloride	**153**	1548
Anisidines	**153**	2431
Anisole	**128**	2222
Anisoyl chloride	**156**	1729
Antimony compound, inorganic, liquid, n.o.s.	**157**	3141
Antimony compound, inorganic, solid, n.o.s.	**157**	1549
Antimony lactate	**151**	1550
Antimony pentachloride, liquid	**157**	1730
Antimony pentachloride, solution	**157**	1731
Antimony pentafluoride	**157**	1732
Antimony potassium tartrate	**151**	1551
Antimony powder	**170**	2871
Antimony trichloride	**157**	1733
Antimony trichloride, liquid	**157**	1733
Antimony trichloride, solid	**157**	1733
Aqua regia	**157**	1798
Argon	**120**	1006
Argon, compressed	**120**	1006
Argon, refrigerated liquid (cryogenic liquid)	**120**	1951
Arsenic	**152**	1558

Name of Material	Guide No.	ID No.
Arsenic acid, liquid	**154**	1553
Arsenic acid, solid	**154**	1554
Arsenical dust	**152**	1562
Arsenical pesticide, liquid, flammable, poisonous	**131**	2760
Arsenical pesticide, liquid, flammable, toxic	**131**	2760
Arsenical pesticide, liquid, poisonous	**151**	2994
Arsenical pesticide, liquid, poisonous, flammable	**131**	2993
Arsenical pesticide, liquid, toxic	**151**	2994
Arsenical pesticide, liquid, toxic, flammable	**131**	2993
Arsenical pesticide, solid, poisonous	**151**	2759
Arsenical pesticide, solid, toxic	**151**	2759
Arsenic bromide	**151**	1555
Arsenic chloride	**157**	1560
Arsenic compound, liquid, n.o.s.	**152**	1556
Arsenic compound, solid, n.o.s.	**152**	1557
Arsenic pentoxide	**151**	1559
Arsenic trichloride	**157**	1560
Arsenic trioxide	**151**	1561
Arsine	**119**	2188
Arsine, adsorbed	**173**	3522
Articles containing a substance liable to spontaneous combustion, n.o.s.	**135**	3542
Articles containing a substance which emits flammable gas in contact with water, n.o.s.	**138**	3543
Articles containing corrosive substance, n.o.s.	**154**	3547

Name of Material	Guide No.	ID No.
Articles containing flammable gas, n.o.s.	**115**	3537
Articles containing flammable liquid, n.o.s.	**127**	3540
Articles containing flammable solid, n.o.s.	**133**	3541
Articles containing miscellaneous dangerous goods, n.o.s.	**171**	3548
Articles containing non-flammable, non-toxic gas, n.o.s.	**120**	3538
Articles containing oxidizing substance, n.o.s.	**140**	3544
Articles containing organic peroxide, n.o.s.	**145**	3545
Articles containing Polychlorinated biphenyls (PCB)	**171**	2315
Articles containing toxic gas, n.o.s.	**123**	3539
Articles containing toxic substance, n.o.s.	**151**	3546
Articles, pressurized, hydraulic (containing non-flammable gas)	**126**	3164
Articles, pressurized, pneumatic (containing non-flammable gas)	**126**	3164
Aryl sulfonic acids, liquid, with more than 5% free Sulfuric acid	**153**	2584
Aryl sulfonic acids, liquid, with not more than 5% free Sulfuric acid	**153**	2586
Aryl sulfonic acids, solid, with more than 5% free Sulfuric acid	**153**	2583
Aryl sulfonic acids, solid, with not more than 5% free Sulfuric acid	**153**	2585

Name of Material	Guide No.	ID No.
Aryl sulphonic acids, liquid, with more than 5% free Sulphuric acid	**153**	2584
Aryl sulphonic acids, liquid, with not more than 5% free Sulphuric acid	**153**	2586
Aryl sulphonic acids, solid, with more than 5% free Sulphuric acid	**153**	2583
Aryl sulphonic acids, solid, with not more than 5% free Sulphuric acid	**153**	2585
Asbestos	**171**	2212
Asbestos, amphibole	**171**	2212
Asbestos, blue	**171**	2212
Asbestos, brown	**171**	2212
Asbestos, chrysotile	**171**	2590
Asbestos, white	**171**	2590
Asphalt	**130**	1999
Asphalt, cut back	**130**	1999
Aviation regulated liquid, n.o.s.	**171**	3334
Aviation regulated solid, n.o.s.	**171**	3335
Azodicarbonamide	**149**	3242
Barium	**138**	1400
Barium alloys, pyrophoric	**135**	1854
Barium azide, wetted with not less than 50% water	**113**	1571
Barium bromate	**141**	2719
Barium chlorate, solid	**141**	1445
Barium chlorate, solution	**141**	3405
Barium compound, n.o.s.	**154**	1564
Barium cyanide	**157**	1565
Barium hypochlorite, with more than 22% available Chlorine	**141**	2741
Barium nitrate	**141**	1446
Barium oxide	**157**	1884
Barium perchlorate, solid	**141**	1447
Barium perchlorate, solution	**141**	3406
Barium permanganate	**141**	1448
Barium peroxide	**141**	1449
Batteries, containing Sodium	**138**	3292
Batteries, dry, containing Potassium hydroxide solid	**154**	3028
Batteries, nickel-metal hydride	**171**	3496
Batteries, wet, filled with acid	**154**	2794
Batteries, wet, filled with alkali	**154**	2795
Batteries, wet, non-spillable	**154**	2800
Battery fluid, acid	**157**	2796
Battery fluid, alkali	**154**	2797
Battery-powered equipment (wet battery)	**154**	3171
Battery-powered equipment (with lithium ion batteries)	**147**	3171
Battery-powered equipment (with lithium metal batteries)	**138**	3171
Battery-powered equipment (with sodium batteries)	**138**	3171
Battery-powered vehicle (wet battery)	**154**	3171
Battery-powered vehicle (with lithium ion batteries)	**147**	3171
Battery-powered vehicle (with sodium batteries)	**138**	3171
Benzaldehyde	**171**	1990
Benzene	**130**	1114
Benzene phosphorus dichloride	**137**	2798
Benzene phosphorus thiodichloride	**137**	2799
Benzenesulfonyl chloride	**156**	2225
Benzenesulphonyl chloride	**156**	2225
Benzidine	**153**	1885
Benzonitrile	**152**	2224

Name of Material	Guide No.	ID No.
Benzoquinone	**153**	2587
Benzotrichloride	**156**	2226
Benzotrifluoride	**127**	2338
Benzoyl chloride	**137**	1736
Benzyl bromide	**156**	1737
Benzyl chloride	**156**	1738
Benzyl chloroformate	**137**	1739
Benzyldimethylamine	**132**	2619
Benzylidene chloride	**156**	1886
Benzyl iodide	**156**	2653
Beryllium compound, n.o.s.	**154**	1566
Beryllium nitrate	**141**	2464
Beryllium powder	**134**	1567
beta-Naphthylamine, solid	**153**	1650
beta-Naphthylamine, solution	**153**	3411
Bhusa, wet, damp or contaminated with oil	**133**	1327
Bicyclo[2.2.1]hepta-2,5-diene, stabilized	**128P**	2251
Biological agents	**158**	——
Biological substance, category B	**158**	3373
(Bio)Medical waste, n.o.s.	**158**	3291
Bipyridilium pesticide, liquid, flammable, poisonous	**131**	2782
Bipyridilium pesticide, liquid, flammable, toxic	**131**	2782
Bipyridilium pesticide, liquid, poisonous	**151**	3016
Bipyridilium pesticide, liquid, poisonous, flammable	**131**	3015
Bipyridilium pesticide, liquid, toxic	**151**	3016
Bipyridilium pesticide, liquid, toxic, flammable	**131**	3015

Name of Material	Guide No.	ID No.
Bipyridilium pesticide, solid, poisonous	**151**	2781
Bipyridilium pesticide, solid, toxic	**151**	2781
Bisulfates, aqueous solution	**154**	2837
Bisulfites, aqueous solution, n.o.s.	**154**	2693
Bisulphates, aqueous solution	**154**	2837
Bisulphites, aqueous solution, n.o.s.	**154**	2693
Blasting agent, n.o.s.	**112**	——
Bleaching powder	**140**	2208
Blue asbestos	**171**	2212
Bombs, smoke, non-explosive, with corrosive liquid, without initiating device	**153**	2028
Borate and Chlorate mixture	**140**	1458
Borneol	**133**	1312
Boron tribromide	**157**	2692
Boron trichloride	**125**	1741
Boron trifluoride	**125**	1008
Boron trifluoride, adsorbed	**173**	3519
Boron trifluoride, compressed	**125**	1008
Boron trifluoride, dihydrate	**157**	2851
Boron trifluoride acetic acid complex, liquid	**157**	1742
Boron trifluoride acetic acid complex, solid	**157**	3419
Boron trifluoride diethyl etherate	**132**	2604
Boron trifluoride dimethyl etherate	**139**	2965
Boron trifluoride propionic acid complex, liquid	**157**	1743
Boron trifluoride propionic acid complex, solid	**157**	3420

Name of Material	Guide No.	ID No.
Bromates, inorganic, aqueous solution, n.o.s.	**140**	3213
Bromates, inorganic, n.o.s.	**140**	1450
Bromine	**154**	1744
Bromine, solution	**154**	1744
Bromine, solution (Inhalation Hazard Zone A)	**154**	1744
Bromine, solution (Inhalation Hazard Zone B)	**154**	1744
Bromine chloride	**124**	2901
Bromine pentafluoride	**144**	1745
Bromine trifluoride	**144**	1746
Bromoacetic acid, solid	**156**	3425
Bromoacetic acid, solution	**156**	1938
Bromoacetone	**131**	1569
Bromoacetyl bromide	**156**	2513
Bromobenzene	**130**	2514
Bromobenzyl cyanides, liquid	**159**	1694
Bromobenzyl cyanides, solid	**159**	3449
1-Bromobutane	**130**	1126
2-Bromobutane	**130**	2339
Bromochloromethane	**160**	1887
1-Bromo-3-chloropropane	**159**	2688
2-Bromoethyl ethyl ether	**130**	2340
Bromoform	**159**	2515
1-Bromo-3-methylbutane	**130**	2341
Bromomethylpropanes	**130**	2342
2-Bromo-2-nitropropane-1,3-diol	**133**	3241
2-Bromopentane	**130**	2343
Bromopropanes	**129**	2344
3-Bromopropyne	**130**	2345
Bromotrifluoroethylene	**116**	2419

Name of Material	Guide No.	ID No.
Bromotrifluoromethane	**126**	1009
Brown asbestos	**171**	2212
Brucine	**152**	1570
Butadienes, stabilized	**116P**	1010
Butadienes and hydrocarbon mixture, stabilized	**116P**	1010
Butane	**115**	1011
Butane	**115**	1075
Butanedione	**127**	2346
Butanols	**129**	1120
Butyl acetates	**129**	1123
Butyl acid phosphate	**153**	1718
Butyl acrylates, stabilized	**129P**	2348
n-Butylamine	**132**	1125
N-Butylaniline	**153**	2738
Butylbenzenes	**128**	2709
n-Butyl bromide	**130**	1126
n-Butyl chloride	**130**	1127
n-Butyl chloroformate	**155**	2743
sec-Butyl chloroformate	**155**	2742
tert-Butylcyclohexyl chloroformate	**156**	2747
Butylene	**115**	1012
Butylene	**115**	1075
1,2-Butylene oxide, stabilized	**127P**	3022
Butyl ethers	**128**	1149
n-Butyl formate	**129**	1128
tert-Butyl hypochlorite	**135**	3255
N,n-Butylimidazole	**152**	2690
n-Butyl isocyanate	**155P**	2485
tert-Butyl isocyanate	**155**	2484
Butyl mercaptan	**130**	2347

Name of Material	Guide No.	ID No.
n-Butyl methacrylate, stabilized	**130P**	2227
Butyl methyl ether	**127**	2350
Butyl nitrites	**129**	2351
Butyl propionates	**130**	1914
Butyltoluenes	**152**	2667
Butyltrichlorosilane	**155**	1747
5-tert-Butyl-2,4,6-trinitro-m-xylene	**149**	2956
Butyl vinyl ether, stabilized	**127P**	2352
1,4-Butynediol	**153**	2716
Butyraldehyde	**129P**	1129
Butyraldoxime	**129**	2840
Butyric acid	**153**	2820
Butyric anhydride	**156**	2739
Butyronitrile	**131**	2411
Butyryl chloride	**132**	2353
Buzz	**153**	—
BZ	**153**	—
CA	**159**	—
Cacodylic acid	**151**	1572
Cadmium compound	**154**	2570
Caesium	**138**	1407
Caesium hydroxide	**157**	2682
Caesium hydroxide, solution	**154**	2681
Caesium nitrate	**140**	1451
Calcium	**138**	1401
Calcium, pyrophoric	**135**	1855
Calcium alloys, pyrophoric	**135**	1855
Calcium arsenate	**151**	1573
Calcium arsenate and Calcium arsenite mixture, solid	**151**	1574

Name of Material	Guide No.	ID No.
Calcium arsenite and Calcium arsenate mixture, solid	**151**	1574
Calcium carbide	**138**	1402
Calcium chlorate	**140**	1452
Calcium chlorate, aqueous solution	**140**	2429
Calcium chlorite	**140**	1453
Calcium cyanamide, with more than 0.1% Calcium carbide	**138**	1403
Calcium cyanide	**157**	1575
Calcium dithionite	**135**	1923
Calcium hydride	**138**	1404
Calcium hydrosulfite	**135**	1923
Calcium hydrosulphite	**135**	1923
Calcium hypochlorite, dry	**140**	1748
Calcium hypochlorite, dry, corrosive, with more than 39% available chlorine (8.8% available oxygen)	**140**	3485
Calcium hypochlorite, hydrated, corrosive, with not less than 5.5% but not more than 16% water	**140**	3487
Calcium hypochlorite, hydrated, with not less than 5.5% but not more than 16% water	**140**	2880
Calcium hypochlorite, hydrated mixture, corrosive, with not less than 5.5% but not more than 16% water	**140**	3487
Calcium hypochlorite, hydrated mixture, with not less than 5.5% but not more than 16% water	**140**	2880
Calcium hypochlorite mixture, dry, corrosive, with more than 10% but not more than 39% available chlorine	**140**	3486

Name of Material	Guide No.	ID No.
Calcium hypochlorite mixture, dry, corrosive, with more than 39% available chlorine (8.8% available oxygen)	**140**	3485
Calcium hypochlorite mixture, dry, with more than 10% but not more than 39% available Chlorine	**140**	2208
Calcium hypochlorite mixture, dry, with more than 39% available Chlorine (8.8% available Oxygen)	**140**	1748
Calcium manganese silicon	**138**	2844
Calcium nitrate	**140**	1454
Calcium oxide	**157**	1910
Calcium perchlorate	**140**	1455
Calcium permanganate	**140**	1456
Calcium peroxide	**140**	1457
Calcium phosphide	**139**	1360
Calcium resinate	**133**	1313
Calcium resinate, fused	**133**	1314
Calcium silicide	**138**	1405
Camphor, synthetic	**133**	2717
Camphor oil	**128**	1130
Capacitor, asymmetric	**171**	3508
Capacitor, electric double layer	**171**	3499
Caproic acid	**153**	2829
Carbamate pesticide, liquid, flammable, poisonous	**131**	2758
Carbamate pesticide, liquid, flammable, toxic	**131**	2758
Carbamate pesticide, liquid, poisonous	**151**	2992
Carbamate pesticide, liquid, poisonous, flammable	**131**	2991
Carbamate pesticide, liquid, toxic	**151**	2992

Name of Material	Guide No.	ID No.
Carbamate pesticide, liquid, toxic, flammable	**131**	2991
Carbamate pesticide, solid, poisonous	**151**	2757
Carbamate pesticide, solid, toxic	**151**	2757
Carbon, activated	**133**	1362
Carbon, animal or vegetable origin	**133**	1361
Carbon bisulfide	**131**	1131
Carbon bisulphide	**131**	1131
Carbon dioxide	**120**	1013
Carbon dioxide, compressed	**120**	1013
Carbon dioxide, refrigerated liquid	**120**	2187
Carbon dioxide, solid	**120**	1845
Carbon dioxide and Ethylene oxide mixture, with more than 9% but not more than 87% Ethylene oxide	**115**	1041
Carbon dioxide and Ethylene oxide mixture, with more than 87% Ethylene oxide	**119P**	3300
Carbon dioxide and Ethylene oxide mixtures, with not more than 9% Ethylene oxide	**126**	1952
Carbon dioxide and Nitrous oxide mixture	**126**	1015
Carbon dioxide and Oxygen mixture, compressed	**122**	1014
Carbon disulfide	**131**	1131
Carbon disulphide	**131**	1131
Carbon monoxide	**119**	1016
Carbon monoxide, compressed	**119**	1016
Carbon monoxide, refrigerated liquid (cryogenic liquid)	**168**	9202
Carbon tetrabromide	**151**	2516
Carbon tetrachloride	**151**	1846

Name of Material	Guide No.	ID No.
Carbonyl fluoride	**125**	2417
Carbonyl fluoride, compressed	**125**	2417
Carbonyl sulfide	**119**	2204
Carbonyl sulphide	**119**	2204
Castor beans, meal, pomace or flake	**171**	2969
Caustic alkali liquid, n.o.s.	**154**	1719
Caustic potash, solid	**154**	1813
Caustic potash, solution	**154**	1814
Caustic soda, solid	**154**	1823
Caustic soda, solution	**154**	1824
Cells, containing Sodium	**138**	3292
Celluloid, in blocks, rods, rolls, sheets, tubes, etc., except scrap	**133**	2000
Celluloid, scrap	**135**	2002
Cerium, slabs, ingots or rods	**170**	1333
Cerium, turnings or gritty powder	**138**	3078
Cesium	**138**	1407
Cesium hydroxide	**157**	2682
Cesium hydroxide, solution	**154**	2681
Cesium nitrate	**140**	1451
CG	**125**	—
Charcoal	**133**	1361
Chemical kit	**154**	1760
Chemical kit	**171**	3316
Chemical sample, poisonous	**151**	3315
Chemical sample, toxic	**151**	3315
Chemical under pressure, corrosive, n.o.s.	**125**	3503
Chemical under pressure, flammable, corrosive, n.o.s.	**118**	3505
Chemical under pressure, flammable, n.o.s.	**115**	3501

Name of Material	Guide No.	ID No.
Chemical under pressure, flammable, poisonous, n.o.s.	**119**	3504
Chemical under pressure, flammable, toxic, n.o.s.	**119**	3504
Chemical under pressure, n.o.s.	**126**	3500
Chemical under pressure, poisonous, n.o.s.	**123**	3502
Chemical under pressure, toxic, n.o.s.	**123**	3502
Chloral, anhydrous, stabilized	**153**	2075
Chlorate and Borate mixture	**140**	1458
Chlorate and Magnesium chloride mixture, solid	**140**	1459
Chlorate and Magnesium chloride mixture, solution	**140**	3407
Chlorates, inorganic, aqueous solution, n.o.s.	**140**	3210
Chlorates, inorganic, n.o.s.	**140**	1461
Chloric acid, aqueous solution, with not more than 10% Chloric acid	**140**	2626
Chlorine	**124**	1017
Chlorine, adsorbed	**173**	3520
Chlorine dioxide, hydrate, frozen	**143**	9191
Chlorine pentafluoride	**124**	2548
Chlorine trifluoride	**124**	1749
Chlorite solution	**154**	1908
Chlorites, inorganic, n.o.s.	**143**	1462
Chloroacetaldehyde	**153**	2232
Chloroacetic acid, molten	**153**	3250
Chloroacetic acid, solid	**153**	1751
Chloroacetic acid, solution	**153**	1750
Chloroacetone, stabilized	**131**	1695
Chloroacetonitrile	**131**	2668

Name of Material	Guide No.	ID No.
Chloroacetophenone, liquid	**153**	3416
Chloroacetophenone, solid	**153**	1697
Chloroacetyl chloride	**156**	1752
Chloroanilines, liquid	**152**	2019
Chloroanilines, solid	**152**	2018
Chloroanisidines	**152**	2233
Chlorobenzene	**130**	1134
Chlorobenzotrifluorides	**130**	2234
Chlorobenzyl chlorides, liquid	**153**	2235
Chlorobenzyl chlorides, solid	**153**	3427
Chlorobutanes	**130**	1127
Chlorocresols, solid	**152**	3437
Chlorocresols, solution	**152**	2669
Chlorodifluorobromomethane	**126**	1974
1-Chloro-1,1-difluoroethane	**115**	2517
Chlorodifluoromethane	**126**	1018
Chlorodifluoromethane and Chloropentafluoroethane mixture	**126**	1973
Chlorodinitrobenzenes, liquid	**153**	1577
Chlorodinitrobenzenes, solid	**153**	3441
2-Chloroethanal	**153**	2232
Chloroform	**151**	1888
Chloroformates, poisonous, corrosive, flammable, n.o.s.	**155**	2742
Chloroformates, poisonous, corrosive, n.o.s.	**154**	3277
Chloroformates, toxic, corrosive, flammable, n.o.s.	**155**	2742
Chloroformates, toxic, corrosive, n.o.s.	**154**	3277
Chloromethyl chloroformate	**157**	2745
Chloromethyl ethyl ether	**131**	2354
3-Chloro-4-methylphenyl isocyanate, liquid	**156**	2236
3-Chloro-4-methylphenyl isocyanate, solid	**156**	3428
Chloronitroanilines	**153**	2237
Chloronitrobenzenes, liquid	**152**	3409
Chloronitrobenzenes, solid	**152**	1578
Chloronitrotoluenes, liquid	**152**	2433
Chloronitrotoluenes, solid	**152**	3457
Chloropentafluoroethane	**126**	1020
Chloropentafluoroethane and Chlorodifluoromethane mixture	**126**	1973
Chlorophenolates, liquid	**154**	2904
Chlorophenolates, solid	**154**	2905
Chlorophenols, liquid	**153**	2021
Chlorophenols, solid	**153**	2020
Chlorophenyltrichlorosilane	**156**	1753
Chloropicrin	**154**	1580
Chloropicrin and Methyl bromide mixture	**123**	1581
Chloropicrin and Methyl chloride mixture	**119**	1582
Chloropicrin mixture, n.o.s.	**154**	1583
Chloropivaloyl chloride	**156**	9263
Chloroplatinic acid, solid	**154**	2507
Chloroprene, stabilized	**131P**	1991
1-Chloropropane	**129**	1278
2-Chloropropane	**129**	2356
3-Chloropropanol-1	**153**	2849
2-Chloropropene	**130P**	2456
2-Chloropropionic acid	**153**	2511
2-Chloropyridine	**153**	2822
Chlorosilanes, corrosive, flammable, n.o.s.	**155**	2986
Chlorosilanes, corrosive, n.o.s.	**156**	2987

Name of Material	Guide No.	ID No.
Chlorosilanes, flammable, corrosive, n.o.s.	**155**	2985
Chlorosilanes, poisonous, corrosive, flammable, n.o.s.	**155**	3362
Chlorosilanes, poisonous, corrosive, n.o.s.	**156**	3361
Chlorosilanes, toxic, corrosive, flammable, n.o.s.	**155**	3362
Chlorosilanes, toxic, corrosive, n.o.s.	**156**	3361
Chlorosilanes, water-reactive, flammable, corrosive, n.o.s.	**139**	2988
Chlorosulfonic acid (with or without sulfur trioxide)	**137**	1754
Chlorosulphonic acid (with or without sulphur trioxide)	**137**	1754
1-Chloro-1,2,2,2-tetrafluoroethane	**126**	1021
Chlorotetrafluoroethane and Ethylene oxide mixture, with not more than 8.8% Ethylene oxide	**126**	3297
Chlorotoluenes	**129**	2238
4-Chloro-o-toluidine hydrochloride, solid	**153**	1579
4-Chloro-o-toluidine hydrochloride, solution	**153**	3410
Chlorotoluidines, liquid	**153**	3429
Chlorotoluidines, solid	**153**	2239
1-Chloro-2,2,2-trifluoroethane	**126**	1983
Chlorotrifluoromethane	**126**	1022
Chlorotrifluoromethane and Trifluoromethane azeotropic mixture with approximately 60% Chlorotrifluoromethane	**126**	2599
Chromic acid, solution	**154**	1755
Chromic fluoride, solid	**154**	1756
Chromic fluoride, solution	**154**	1757
Chromium nitrate	**141**	2720

Name of Material	Guide No.	ID No.
Chromium oxychloride	**137**	1758
Chromium trioxide, anhydrous	**141**	1463
Chromosulfuric acid	**154**	2240
Chromosulphuric acid	**154**	2240
CK	**125**	—
Clinical waste, unspecified, n.o.s.	**158**	3291
CN	**153**	—
Coal gas	**119**	1023
Coal gas, compressed	**119**	1023
Coal tar distillates, flammable	**128**	1136
Coating solution	**127**	1139
Cobalt naphthenates, powder	**133**	2001
Cobalt resinate, precipitated	**133**	1318
Combustible liquid, n.o.s.	**128**	1993
Compounds, cleaning liquid (corrosive)	**154**	1760
Compounds, cleaning liquid (flammable)	**128**	1993
Compounds, tree or weed killing, liquid (corrosive)	**154**	1760
Compounds, tree or weed killing, liquid (flammable)	**128**	1993
Compounds, tree or weed killing, liquid (toxic)	**153**	2810
Compressed gas, flammable, n.o.s.	**115**	1954
Compressed gas, n.o.s.	**126**	1956
Compressed gas, oxidizing, n.o.s.	**122**	3156
Compressed gas, poisonous, corrosive, n.o.s.	**125**	3304
Compressed gas, poisonous, corrosive, n.o.s. (Inhalation Hazard Zone A)	**125**	3304

Name of Material	Guide No.	ID No.
Compressed gas, poisonous, corrosive, n.o.s. (Inhalation Hazard Zone B)	**125**	3304
Compressed gas, poisonous, corrosive, n.o.s. (Inhalation Hazard Zone C)	**125**	3304
Compressed gas, poisonous, corrosive, n.o.s. (Inhalation Hazard Zone D)	**125**	3304
Compressed gas, poisonous, flammable, corrosive, n.o.s.	**119**	3305
Compressed gas, poisonous, flammable, corrosive, n.o.s. (Inhalation Hazard Zone A)	**119**	3305
Compressed gas, poisonous, flammable, corrosive, n.o.s. (Inhalation Hazard Zone B)	**119**	3305
Compressed gas, poisonous, flammable, corrosive, n.o.s. (Inhalation Hazard Zone C)	**119**	3305
Compressed gas, poisonous, flammable, corrosive, n.o.s. (Inhalation Hazard Zone D)	**119**	3305
Compressed gas, poisonous, flammable, n.o.s.	**119**	1953
Compressed gas, poisonous, flammable, n.o.s. (Inhalation Hazard Zone A)	**119**	1953
Compressed gas, poisonous, flammable, n.o.s. (Inhalation Hazard Zone B)	**119**	1953
Compressed gas, poisonous, flammable, n.o.s. (Inhalation Hazard Zone C)	**119**	1953
Compressed gas, poisonous, flammable, n.o.s. (Inhalation Hazard Zone D)	**119**	1953
Compressed gas, poisonous, n.o.s.	**123**	1955
Compressed gas, poisonous, n.o.s. (Inhalation Hazard Zone A)	**123**	1955

Name of Material	Guide No.	ID No.
Compressed gas, poisonous, n.o.s. (Inhalation Hazard Zone B)	**123**	1955
Compressed gas, poisonous, n.o.s. (Inhalation Hazard Zone C)	**123**	1955
Compressed gas, poisonous, n.o.s. (Inhalation Hazard Zone D)	**123**	1955
Compressed gas, poisonous, oxidizing, corrosive, n.o.s.	**124**	3306
Compressed gas, poisonous, oxidizing, corrosive, n.o.s. (Inhalation Hazard Zone A)	**124**	3306
Compressed gas, poisonous, oxidizing, corrosive, n.o.s. (Inhalation Hazard Zone B)	**124**	3306
Compressed gas, poisonous, oxidizing, corrosive, n.o.s. (Inhalation Hazard Zone C)	**124**	3306
Compressed gas, poisonous, oxidizing, corrosive, n.o.s. (Inhalation Hazard Zone D)	**124**	3306
Compressed gas, poisonous, oxidizing, n.o.s.	**124**	3303
Compressed gas, poisonous, oxidizing, n.o.s. (Inhalation Hazard Zone A)	**124**	3303
Compressed gas, poisonous, oxidizing, n.o.s. (Inhalation Hazard Zone B)	**124**	3303
Compressed gas, poisonous, oxidizing, n.o.s. (Inhalation Hazard Zone C)	**124**	3303
Compressed gas, poisonous, oxidizing, n.o.s. (Inhalation Hazard Zone D)	**124**	3303
Compressed gas, toxic, corrosive, n.o.s.	**125**	3304
Compressed gas, toxic, corrosive, n.o.s. (Inhalation Hazard Zone A)	**125**	3304

Name of Material	Guide No.	ID No.
Compressed gas, toxic, corrosive, n.o.s. (Inhalation Hazard Zone B)	**125**	3304
Compressed gas, toxic, corrosive, n.o.s. (Inhalation Hazard Zone C)	**125**	3304
Compressed gas, toxic, corrosive, n.o.s. (Inhalation Hazard Zone D)	**125**	3304
Compressed gas, toxic, flammable, corrosive, n.o.s.	**119**	3305
Compressed gas, toxic, flammable, corrosive, n.o.s. (Inhalation Hazard Zone A)	**119**	3305
Compressed gas, toxic, flammable, corrosive, n.o.s. (Inhalation Hazard Zone B)	**119**	3305
Compressed gas, toxic, flammable, corrosive, n.o.s. (Inhalation Hazard Zone C)	**119**	3305
Compressed gas, toxic, flammable, corrosive, n.o.s. (Inhalation Hazard Zone D)	**119**	3305
Compressed gas, toxic, flammable, n.o.s.	**119**	1953
Compressed gas, toxic, flammable, n.o.s. (Inhalation Hazard Zone A)	**119**	1953
Compressed gas, toxic, flammable, n.o.s. (Inhalation Hazard Zone B)	**119**	1953
Compressed gas, toxic, flammable, n.o.s. (Inhalation Hazard Zone C)	**119**	1953
Compressed gas, toxic, flammable, n.o.s. (Inhalation Hazard Zone D)	**119**	1953
Compressed gas, toxic, n.o.s.	**123**	1955
Compressed gas, toxic, n.o.s. (Inhalation Hazard Zone A)	**123**	1955
Compressed gas, toxic, n.o.s. (Inhalation Hazard Zone B)	**123**	1955

Name of Material	Guide No.	ID No.
Compressed gas, toxic, n.o.s. (Inhalation Hazard Zone C)	**123**	1955
Compressed gas, toxic, n.o.s. (Inhalation Hazard Zone D)	**123**	1955
Compressed gas, toxic, oxidizing, corrosive, n.o.s.	**124**	3306
Compressed gas, toxic, oxidizing, corrosive, n.o.s. (Inhalation Hazard Zone A)	**124**	3306
Compressed gas, toxic, oxidizing, corrosive, n.o.s. (Inhalation Hazard Zone B)	**124**	3306
Compressed gas, toxic, oxidizing, corrosive, n.o.s. (Inhalation Hazard Zone C)	**124**	3306
Compressed gas, toxic, oxidizing, corrosive, n.o.s. (Inhalation Hazard Zone D)	**124**	3306
Compressed gas, toxic, oxidizing, n.o.s.	**124**	3303
Compressed gas, toxic, oxidizing, n.o.s. (Inhalation Hazard Zone A)	**124**	3303
Compressed gas, toxic, oxidizing, n.o.s. (Inhalation Hazard Zone B)	**124**	3303
Compressed gas, toxic, oxidizing, n.o.s. (Inhalation Hazard Zone C)	**124**	3303
Compressed gas, toxic, oxidizing, n.o.s. (Inhalation Hazard Zone D)	**124**	3303
Compressed gas and hexaethyl tetraphosphate mixture	**123**	1612
Consumer commodity	**171**	8000
Copper acetoarsenite	**151**	1585
Copper arsenite	**151**	1586
Copper based pesticide, liquid, flammable, poisonous	**131**	2776
Copper based pesticide, liquid, flammable, toxic	**131**	2776

Name of Material	Guide No.	ID No.
Copper based pesticide, liquid, poisonous	**151**	3010
Copper based pesticide, liquid, poisonous, flammable	**131**	3009
Copper based pesticide, liquid, toxic	**151**	3010
Copper based pesticide, liquid, toxic, flammable	**131**	3009
Copper based pesticide, solid, poisonous	**151**	2775
Copper based pesticide, solid, toxic	**151**	2775
Copper chlorate	**140**	2721
Copper chloride	**154**	2802
Copper cyanide	**151**	1587
Copra	**135**	1363
Corrosive liquid, acidic, inorganic, n.o.s.	**154**	3264
Corrosive liquid, acidic, organic, n.o.s.	**153**	3265
Corrosive liquid, basic, inorganic, n.o.s.	**154**	3266
Corrosive liquid, basic, organic, n.o.s.	**153**	3267
Corrosive liquid, flammable, n.o.s.	**132**	2920
Corrosive liquid, n.o.s.	**154**	1760
Corrosive liquid, oxidizing, n.o.s.	**157**	3093
Corrosive liquid, poisonous, n.o.s.	**154**	2922
Corrosive liquid, self-heating, n.o.s.	**136**	3301
Corrosive liquid, toxic, n.o.s.	**154**	2922
Corrosive liquid, water-reactive, n.o.s.	**138**	3094
Corrosive solid, acidic, inorganic, n.o.s.	**154**	3260
Corrosive solid, acidic, organic, n.o.s.	**154**	3261
Corrosive solid, basic, inorganic, n.o.s.	**154**	3262
Corrosive solid, basic, organic, n.o.s.	**154**	3263
Corrosive solid, flammable, n.o.s.	**134**	2921
Corrosive solid, n.o.s.	**154**	1759
Corrosive solid, oxidizing, n.o.s.	**157**	3084
Corrosive solid, poisonous, n.o.s.	**154**	2923
Corrosive solid, self-heating, n.o.s.	**136**	3095
Corrosive solid, toxic, n.o.s.	**154**	2923
Corrosive solid, water-reactive, n.o.s.	**138**	3096
Cotton	**133**	1365
Cotton, wet	**133**	1365
Cotton waste, oily	**133**	1364
Coumarin derivative pesticide, liquid, flammable, poisonous	**131**	3024
Coumarin derivative pesticide, liquid, flammable, toxic	**131**	3024
Coumarin derivative pesticide, liquid, poisonous	**151**	3026
Coumarin derivative pesticide, liquid, poisonous, flammable	**131**	3025
Coumarin derivative pesticide, liquid, toxic	**151**	3026
Coumarin derivative pesticide, liquid, toxic, flammable	**131**	3025
Coumarin derivative pesticide, solid, poisonous	**151**	3027
Coumarin derivative pesticide, solid, toxic	**151**	3027
Cresols, liquid	**153**	2076

Name of Material	Guide No.	ID No.
Cresols, solid	**153**	3455
Cresylic acid	**153**	2022
Crotonaldehyde	**131P**	1143
Crotonaldehyde, stabilized	**131P**	1143
Crotonic acid, liquid	**153**	3472
Crotonic acid, solid	**153**	2823
Crotonylene	**128**	1144
CS	**153**	—
Cumene	**130**	1918
Cupriethylenediamine, solution	**154**	1761
CX	**154**	—
Cyanide solution, n.o.s.	**157**	1935
Cyanides, inorganic, solid, n.o.s.	**157**	1588
Cyanogen	**119**	1026
Cyanogen bromide	**157**	1889
Cyanogen chloride, stabilized	**125**	1589
Cyanuric chloride	**157**	2670
Cyclobutane	**115**	2601
Cyclobutyl chloroformate	**155**	2744
1,5,9-Cyclododecatriene	**153**	2518
Cycloheptane	**128**	2241
Cycloheptatriene	**131**	2603
Cycloheptene	**128**	2242
Cyclohexane	**128**	1145
Cyclohexanethiol	**129**	3054
Cyclohexanone	**127**	1915
Cyclohexene	**130**	2256
Cyclohexenyltrichlorosilane	**156**	1762
Cyclohexyl acetate	**130**	2243
Cyclohexylamine	**132**	2357
Cyclohexyl isocyanate	**155**	2488

Name of Material	Guide No.	ID No.
Cyclohexyl mercaptan	**129**	3054
Cyclohexyltrichlorosilane	**156**	1763
Cyclooctadiene phosphines	**135**	2940
Cyclooctadienes	**130P**	2520
Cyclooctatetraene	**128P**	2358
Cyclopentane	**128**	1146
Cyclopentanol	**129**	2244
Cyclopentanone	**128**	2245
Cyclopentene	**128**	2246
Cyclopropane	**115**	1027
Cymenes	**130**	2046
DA	**151**	—
Dangerous goods in apparatus	**171**	3363
Dangerous goods in articles	**171**	3363
Dangerous goods in machinery	**171**	3363
DC	**153**	—
Decaborane	**134**	1868
Decahydronaphthalene	**130**	1147
n-Decane	**128**	2247
Denatured alcohol	**127**	1987
Desensitized explosive, liquid, n.o.s.	**113**	3379
Desensitized explosive, solid, n.o.s.	**113**	3380
Deuterium	**115**	1957
Deuterium, compressed	**115**	1957
Devices, small, hydrocarbon gas powered, with release device	**115**	3150
Diacetone alcohol	**129**	1148
Diacetyl	**127**	2346
Diallylamine	**132**	2359
Diallyl ether	**131P**	2360
4,4'-Diaminodiphenylmethane	**153**	2651

Name of Material	Guide No.	ID No.
Di-n-amylamine	**131**	2841
Dibenzyldichlorosilane	**156**	2434
Diborane	**119**	1911
Diborane, compressed	**119**	1911
Diborane mixtures	**119**	1911
1,2-Dibromobutan-3-one	**154**	2648
Dibromochloropropanes	**159**	2872
Dibromodifluoromethane	**171**	1941
Dibromomethane	**160**	2664
Di-n-butylamine	**132**	2248
Dibutylaminoethanol	**153**	2873
Dibutyl ethers	**128**	1149
Dichloroacetic acid	**153**	1764
1,3-Dichloroacetone	**153**	2649
Dichloroacetyl chloride	**156**	1765
Dichloroanilines, liquid	**153**	1590
Dichloroanilines, solid	**153**	3442
o-Dichlorobenzene	**152**	1591
2,2'-Dichlorodiethyl ether	**152**	1916
Dichlorodifluoromethane	**126**	1028
Dichlorodifluoromethane and Difluoroethane azeotropic mixture with approximately 74% Dichlorodifluoromethane	**126**	2602
Dichlorodifluoromethane and Ethylene oxide mixture, with not more than 12.5% Ethylene oxide	**126**	3070
Dichlorodimethyl ether, symmetrical	**131**	2249
1,1-Dichloroethane	**130**	2362
1,2-Dichloroethylene	**130P**	1150
Dichloroethyl ether	**152**	1916
Dichlorofluoromethane	**126**	1029

Name of Material	Guide No.	ID No.
Dichloroisocyanuric acid, dry	**140**	2465
Dichloroisocyanuric acid salts	**140**	2465
Dichloroisopropyl ether	**153**	2490
Dichloromethane	**160**	1593
1,1-Dichloro-1-nitroethane	**153**	2650
Dichloropentanes	**130**	1152
Dichlorophenyl isocyanates	**156**	2250
Dichlorophenyltrichlorosilane	**156**	1766
1,2-Dichloropropane	**130**	1279
1,3-Dichloropropanol-2	**153**	2750
Dichloropropenes	**129**	2047
Dichlorosilane	**119**	2189
1,2-Dichloro-1,1,2,2-tetrafluoroethane	**126**	1958
3,5-Dichloro-2,4,6-trifluoropyridine	**151**	9264
Dicyclohexylamine	**153**	2565
Dicyclohexylammonium nitrite	**133**	2687
Dicyclopentadiene	**130P**	2048
1,2-Di-(dimethylamino)ethane	**129**	2372
Didymium nitrate	**140**	1465
Diesel fuel	**128**	1202
Diesel fuel	**128**	1993
Diethoxymethane	**127**	2373
3,3-Diethoxypropene	**127**	2374
Diethylamine	**132**	1154
2-Diethylaminoethanol	**132**	2686
3-Diethylaminopropylamine	**132**	2684
N,N-Diethylaniline	**153**	2432
Diethylbenzene	**130**	2049
Diethyl carbonate	**128**	2366
Diethyldichlorosilane	**155**	1767
Diethylenetriamine	**154**	2079

Name of Material	Guide No.	ID No.
Diethyl ether	**127**	1155
N,N-Diethylethylenediamine	**132**	2685
Diethyl ketone	**127**	1156
Diethyl sulfate	**152**	1594
Diethyl sulfide	**129**	2375
Diethyl sulphate	**152**	1594
Diethyl sulphide	**129**	2375
Diethylthiophosphoryl chloride	**155**	2751
Diethylzinc	**135**	1366
Difluorochloroethanes	**115**	2517
1,1-Difluoroethane	**115**	1030
Difluoroethane and Dichlorodifluoromethane azeotropic mixture with approximately 74% Dichlorodifluoromethane	**126**	2602
1,1-Difluoroethylene	**116P**	1959
Difluoromethane	**115**	3252
Difluorophosphoric acid, anhydrous	**154**	1768
2,3-Dihydropyran	**127**	2376
Diisobutylamine	**132**	2361
Diisobutylene, isomeric compounds	**128**	2050
Diisobutyl ketone	**128**	1157
Diisooctyl acid phosphate	**153**	1902
Diisopropylamine	**132**	1158
Diisopropyl ether	**127**	1159
Diketene, stabilized	**131P**	2521
1,1-Dimethoxyethane	**127**	2377
1,2-Dimethoxyethane	**127**	2252
Dimethylamine, anhydrous	**118**	1032
Dimethylamine, aqueous solution	**132**	1160
Dimethylamine, solution	**132**	1160

Name of Material	Guide No.	ID No.
2-Dimethylaminoacetonitrile	**131**	2378
2-Dimethylaminoethanol	**132**	2051
2-Dimethylaminoethyl acrylate	**152**	3302
2-Dimethylaminoethyl methacrylate	**153P**	2522
N,N-Dimethylaniline	**153**	2253
2,3-Dimethylbutane	**128**	2457
1,3-Dimethylbutylamine	**132**	2379
Dimethylcarbamoyl chloride	**156**	2262
Dimethyl carbonate	**129**	1161
Dimethylcyclohexanes	**128**	2263
N,N-Dimethylcyclohexylamine	**132**	2264
Dimethylcyclohexylamine	**132**	2264
Dimethyldichlorosilane	**155**	1162
Dimethyldiethoxysilane	**127**	2380
Dimethyldioxanes	**127**	2707
Dimethyl disulfide	**131**	2381
Dimethyl disulphide	**131**	2381
Dimethyl ether	**115**	1033
N,N-Dimethylformamide	**129**	2265
Dimethylhydrazine, symmetrical	**131**	2382
Dimethylhydrazine, unsymmetrical	**131**	1163
2,2-Dimethylpropane	**115**	2044
Dimethyl-N-propylamine	**132**	2266
Dimethyl sulfate	**156**	1595
Dimethyl sulfide	**130**	1164
Dimethyl sulphate	**156**	1595
Dimethyl sulphide	**130**	1164
Dimethyl thiophosphoryl chloride	**156**	2267
Dimethylzinc	**135**	1370

Name of Material	Guide No.	ID No.
Dinitroanilines	**153**	1596
Dinitrobenzenes, liquid	**152**	1597
Dinitrobenzenes, solid	**152**	3443
Dinitro-o-cresol	**153**	1598
Dinitrogen tetroxide	**124**	1067
Dinitrogen tetroxide and Nitric oxide mixture	**124**	1975
Dinitrophenol, solution	**153**	1599
Dinitrophenol, wetted with not less than 15% water	**113**	1320
Dinitrophenolates, wetted with not less than 15% water	**113**	1321
Dinitroresorcinol, wetted with not less than 15% water	**113**	1322
Dinitrotoluenes, liquid	**152**	2038
Dinitrotoluenes, molten	**152**	1600
Dinitrotoluenes, solid	**152**	3454
Dioxane	**127**	1165
Dioxolane	**127**	1166
Dipentene	**128**	2052
Diphenylamine chloroarsine	**154**	1698
Diphenylchloroarsine, liquid	**151**	1699
Diphenylchloroarsine, solid	**151**	3450
Diphenyldichlorosilane	**156**	1769
Diphenylmethyl bromide	**153**	1770
Dipicryl sulfide, wetted with not less than 10% water	**113**	2852
Dipicryl sulphide, wetted with not less than 10% water	**113**	2852
Dipropylamine	**132**	2383
Di-n-propyl ether	**127**	2384
Dipropyl ketone	**128**	2710
Disinfectant, liquid, corrosive, n.o.s.	**153**	1903

Name of Material	Guide No.	ID No.
Disinfectant, liquid, poisonous, n.o.s.	**151**	3142
Disinfectant, liquid, toxic, n.o.s.	**151**	3142
Disinfectant, solid, poisonous, n.o.s.	**151**	1601
Disinfectant, solid, toxic, n.o.s.	**151**	1601
Disodium trioxosilicate	**154**	3253
Dispersant gas, n.o.s.	**126**	1078
Dispersant gases, n.o.s. (flammable)	**115**	1954
Divinyl ether, stabilized	**128P**	1167
DM	**154**	—
Dodecyltrichlorosilane	**156**	1771
DP	**125**	—
Dry ice	**120**	1845
Dye, liquid, corrosive, n.o.s.	**154**	2801
Dye, liquid, poisonous, n.o.s.	**151**	1602
Dye, liquid, toxic, n.o.s.	**151**	1602
Dye, solid, corrosive, n.o.s.	**154**	3147
Dye, solid, poisonous, n.o.s.	**151**	3143
Dye, solid, toxic, n.o.s.	**151**	3143
Dye intermediate, liquid, corrosive, n.o.s.	**154**	2801
Dye intermediate, liquid, poisonous, n.o.s.	**151**	1602
Dye intermediate, liquid, toxic, n.o.s.	**151**	1602
Dye intermediate, solid, corrosive, n.o.s.	**154**	3147
Dye intermediate, solid, poisonous, n.o.s.	**151**	3143
Dye intermediate, solid, toxic, n.o.s.	**151**	3143
ED	**151**	—

Name of Material	Guide No.	ID No.
Elevated temperature liquid, flammable, n.o.s., with flash point above 37.8°C (100°F), at or above its flash point	**128**	3256
Elevated temperature liquid, flammable, n.o.s., with flash point above 60°C (140°F), at or above its flash point	**128**	3256
Elevated temperature liquid, n.o.s., at or above 100°C (212°F), and below its flash point	**171**	3257
Elevated temperature solid, n.o.s., at or above 240°C (464°F)	**171**	3258
Engine, fuel cell, flammable gas powered	**115**	3166
Engine, fuel cell, flammable gas powered	**115**	3529
Engine, fuel cell, flammable liquid powered	**128**	3166
Engine, fuel cell, flammable liquid powered	**128**	3528
Engine, internal combustion	**128**	3166
Engine, internal combustion	**171**	3530
Engine, internal combustion, flammable gas powered	**115**	3529
Engine, internal combustion, flammable liquid powered	**128**	3528
Engines, internal combustion, flammable gas powered	**115**	3166
Engines, internal combustion, flammable liquid powered	**128**	3166
Environmentally hazardous substance, liquid, n.o.s.	**171**	3082
Environmentally hazardous substance, solid, n.o.s.	**171**	3077
Epibromohydrin	**131**	2558
Epichlorohydrin	**131P**	2023
1,2-Epoxy-3-ethoxypropane	**127**	2752

Name of Material	Guide No.	ID No.
Esters, n.o.s.	**127**	3272
Ethane	**115**	1035
Ethane, compressed	**115**	1035
Ethane, refrigerated liquid	**115**	1961
Ethane-Propane mixture, refrigerated liquid	**115**	1961
Ethanol	**127**	1170
Ethanol and gasoline mixture, with more than 10% ethanol	**127**	3475
Ethanol and motor spirit mixture, with more than 10% ethanol	**127**	3475
Ethanol and petrol mixture, with more than 10% ethanol	**127**	3475
Ethanol, solution	**127**	1170
Ethanolamine	**153**	2491
Ethanolamine, solution	**153**	2491
Ethers, n.o.s.	**127**	3271
Ethyl acetate	**129**	1173
Ethylacetylene, stabilized	**116P**	2452
Ethyl acrylate, stabilized	**129P**	1917
Ethyl alcohol	**127**	1170
Ethyl alcohol, solution	**127**	1170
Ethylamine	**118**	1036
Ethylamine, aqueous solution, with not less than 50% but not more than 70% Ethylamine	**132**	2270
Ethyl amyl ketone	**128**	2271
2-Ethylaniline	**153**	2273
N-Ethylaniline	**153**	2272
Ethylbenzene	**130**	1175
N-Ethyl-N-benzylaniline	**153**	2274
N-Ethylbenzyltoluidines, liquid	**153**	2753
N-Ethylbenzyltoluidines, solid	**153**	3460

Name of Material	Guide No.	ID No.
Ethyl borate	**129**	1176
Ethyl bromide	**131**	1891
Ethyl bromoacetate	**155**	1603
2-Ethylbutanol	**129**	2275
2-Ethylbutyl acetate	**130**	1177
Ethyl butyl ether	**127**	1179
2-Ethylbutyraldehyde	**130**	1178
Ethyl butyrate	**130**	1180
Ethyl chloride	**115**	1037
Ethyl chloroacetate	**155**	1181
Ethyl chloroformate	**155**	1182
Ethyl 2-chloropropionate	**129**	2935
Ethyl chlorothioformate	**155**	2826
Ethyl crotonate	**130**	1862
Ethyldichloroarsine	**151**	1892
Ethyldichlorosilane	**139**	1183
Ethylene	**116P**	1962
Ethylene, Acetylene and Propylene in mixture, refrigerated liquid containing at least 71.5% Ethylene with not more than 22.5% Acetylene and not more than 6% Propylene	**115**	3138
Ethylene, compressed	**116P**	1962
Ethylene, refrigerated liquid (cryogenic liquid)	**115**	1038
Ethylene chlorohydrin	**131**	1135
Ethylenediamine	**132**	1604
Ethylene dibromide	**154**	1605
Ethylene dibromide and Methyl bromide mixture, liquid	**151**	1647
Ethylene dichloride	**131**	1184
Ethylene glycol diethyl ether	**127**	1153
Ethylene glycol monoethyl ether	**127**	1171
Ethylene glycol monoethyl ether acetate	**129**	1172
Ethylene glycol monomethyl ether	**127**	1188
Ethylene glycol monomethyl ether acetate	**129**	1189
Ethyleneimine, stabilized	**131P**	1185
Ethylene oxide	**119P**	1040
Ethylene oxide and Carbon dioxide mixture, with more than 9% but not more than 87% Ethylene oxide	**115**	1041
Ethylene oxide and Carbon dioxide mixture, with more than 87% Ethylene oxide	**119P**	3300
Ethylene oxide and Carbon dioxide mixtures, with not more than 9% Ethylene oxide	**126**	1952
Ethylene oxide and Chlorotetrafluoroethane mixture, with not more than 8.8% Ethylene oxide	**126**	3297
Ethylene oxide and Dichlorodifluoromethane mixture, with not more than 12.5% Ethylene oxide	**126**	3070
Ethylene oxide and Pentafluoroethane mixture, with not more than 7.9% Ethylene oxide	**126**	3298
Ethylene oxide and Propylene oxide mixture, with not more than 30% Ethylene oxide	**131P**	2983
Ethylene oxide and Tetrafluoroethane mixture, with not more than 5.6% Ethylene oxide	**126**	3299
Ethylene oxide with Nitrogen	**119P**	1040
Ethyl ether	**127**	1155
Ethyl fluoride	**115**	2453

Name of Material	Guide No.	ID No.
Ethyl formate	**129**	1190
Ethylhexaldehydes	**129**	1191
2-Ethylhexylamine	**132**	2276
2-Ethylhexyl chloroformate	**156**	2748
Ethyl isobutyrate	**129**	2385
Ethyl isocyanate	**155**	2481
Ethyl lactate	**129**	1192
Ethyl mercaptan	**129**	2363
Ethyl methacrylate, stabilized	**130P**	2277
Ethyl methyl ether	**115**	1039
Ethyl methyl ketone	**127**	1193
Ethyl nitrite, solution	**131**	1194
Ethyl orthoformate	**129**	2524
Ethyl oxalate	**156**	2525
Ethylphenyldichlorosilane	**156**	2435
Ethyl phosphonothioic dichloride, anhydrous	**154**	2927
Ethyl phosphonous dichloride, anhydrous	**135**	2845
Ethyl phosphorodichloridate	**154**	2927
1-Ethylpiperidine	**132**	2386
Ethyl propionate	**129**	1195
Ethyl propyl ether	**127**	2615
Ethyl silicate	**129**	1292
N-Ethyltoluidines	**153**	2754
Ethyltrichlorosilane	**155**	1196
Explosives, division 1.1, 1.2, 1.3 or 1.5	**112**	—
Explosives, division 1.4 or 1.6	**114**	—
Extracts, aromatic, liquid	**127**	1169
Extracts, flavoring, liquid	**127**	1197
Extracts, flavouring, liquid	**127**	1197
Fabrics, animal or vegetable or synthetic, n.o.s. with oil	**133**	1373
Fabrics impregnated with weakly nitrated Nitrocellulose, n.o.s.	**133**	1353
Ferric arsenate	**151**	1606
Ferric arsenite	**151**	1607
Ferric chloride, anhydrous	**157**	1773
Ferric chloride, solution	**154**	2582
Ferric nitrate	**140**	1466
Ferrocerium	**170**	1323
Ferrosilicon	**139**	1408
Ferrous arsenate	**151**	1608
Ferrous chloride, solid	**154**	1759
Ferrous chloride, solution	**154**	1760
Ferrous metal borings, shavings, turnings or cuttings	**170**	2793
Fertilizer, ammoniating solution, with free Ammonia	**125**	1043
Fibers, animal or vegetable, burnt, wet or damp	**133**	1372
Fibers, animal or vegetable or synthetic, n.o.s. with oil	**133**	1373
Fibers, vegetable, dry	**133**	3360
Fibers impregnated with weakly nitrated Nitrocellulose, n.o.s.	**133**	1353
Fibres, animal or vegetable, burnt, wet or damp	**133**	1372
Fibres, animal or vegetable or synthetic, n.o.s. with oil	**133**	1373
Fibres, vegetable, dry	**133**	3360
Fibres impregnated with weakly nitrated Nitrocellulose, n.o.s.	**133**	1353
Films, nitrocellulose base	**133**	1324
Fire extinguisher charges, corrosive liquid	**154**	1774

Name of Material	Guide No.	ID No.
Fire extinguishers with compressed or liquefied gas	**126**	1044
Firelighters, solid, with flammable liquid	**133**	2623
First aid kit	**171**	3316
Fish meal, stabilized	**171**	2216
Fish meal, unstabilized	**133**	1374
Fish scrap, stabilized	**171**	2216
Fish scrap, unstabilized	**133**	1374
Flammable liquid, corrosive, n.o.s	**132**	2924
Flammable liquid, n.o.s.	**128**	1993
Flammable liquid, poisonous, corrosive, n.o.s.	**131**	3286
Flammable liquid, poisonous, n.o.s.	**131**	1992
Flammable liquid, toxic, corrosive, n.o.s.	**131**	3286
Flammable liquid, toxic, n.o.s.	**131**	1992
Flammable solid, corrosive, inorganic, n.o.s.	**134**	3180
Flammable solid, corrosive, organic, n.o.s.	**134**	2925
Flammable solid, inorganic, n.o.s.	**133**	3178
Flammable solid, organic, molten, n.o.s.	**133**	3176
Flammable solid, organic, n.o.s.	**133**	1325
Flammable solid, oxidizing, n.o.s.	**140**	3097
Flammable solid, poisonous, inorganic, n.o.s.	**134**	3179
Flammable solid, poisonous, organic, n.o.s.	**134**	2926
Flammable solid, toxic, inorganic, n.o.s.	**134**	3179

Name of Material	Guide No.	ID No.
Flammable solid, toxic, organic, n.o.s.	**134**	2926
Fluorine	**124**	1045
Fluorine, compressed	**124**	1045
Fluoroacetic acid	**154**	2642
Fluoroanilines	**153**	2941
Fluorobenzene	**130**	2387
Fluoroboric acid	**154**	1775
Fluorophosphoric acid, anhydrous	**154**	1776
Fluorosilicates, n.o.s.	**151**	2856
Fluorosilicic acid	**154**	1778
Fluorosulfonic acid	**137**	1777
Fluorosulphonic acid	**137**	1777
Fluorotoluenes	**130**	2388
Formaldehyde, solution (corrosive)	**153**	2209
Formaldehyde, solution, flammable	**132**	1198
Formalin (corrosive)	**153**	2209
Formalin (flammable)	**132**	1198
Formic acid	**153**	1779
Formic acid, with more than 85% acid	**153**	1779
Formic acid, with not less than 5% but less than 10% acid	**153**	3412
Formic acid, with not less than 10% but not more than 85% acid	**153**	3412
Fuel, aviation, turbine engine	**128**	1863
Fuel cell cartridges, containing corrosive substances	**153**	3477
Fuel cell cartridges, containing flammable liquids	**128**	3473
Fuel cell cartridges, containing hydrogen in metal hydride	**115**	3479

Name of Material	Guide No.	ID No.
Fuel cell cartridges, containing liquefied flammable gas	**115**	3478
Fuel cell cartridges, containing water-reactive substances	**138**	3476
Fuel cell cartridges contained in equipment, containing corrosive substances	**153**	3477
Fuel cell cartridges contained in equipment, containing flammable liquids	**128**	3473
Fuel cell cartridges contained in equipment, containing hydrogen in metal hydride	**115**	3479
Fuel cell cartridges contained in equipment, containing liquefied flammable gas	**115**	3478
Fuel cell cartridges contained in equipment, containing water-reactive substances	**138**	3476
Fuel cell cartridges packed with equipment, containing corrosive substances	**153**	3477
Fuel cell cartridges packed with equipment, containing flammable liquids	**128**	3473
Fuel cell cartridges packed with equipment, containing hydrogen in metal hydride	**115**	3479
Fuel cell cartridges packed with equipment, containing liquefied flammable gas	**115**	3478
Fuel cell cartridges packed with equipment, containing water-reactive substances	**138**	3476
Fuel oil	**128**	1202
Fuel oil	**128**	1993
Fumaryl chloride	**156**	1780
Fumigated cargo transport unit	**171**	3359
Furaldehydes	**153P**	1199
Furan	**128**	2389
Furfuryl alcohol	**153**	2874

Name of Material	Guide No.	ID No.
Furfurylamine	**132**	2526
Fusee (railway or highway)	**133**	1325
Fusel oil	**127**	1201
GA	**153**	—
Gallium	**172**	2803
Gas, refrigerated liquid, flammable, n.o.s.	**115**	3312
Gas, refrigerated liquid, n.o.s.	**120**	3158
Gas, refrigerated liquid, oxidizing, n.o.s.	**122**	3311
Gas cartridges	**115**	2037
Gas identification set	**123**	9035
Gasohol	**128**	1203
Gas oil	**128**	1202
Gasoline	**128**	1203
Gasoline and ethanol mixture, with more than 10% ethanol	**127**	3475
Gas sample, non-pressurized, flammable, n.o.s., not refrigerated liquid	**115**	3167
Gas sample, non-pressurized, poisonous, flammable, n.o.s., not refrigerated liquid	**119**	3168
Gas sample, non-pressurized, poisonous, n.o.s., not refrigerated liquid	**123**	3169
Gas sample, non-pressurized, toxic, flammable, n.o.s., not refrigerated liquid	**119**	3168
Gas sample, non-pressurized, toxic, n.o.s., not refrigerated liquid	**123**	3169
GB	**153**	—
GD	**153**	—
Genetically modified micro-organisms	**171**	3245
Genetically modified organisms	**171**	3245

Name of Material	Guide No.	ID No.
Germane	119	2192
Germane, adsorbed	173	3523
GF	153	—
Glycerol alpha-monochlorohydrin	153	2689
Glycidaldehyde	131P	2622
Guanidine nitrate	143	1467
H	153	—
Hafnium powder, dry	135	2545
Hafnium powder, wetted with not less than 25% water	170	1326
Halogenated monomethyldiphenylmethanes, liquid	171	3151
Halogenated monomethyldiphenylmethanes, solid	171	3152
Hay, wet, damp or contaminated with oil	133	1327
Hazardous waste, liquid, n.o.s.	171	3082
Hazardous waste, solid, n.o.s.	171	3077
HD	153	—
Heating oil, light	128	1202
Helium	120	1046
Helium, compressed	120	1046
Helium, refrigerated liquid (cryogenic liquid)	120	1963
Heptafluoropropane	126	3296
n-Heptaldehyde	129	3056
Heptanes	128	1206
n-Heptene	128	2278
Hexachloroacetone	153	2661
Hexachlorobenzene	152	2729
Hexachlorobutadiene	151	2279
Hexachlorocyclopentadiene	151	2646

Name of Material	Guide No.	ID No.
Hexachlorophene	151	2875
Hexadecyltrichlorosilane	156	1781
Hexadiene	130	2458
Hexaethyl tetraphosphate	151	1611
Hexaethyl tetraphosphate and compressed gas mixture	123	1612
Hexafluoroacetone	125	2420
Hexafluoroacetone hydrate, liquid	151	2552
Hexafluoroacetone hydrate, solid	151	3436
Hexafluoroethane	126	2193
Hexafluoroethane, compressed	126	2193
Hexafluorophosphoric acid	154	1782
Hexafluoropropylene	126	1858
Hexafluoropropylene, compressed	126	1858
Hexaldehyde	130	1207
Hexamethylenediamine, solid	153	2280
Hexamethylenediamine, solution	153	1783
Hexamethylene diisocyanate	156	2281
Hexamethyleneimine	132	2493
Hexamethylenetetramine	133	1328
Hexanes	128	1208
Hexanoic acid	153	2829
Hexanols	129	2282
1-Hexene	128	2370
Hexyltrichlorosilane	156	1784
HL	153	—
HN-1	153	—
HN-2	153	—
HN-3	153	—
Hydrazine, anhydrous	132	2029

Name of Material	Guide No.	ID No.
Hydrazine aqueous solution, flammable, with more than 37% hydrazine, by mass	**132**	3484
Hydrazine, aqueous solution, with more than 37% Hydrazine	**153**	2030
Hydrazine, aqueous solution, with not more than 37% Hydrazine	**152**	3293
Hydriodic acid	**154**	1787
Hydrobromic acid	**154**	1788
Hydrocarbon and butadienes mixture, stabilized	**116P**	1010
Hydrocarbon gas mixture, compressed, n.o.s.	**115**	1964
Hydrocarbon gas mixture, liquefied, n.o.s.	**115**	1965
Hydrocarbon gas refills for small devices, with release device	**115**	3150
Hydrocarbons, liquid, n.o.s.	**128**	3295
Hydrochloric acid	**157**	1789
Hydrocyanic acid, aqueous solution, with less than 5% Hydrogen cyanide	**154**	1613
Hydrocyanic acid, aqueous solution, with not more than 20% Hydrogen cyanide	**154**	1613
Hydrofluoric acid	**157**	1790
Hydrofluoric acid and Sulfuric acid mixture	**157**	1786
Hydrofluoric acid and Sulphuric acid mixture	**157**	1786
Hydrofluorosilicic acid	**154**	1778
Hydrogen	**115**	1049
Hydrogen, compressed	**115**	1049
Hydrogen in a metal hydride storage system	**115**	3468
Hydrogen in a metal hydride storage system contained in equipment	**115**	3468
Hydrogen in a metal hydride storage system packed with equipment	**115**	3468
Hydrogen, refrigerated liquid (cryogenic liquid)	**115**	1966
Hydrogen and Methane mixture, compressed	**115**	2034
Hydrogen bromide, anhydrous	**125**	1048
Hydrogen chloride, anhydrous	**125**	1050
Hydrogen chloride, refrigerated liquid	**125**	2186
Hydrogen cyanide, anhydrous, stabilized	**117P**	1051
Hydrogen cyanide, aqueous solution, with not more than 20% Hydrogen cyanide	**154**	1613
Hydrogen cyanide, solution in alcohol, with not more than 45% Hydrogen cyanide	**131**	3294
Hydrogen cyanide, stabilized	**117P**	1051
Hydrogen cyanide, stabilized (absorbed)	**152**	1614
Hydrogendifluorides, solid, n.o.s.	**154**	1740
Hydrogendifluorides, solution, n.o.s.	**154**	3471
Hydrogen fluoride, anhydrous	**125**	1052
Hydrogen iodide, anhydrous	**125**	2197
Hydrogen peroxide, aqueous solution, stabilized, with more than 60% Hydrogen peroxide	**143**	2015
Hydrogen peroxide, aqueous solution, with not less than 8% but less than 20% Hydrogen peroxide	**140**	2984

Name of Material	Guide No.	ID No.
Hydrogen peroxide, aqueous solution, with not less than 20% but not more than 60% Hydrogen peroxide (stabilized as necessary)	**140**	2014
Hydrogen peroxide, stabilized	**143**	2015
Hydrogen peroxide and Peroxyacetic acid mixture, with acid(s), water and not more than 5% Peroxyacetic acid, stabilized	**140**	3149
Hydrogen selenide, adsorbed	**173**	3526
Hydrogen selenide, anhydrous	**117**	2202
Hydrogen sulfide	**117**	1053
Hydrogen sulphide	**117**	1053
1-Hydroxybenzotriazole, anhydrous, wetted with not less than 20% water	**113**	3474
1-Hydroxybenzotriazole, monohydrate	**113**	3474
Hydroxylamine sulfate	**154**	2865
Hydroxylamine sulphate	**154**	2865
Hypochlorite solution	**154**	1791
Hypochlorites, inorganic, n.o.s.	**140**	3212
3,3'-Iminodipropylamine	**153**	2269
Infectious substance, affecting animals only	**158**	2900
Infectious substance, affecting humans	**158**	2814
Ink, printer's, flammable	**129**	1210
Insecticide gas, flammable, n.o.s.	**115**	3354
Insecticide gas, n.o.s.	**126**	1968
Insecticide gas, poisonous, flammable, n.o.s.	**119**	3355
Insecticide gas, poisonous, flammable, n.o.s. (Inhalation Hazard Zone A)	**119**	3355
Insecticide gas, poisonous, flammable, n.o.s. (Inhalation Hazard Zone B)	**119**	3355
Insecticide gas, poisonous, flammable, n.o.s. (Inhalation Hazard Zone C)	**119**	3355
Insecticide gas, poisonous, flammable, n.o.s. (Inhalation Hazard Zone D)	**119**	3355
Insecticide gas, poisonous, n.o.s.	**123**	1967
Insecticide gas, toxic, flammable, n.o.s.	**119**	3355
Insecticide gas, toxic, flammable, n.o.s. (Inhalation Hazard Zone A)	**119**	3355
Insecticide gas, toxic, flammable, n.o.s. (Inhalation Hazard Zone B)	**119**	3355
Insecticide gas, toxic, flammable, n.o.s. (Inhalation Hazard Zone C)	**119**	3355
Insecticide gas, toxic, flammable, n.o.s. (Inhalation Hazard Zone D)	**119**	3355
Insecticide gas, toxic, n.o.s.	**123**	1967
Iodine	**154**	3495
Iodine monochloride, liquid	**157**	3498
Iodine monochloride, solid	**157**	1792
Iodine pentafluoride	**144**	2495
2-Iodobutane	**129**	2390
Iodomethylpropanes	**129**	2391
Iodopropanes	**129**	2392
Iron oxide, spent	**135**	1376
Iron pentacarbonyl	**136**	1994
Iron sponge, spent	**135**	1376
Isobutane	**115**	1075
Isobutane	**115**	1969

Name of Material	Guide No.	ID No.
Isobutanol	**129**	1212
Isobutyl acetate	**129**	1213
Isobutyl acrylate, stabilized	**129P**	2527
Isobutyl alcohol	**129**	1212
Isobutyl aldehyde	**130**	2045
Isobutylamine	**132**	1214
Isobutyl chloroformate	**155**	2742
Isobutylene	**115**	1055
Isobutylene	**115**	1075
Isobutyl formate	**129**	2393
Isobutyl isobutyrate	**130**	2528
Isobutyl isocyanate	**155P**	2486
Isobutyl methacrylate, stabilized	**130P**	2283
Isobutyl propionate	**129**	2394
Isobutyraldehyde	**130**	2045
Isobutyric acid	**132**	2529
Isobutyronitrile	**131**	2284
Isobutyryl chloride	**132**	2395
Isocyanate solution, flammable, poisonous, n.o.s.	**155**	2478
Isocyanate solution, flammable, toxic, n.o.s.	**155**	2478
Isocyanate solution, poisonous, flammable, n.o.s.	**155**	3080
Isocyanate solution, poisonous, n.o.s.	**155**	2206
Isocyanate solution, toxic, flammable, n.o.s.	**155**	3080
Isocyanate solution, toxic, n.o.s.	**155**	2206
Isocyanates, flammable, poisonous, n.o.s.	**155**	2478
Isocyanates, flammable, toxic, n.o.s.	**155**	2478
Isocyanates, poisonous, flammable, n.o.s.	**155**	3080
Isocyanates, poisonous, n.o.s.	**155**	2206
Isocyanates, toxic, flammable, n.o.s.	**155**	3080
Isocyanates, toxic, n.o.s.	**155**	2206
Isocyanatobenzotrifluorides	**156**	2285
Isoheptenes	**128**	2287
Isohexenes	**128**	2288
Isooctane	**128**	1262
Isooctenes	**128**	1216
Isopentane	**128**	1265
Isopentenes	**128**	2371
Isophoronediamine	**153**	2289
Isophorone diisocyanate	**156**	2290
Isoprene, stabilized	**130P**	1218
Isopropanol	**129**	1219
Isopropenyl acetate	**129P**	2403
Isopropenylbenzene	**128**	2303
Isopropyl acetate	**129**	1220
Isopropyl acid phosphate	**153**	1793
Isopropyl alcohol	**129**	1219
Isopropylamine	**132**	1221
Isopropylbenzene	**130**	1918
Isopropyl butyrate	**129**	2405
Isopropyl chloroacetate	**155**	2947
Isopropyl chloroformate	**155**	2407
Isopropyl 2-chloropropionate	**129**	2934
Isopropyl isobutyrate	**127**	2406
Isopropyl isocyanate	**155P**	2483
Isopropyl nitrate	**130**	1222
Isopropyl propionate	**129**	2409
Isosorbide dinitrate mixture	**133**	2907

Name of Material	Guide No.	ID No.
Isosorbide-5-mononitrate	**133**	3251
Kerosene	**128**	1223
Ketones, liquid, n.o.s.	**127**	1224
Krill meal	**133**	3497
Krypton	**120**	1056
Krypton, compressed	**120**	1056
Krypton, refrigerated liquid (cryogenic liquid)	**120**	1970
L (Lewisite)	**153**	—
Lead acetate	**151**	1616
Lead arsenates	**151**	1617
Lead arsenites	**151**	1618
Lead compound, soluble, n.o.s.	**151**	2291
Lead cyanide	**151**	1620
Lead dioxide	**140**	1872
Lead nitrate	**141**	1469
Lead perchlorate, solid	**141**	1470
Lead perchlorate, solution	**141**	3408
Lead phosphite, dibasic	**133**	2989
Lead sulfate, with more than 3% free acid	**154**	1794
Lead sulphate, with more than 3% free acid	**154**	1794
Lewisite	**153**	—
Life-saving appliances, not self-inflating	**171**	3072
Life-saving appliances, self-inflating	**171**	2990
Lighter refills containing flammable gas	**115**	1057
Lighters containing flammable gas	**115**	1057
Lighters, non-pressurized, containing flammable liquid	**128**	1057

Name of Material	Guide No.	ID No.
Liquefied gas, flammable, n.o.s.	**115**	3161
Liquefied gas, n.o.s.	**126**	3163
Liquefied gas, oxidizing, n.o.s.	**122**	3157
Liquefied gas, poisonous, corrosive, n.o.s.	**125**	3308
Liquefied gas, poisonous, corrosive, n.o.s. (Inhalation Hazard Zone A)	**125**	3308
Liquefied gas, poisonous, corrosive, n.o.s. (Inhalation Hazard Zone B)	**125**	3308
Liquefied gas, poisonous, corrosive, n.o.s. (Inhalation Hazard Zone C)	**125**	3308
Liquefied gas, poisonous, corrosive, n.o.s. (Inhalation Hazard Zone D)	**125**	3308
Liquefied gas, poisonous, flammable, corrosive, n.o.s.	**119**	3309
Liquefied gas, poisonous, flammable, corrosive, n.o.s. (Inhalation Hazard Zone A)	**119**	3309
Liquefied gas, poisonous, flammable, corrosive, n.o.s. (Inhalation Hazard Zone B)	**119**	3309
Liquefied gas, poisonous, flammable, corrosive, n.o.s. (Inhalation Hazard Zone C)	**119**	3309
Liquefied gas, poisonous, flammable, corrosive, n.o.s. (Inhalation Hazard Zone D)	**119**	3309
Liquefied gas, poisonous, flammable, n.o.s.	**119**	3160
Liquefied gas, poisonous, flammable, n.o.s. (Inhalation Hazard Zone A)	**119**	3160
Liquefied gas, poisonous, flammable, n.o.s. (Inhalation Hazard Zone B)	**119**	3160

Name of Material	Guide No.	ID No.
Liquefied gas, poisonous, flammable, n.o.s. (Inhalation Hazard Zone C)	**119**	3160
Liquefied gas, poisonous, flammable, n.o.s. (Inhalation Hazard Zone D)	**119**	3160
Liquefied gas, poisonous, n.o.s.	**123**	3162
Liquefied gas, poisonous, n.o.s. (Inhalation Hazard Zone A)	**123**	3162
Liquefied gas, poisonous, n.o.s. (Inhalation Hazard Zone B)	**123**	3162
Liquefied gas, poisonous, n.o.s. (Inhalation Hazard Zone C)	**123**	3162
Liquefied gas, poisonous, n.o.s. (Inhalation Hazard Zone D)	**123**	3162
Liquefied gas, poisonous, oxidizing, corrosive, n.o.s.	**124**	3310
Liquefied gas, poisonous, oxidizing, corrosive, n.o.s. (Inhalation Hazard Zone A)	**124**	3310
Liquefied gas, poisonous, oxidizing, corrosive, n.o.s. (Inhalation Hazard Zone B)	**124**	3310
Liquefied gas, poisonous, oxidizing, corrosive, n.o.s. (Inhalation Hazard Zone C)	**124**	3310
Liquefied gas, poisonous, oxidizing, corrosive, n.o.s. (Inhalation Hazard Zone D)	**124**	3310
Liquefied gas, poisonous, oxidizing, n.o.s.	**124**	3307
Liquefied gas, poisonous, oxidizing, n.o.s. (Inhalation Hazard Zone A)	**124**	3307
Liquefied gas, poisonous, oxidizing, n.o.s. (Inhalation Hazard Zone B)	**124**	3307

Name of Material	Guide No.	ID No.
Liquefied gas, poisonous, oxidizing, n.o.s. (Inhalation Hazard Zone C)	**124**	3307
Liquefied gas, poisonous, oxidizing, n.o.s. (Inhalation Hazard Zone D)	**124**	3307
Liquefied gas, toxic, corrosive, n.o.s.	**125**	3308
Liquefied gas, toxic, corrosive, n.o.s. (Inhalation Hazard Zone A)	**125**	3308
Liquefied gas, toxic, corrosive, n.o.s. (Inhalation Hazard Zone B)	**125**	3308
Liquefied gas, toxic, corrosive, n.o.s. (Inhalation Hazard Zone C)	**125**	3308
Liquefied gas, toxic, corrosive, n.o.s. (Inhalation Hazard Zone D)	**125**	3308
Liquefied gas, toxic, flammable, corrosive, n.o.s.	**119**	3309
Liquefied gas, toxic, flammable, corrosive, n.o.s. (Inhalation Hazard Zone A)	**119**	3309
Liquefied gas, toxic, flammable, corrosive, n.o.s. (Inhalation Hazard Zone B)	**119**	3309
Liquefied gas, toxic, flammable, corrosive, n.o.s. (Inhalation Hazard Zone C)	**119**	3309
Liquefied gas, toxic, flammable, corrosive, n.o.s. (Inhalation Hazard Zone D)	**119**	3309
Liquefied gas, toxic, flammable, n.o.s.	**119**	3160
Liquefied gas, toxic, flammable, n.o.s. (Inhalation Hazard Zone A)	**119**	3160
Liquefied gas, toxic, flammable, n.o.s. (Inhalation Hazard Zone B)	**119**	3160

Name of Material	Guide No.	ID No.
Liquefied gas, toxic, flammable, n.o.s. (Inhalation Hazard Zone C)	**119**	3160
Liquefied gas, toxic, flammable, n.o.s. (Inhalation Hazard Zone D)	**119**	3160
Liquefied gas, toxic, n.o.s.	**123**	3162
Liquefied gas, toxic, n.o.s. (Inhalation Hazard Zone A)	**123**	3162
Liquefied gas, toxic, n.o.s. (Inhalation Hazard Zone B)	**123**	3162
Liquefied gas, toxic, n.o.s. (Inhalation Hazard Zone C)	**123**	3162
Liquefied gas, toxic, n.o.s. (Inhalation Hazard Zone D)	**123**	3162
Liquefied gas, toxic, oxidizing, corrosive, n.o.s.	**124**	3310
Liquefied gas, toxic, oxidizing, corrosive, n.o.s. (Inhalation Hazard Zone A)	**124**	3310
Liquefied gas, toxic, oxidizing, corrosive, n.o.s. (Inhalation Hazard Zone B)	**124**	3310
Liquefied gas, toxic, oxidizing, corrosive, n.o.s. (Inhalation Hazard Zone C)	**124**	3310
Liquefied gas, toxic, oxidizing, corrosive, n.o.s. (Inhalation Hazard Zone D)	**124**	3310
Liquefied gas, toxic, oxidizing, n.o.s.	**124**	3307
Liquefied gas, toxic, oxidizing, n.o.s. (Inhalation Hazard Zone A)	**124**	3307
Liquefied gas, toxic, oxidizing, n.o.s. (Inhalation Hazard Zone B)	**124**	3307
Liquefied gas, toxic, oxidizing, n.o.s. (Inhalation Hazard Zone C)	**124**	3307
Liquefied gas, toxic, oxidizing, n.o.s. (Inhalation Hazard Zone D)	**124**	3307
Liquefied gases, non-flammable, charged with Nitrogen, Carbon dioxide or Air	**120**	1058
Liquefied natural gas (cryogenic liquid)	**115**	1972
Liquefied petroleum gas	**115**	1075
Lithium	**138**	1415
Lithium aluminum hydride	**138**	1410
Lithium aluminum hydride, ethereal	**138**	1411
Lithium batteries	**138**	3090
Lithium batteries contained in equipment	**138**	3091
Lithium batteries installed in cargo transport unit (lithium ion batteries)	**147**	3536
Lithium batteries installed in cargo transport unit (lithium metal batteries)	**138**	3536
Lithium batteries packed with equipment	**138**	3091
Lithium borohydride	**138**	1413
Lithium ferrosilicon	**139**	2830
Lithium hydride	**138**	1414
Lithium hydride, fused solid	**138**	2805
Lithium hydroxide	**154**	2680
Lithium hydroxide, solution	**154**	2679
Lithium hypochlorite, dry	**140**	1471
Lithium hypochlorite mixture	**140**	1471
Lithium hypochlorite mixtures, dry	**140**	1471
Lithium ion batteries (including lithium ion polymer batteries)	**147**	3480

Name of Material	Guide No.	ID No.
Lithium ion batteries contained in equipment (including lithium ion polymer batteries)	**147**	3481
Lithium ion batteries packed with equipment (including lithium ion polymer batteries)	**147**	3481
Lithium metal batteries (including lithium alloy batteries)	**138**	3090
Lithium metal batteries contained in equipment (including lithium alloy batteries)	**138**	3091
Lithium metal batteries packed with equipment (including lithium alloy batteries)	**138**	3091
Lithium nitrate	**140**	2722
Lithium nitride	**139**	2806
Lithium peroxide	**143**	1472
Lithium silicon	**138**	1417
LNG (cryogenic liquid)	**115**	1972
London purple	**151**	1621
LPG	**115**	1075
Machinery, fuel cell, flammable gas powered	**115**	3529
Machinery, fuel cell, flammable liquid powered	**128**	3528
Machinery, internal combustion	**171**	3530
Machinery, internal combustion, flammable gas powered	**115**	3529
Machinery, internal combustion, flammable liquid powered	**128**	3528
Magnesium	**138**	1869
Magnesium, in pellets, turnings or ribbons	**138**	1869
Magnesium alkyls	**135**	3053

Name of Material	Guide No.	ID No.
Magnesium alloys, with more than 50% Magnesium, in pellets, turnings or ribbons	**138**	1869
Magnesium alloys powder	**138**	1418
Magnesium aluminum phosphide	**139**	1419
Magnesium arsenate	**151**	1622
Magnesium bromate	**140**	1473
Magnesium chlorate	**140**	2723
Magnesium chloride and Chlorate mixture, solid	**140**	1459
Magnesium chloride and Chlorate mixture, solution	**140**	3407
Magnesium diamide	**135**	2004
Magnesium diphenyl	**135**	2005
Magnesium fluorosilicate	**151**	2853
Magnesium granules, coated	**138**	2950
Magnesium hydride	**138**	2010
Magnesium nitrate	**140**	1474
Magnesium perchlorate	**140**	1475
Magnesium peroxide	**140**	1476
Magnesium phosphide	**139**	2011
Magnesium powder	**138**	1418
Magnesium silicide	**138**	2624
Magnetized material	**171**	2807
Maleic anhydride	**156**	2215
Maleic anhydride, molten	**156**	2215
Malononitrile	**153**	2647
Maneb	**135**	2210
Maneb, stabilized	**135**	2968
Maneb preparation, stabilized	**135**	2968
Maneb preparation, with not less than 60% Maneb	**135**	2210
Manganese nitrate	**140**	2724

Name of Material	Guide No.	ID No.
Manganese resinate	**133**	1330
Matches, fusee	**133**	2254
Matches, safety	**133**	1944
Matches, "strike anywhere"	**133**	1331
Matches, wax "vesta"	**133**	1945
MD	**152**	—
Medical waste, category A, affecting animals only, solid	**158**	3549
Medical waste, category A, affecting humans, solid	**158**	3549
Medical waste, n.o.s.	**158**	3291
Medicine, liquid, flammable, poisonous, n.o.s.	**131**	3248
Medicine, liquid, flammable, toxic, n.o.s.	**131**	3248
Medicine, liquid, poisonous, n.o.s.	**151**	1851
Medicine, liquid, toxic, n.o.s.	**151**	1851
Medicine, solid, poisonous, n.o.s.	**151**	3249
Medicine, solid, toxic, n.o.s.	**151**	3249
Mercaptan mixture, liquid, flammable, n.o.s.	**130**	3336
Mercaptan mixture, liquid, flammable, poisonous, n.o.s.	**131**	1228
Mercaptan mixture, liquid, flammable, toxic, n.o.s.	**131**	1228
Mercaptan mixture, liquid, poisonous, flammable, n.o.s.	**131**	3071
Mercaptan mixture, liquid, toxic, flammable, n.o.s.	**131**	3071
Mercaptans, liquid, flammable, n.o.s.	**130**	3336
Mercaptans, liquid, flammable, poisonous, n.o.s.	**131**	1228
Mercaptans, liquid, flammable, toxic, n.o.s.	**131**	1228

Name of Material	Guide No.	ID No.
Mercaptans, liquid, poisonous, flammable, n.o.s.	**131**	3071
Mercaptans, liquid, toxic, flammable, n.o.s.	**131**	3071
Mercuric arsenate	**151**	1623
Mercuric chloride	**154**	1624
Mercuric nitrate	**141**	1625
Mercuric potassium cyanide	**157**	1626
Mercurous nitrate	**141**	1627
Mercury	**172**	2809
Mercury acetate	**151**	1629
Mercury ammonium chloride	**151**	1630
Mercury based pesticide, liquid, flammable, poisonous	**131**	2778
Mercury based pesticide, liquid, flammable, toxic	**131**	2778
Mercury based pesticide, liquid, poisonous	**151**	3012
Mercury based pesticide, liquid, poisonous, flammable	**131**	3011
Mercury based pesticide, liquid, toxic	**151**	3012
Mercury based pesticide, liquid, toxic, flammable	**131**	3011
Mercury based pesticide, solid, poisonous	**151**	2777
Mercury based pesticide, solid, toxic	**151**	2777
Mercury benzoate	**154**	1631
Mercury bromides	**154**	1634
Mercury compound, liquid, n.o.s.	**151**	2024
Mercury compound, solid, n.o.s.	**151**	2025
Mercury contained in manufactured articles	**172**	3506
Mercury cyanide	**154**	1636

Name of Material	Guide No.	ID No.
Mercury gluconate	**151**	1637
Mercury iodide	**151**	1638
Mercury nucleate	**151**	1639
Mercury oleate	**151**	1640
Mercury oxide	**151**	1641
Mercury oxycyanide, desensitized	**151**	1642
Mercury potassium iodide	**151**	1643
Mercury salicylate	**151**	1644
Mercury sulfate	**151**	1645
Mercury sulphate	**151**	1645
Mercury thiocyanate	**151**	1646
Mesityl oxide	**129**	1229
Metal carbonyls, liquid, n.o.s.	**151**	3281
Metal carbonyls, solid, n.o.s.	**151**	3466
Metal catalyst, dry	**135**	2881
Metal catalyst, wetted	**170**	1378
Metaldehyde	**133**	1332
Metal hydrides, flammable, n.o.s.	**170**	3182
Metal hydrides, water-reactive, n.o.s.	**138**	1409
Metallic substance, water-reactive, n.o.s.	**138**	3208
Metallic substance, water-reactive, self-heating, n.o.s.	**138**	3209
Metal powder, flammable, n.o.s.	**170**	3089
Metal powder, self-heating, n.o.s.	**135**	3189
Metal salts of organic compounds, flammable, n.o.s.	**133**	3181
Methacrylaldehyde, stabilized	**131P**	2396
Methacrylic acid, stabilized	**153P**	2531
Methacrylonitrile, stabilized	**131P**	3079
Methallyl alcohol	**129**	2614
Methane	**115**	1971
Methane, compressed	**115**	1971
Methane, refrigerated liquid (cryogenic liquid)	**115**	1972
Methane and Hydrogen mixture, compressed	**115**	2034
Methanesulfonyl chloride	**156**	3246
Methanesulphonyl chloride	**156**	3246
Methanol	**131**	1230
Methoxymethyl isocyanate	**155**	2605
4-Methoxy-4-methylpentan-2-one	**128**	2293
1-Methoxy-2-propanol	**129**	3092
Methyl acetate	**129**	1231
Methylacetylene and Propadiene mixture, stabilized	**116P**	1060
Methyl acrylate, stabilized	**129P**	1919
Methylal	**127**	1234
Methyl alcohol	**131**	1230
Methylallyl chloride	**130P**	2554
Methylamine, anhydrous	**118**	1061
Methylamine, aqueous solution	**132**	1235
Methylamyl acetate	**130**	1233
Methylamyl alcohol	**129**	2053
Methyl amyl ketone	**127**	1110
N-Methylaniline	**153**	2294
Methylbenzyl (alpha) alcohol, liquid	**153**	2937
Methylbenzyl (alpha) alcohol, solid	**153**	3438
Methyl bromide	**123**	1062

Name of Material	Guide No.	ID No.
Methyl bromide and Chloropicrin mixture	123	1581
Methyl bromide and Ethylene dibromide mixture, liquid	151	1647
Methyl bromoacetate	155	2643
2-Methylbutanal	129	3371
3-Methylbutan-2-one	127	2397
2-Methyl-1-butene	128	2459
2-Methyl-2-butene	128	2460
3-Methyl-1-butene	128	2561
N-Methylbutylamine	132	2945
Methyl tert-butyl ether	127	2398
Methyl butyrate	129	1237
Methyl chloride	115	1063
Methyl chloride and Chloropicrin mixture	119	1582
Methyl chloride and Methylene chloride mixture	115	1912
Methyl chloroacetate	155	2295
Methyl chloroformate	155	1238
Methyl chloromethyl ether	131	1239
Methyl 2-chloropropionate	129	2933
Methylchlorosilane	119	2534
Methylcyclohexane	128	2296
Methylcyclohexanols	129	2617
Methylcyclohexanone	128	2297
Methylcyclopentane	128	2298
Methyl dichloroacetate	155	2299
Methyldichloroarsine	152	1556
Methyldichlorosilane	139	1242
Methylene chloride	160	1593
Methylene chloride and Methyl chloride mixture	115	1912
Methyl ethyl ether	115	1039

Name of Material	Guide No.	ID No.
Methyl ethyl ketone	127	1193
2-Methyl-5-ethylpyridine	153	2300
Methyl fluoride	115	2454
Methyl formate	129	1243
2-Methylfuran	128	2301
2-Methyl-2-heptanethiol	131	3023
5-Methylhexan-2-one	127	2302
Methylhydrazine	131	1244
Methyl iodide	151	2644
Methyl isobutyl carbinol	129	2053
Methyl isobutyl ketone	127	1245
Methyl isocyanate	155P	2480
Methyl isopropenyl ketone, stabilized	127P	1246
Methyl isothiocyanate	131	2477
Methyl isovalerate	130	2400
Methyl magnesium bromide in Ethyl ether	138	1928
Methyl mercaptan	117	1064
Methyl methacrylate monomer, stabilized	129P	1247
4-Methylmorpholine	132	2535
N-Methylmorpholine	132	2535
Methyl nitrite	116	2455
Methyl orthosilicate	155	2606
Methylpentadiene	128	2461
2-Methylpentan-2-ol	129	2560
Methylphenyldichlorosilane	156	2437
Methyl phosphonic dichloride	137	9206
Methyl phosphonous dichloride	135	2845
1-Methylpiperidine	132	2399
Methyl propionate	129	1248
Methyl propyl ether	127	2612

Name of Material	Guide No.	ID No.
Methyl propyl ketone	**127**	1249
Methyltetrahydrofuran	**127**	2536
Methyl trichloroacetate	**156**	2533
Methyltrichlorosilane	**155**	1250
Methyl valeraldehyde (alpha)	**130**	2367
Methyl vinyl ketone, stabilized	**131P**	1251
Molten sulfur	**133**	2448
Molten sulphur	**133**	2448
Molybdenum pentachloride	**156**	2508
Monoethanolamine	**153**	2491
Mononitrotoluidines	**153**	2660
Morpholine	**132**	2054
Motor fuel anti-knock mixture	**152**	1649
Motor fuel anti-knock mixture, flammable	**131**	3483
Motor spirit	**128**	1203
Motor spirit and ethanol mixture, with more than 10% ethanol	**127**	3475
Muriatic acid	**157**	1789
Musk xylene	**149**	2956
Mustard	**153**	—
Mustard Lewisite	**153**	—
Naphthalene, crude	**133**	1334
Naphthalene, molten	**133**	2304
Naphthalene, refined	**133**	1334
Naphthylamine (alpha)	**153**	2077
Naphthylamine (beta), solid	**153**	1650
Naphthylamine (beta), solution	**153**	3411
Naphthylthiourea	**153**	1651
Naphthylurea	**153**	1652
Natural gas, compressed	**115**	1971

Name of Material	Guide No.	ID No.
Natural gas, refrigerated liquid (cryogenic liquid)	**115**	1972
Neohexane	**128**	1208
Neon	**120**	1065
Neon, compressed	**120**	1065
Neon, refrigerated liquid (cryogenic liquid)	**120**	1913
Nickel carbonyl	**131**	1259
Nickel catalyst, dry	**135**	2881
Nickel cyanide	**151**	1653
Nickel nitrate	**140**	2725
Nickel nitrite	**140**	2726
Nicotine	**151**	1654
Nicotine compound, liquid, n.o.s.	**151**	3144
Nicotine compound, solid, n.o.s.	**151**	1655
Nicotine hydrochloride, liquid	**151**	1656
Nicotine hydrochloride, solid	**151**	3444
Nicotine hydrochloride, solution	**151**	1656
Nicotine preparation, liquid, n.o.s.	**151**	3144
Nicotine preparation, solid, n.o.s.	**151**	1655
Nicotine salicylate	**151**	1657
Nicotine sulfate, solid	**151**	3445
Nicotine sulfate, solution	**151**	1658
Nicotine sulphate, solid	**151**	3445
Nicotine sulphate, solution	**151**	1658
Nicotine tartrate	**151**	1659
Nitrates, inorganic, aqueous solution, n.o.s.	**140**	3218
Nitrates, inorganic, n.o.s.	**140**	1477

Name of Material	Guide No.	ID No.
Nitrating acid mixture with more than 50% nitric acid	**157**	1796
Nitrating acid mixture with not more than 50% nitric acid	**157**	1796
Nitrating acid mixture, spent, with more than 50% nitric acid	**157**	1826
Nitrating acid mixture, spent, with not more than 50% nitric acid	**157**	1826
Nitric acid, other than red fuming, with more than 65% nitric acid	**157**	2031
Nitric acid, other than red fuming, with not more than 65% nitric acid	**157**	2031
Nitric acid, red fuming	**157**	2032
Nitric oxide	**124**	1660
Nitric oxide, compressed	**124**	1660
Nitric oxide and Dinitrogen tetroxide mixture	**124**	1975
Nitric oxide and Nitrogen dioxide mixture	**124**	1975
Nitriles, flammable, poisonous, n.o.s.	**131**	3273
Nitriles, flammable, toxic, n.o.s.	**131**	3273
Nitriles, liquid, poisonous, n.o.s.	**151**	3276
Nitriles, liquid, toxic, n.o.s.	**151**	3276
Nitriles, poisonous, flammable, n.o.s.	**131**	3275
Nitriles, poisonous, liquid, n.o.s.	**151**	3276
Nitriles, poisonous, solid, n.o.s.	**151**	3439
Nitriles, solid, poisonous, n.o.s.	**151**	3439
Nitriles, solid, toxic, n.o.s.	**151**	3439
Nitriles, toxic, flammable, n.o.s.	**131**	3275
Nitriles, toxic, liquid, n.o.s.	**151**	3276
Nitriles, toxic, solid, n.o.s.	**151**	3439
Nitrites, inorganic, aqueous solution, n.o.s.	**140**	3219
Nitrites, inorganic, n.o.s.	**140**	2627
Nitroanilines	**153**	1661
Nitroanisoles, liquid	**152**	2730
Nitroanisoles, solid	**152**	3458
Nitrobenzene	**152**	1662
Nitrobenzenesulfonic acid	**153**	2305
Nitrobenzenesulphonic acid	**153**	2305
Nitrobenzotrifluorides, liquid	**152**	2306
Nitrobenzotrifluorides, solid	**152**	3431
Nitrobromobenzenes, liquid	**152**	2732
Nitrobromobenzenes, solid	**152**	3459
Nitrocellulose membrane filters	**133**	3270
Nitrocellulose mixture, without pigment	**133**	2557
Nitrocellulose mixture, without plasticizer	**133**	2557
Nitrocellulose mixture, with pigment	**133**	2557
Nitrocellulose mixture, with plasticizer	**133**	2557
Nitrocellulose, solution, flammable	**127**	2059
Nitrocellulose with alcohol, not less than 25% alcohol	**113**	2556
Nitrocellulose with water, not less than 25% water	**113**	2555
3-Nitro-4-chlorobenzotrifluoride	**152**	2307
Nitrocresols, liquid	**153**	3434
Nitrocresols, solid	**153**	2446

Name of Material	Guide No.	ID No.
Nitroethane	**129**	2842
Nitrogen	**120**	1066
Nitrogen, compressed	**120**	1066
Nitrogen, refrigerated liquid (cryogenic liquid)	**120**	1977
Nitrogen dioxide	**124**	1067
Nitrogen dioxide and Nitric oxide mixture	**124**	1975
Nitrogen trifluoride	**122**	2451
Nitrogen trifluoride, compressed	**122**	2451
Nitrogen trioxide	**124**	2421
Nitroglycerin, solution in alcohol, with more than 1% but not more than 5% Nitroglycerin	**127**	3064
Nitroglycerin, solution in alcohol, with not more than 1% Nitroglycerin	**127**	1204
Nitroglycerin mixture, desensitized, liquid, flammable, n.o.s., with not more than 30% Nitroglycerin	**113**	3343
Nitroglycerin mixture, desensitized, liquid, n.o.s., with not more than 30% Nitroglycerin	**113**	3357
Nitroglycerin mixture, desensitized, solid, n.o.s., with more than 2% but not more than 10% Nitroglycerin	**113**	3319
Nitroguanidine, wetted with not less than 20% water	**113**	1336
Nitrohydrochloric acid	**157**	1798
Nitromethane	**129**	1261
Nitronaphthalene	**133**	2538
Nitrophenols	**153**	1663
4-Nitrophenylhydrazine, with not less than 30% water	**113**	3376

Name of Material	Guide No.	ID No.
Nitropropanes	**129**	2608
p-Nitrosodimethylaniline	**135**	1369
Nitrostarch, wetted with not less than 20% water	**113**	1337
Nitrosyl chloride	**125**	1069
Nitrosylsulfuric acid, liquid	**157**	2308
Nitrosylsulfuric acid, solid	**157**	3456
Nitrosylsulphuric acid, liquid	**157**	2308
Nitrosylsulphuric acid, solid	**157**	3456
Nitrotoluenes, liquid	**152**	1664
Nitrotoluenes, solid	**152**	3446
Nitrotoluidines (mono)	**153**	2660
Nitrous oxide	**122**	1070
Nitrous oxide, compressed	**122**	1070
Nitrous oxide, refrigerated liquid	**122**	2201
Nitrous oxide and Carbon dioxide mixture	**126**	1015
Nitroxylenes, liquid	**152**	1665
Nitroxylenes, solid	**152**	3447
Nonanes	**128**	1920
Nonyltrichlorosilane	**156**	1799
2,5-Norbornadiene, stabilized	**128P**	2251
Octadecyltrichlorosilane	**156**	1800
Octadiene	**128P**	2309
Octafluorobut-2-ene	**126**	2422
Octafluorocyclobutane	**126**	1976
Octafluoropropane	**126**	2424
Octanes	**128**	1262
Octyl aldehydes	**129**	1191
Octyltrichlorosilane	**156**	1801
Oil, petroleum	**128**	1270
Oil gas	**119**	1071

Name of Material	Guide No.	ID No.
Oil gas, compressed	**119**	1071
Organic peroxide type B, liquid	**146**	3101
Organic peroxide type B, liquid, temperature controlled	**148**	3111
Organic peroxide type B, solid	**146**	3102
Organic peroxide type B, solid, temperature controlled	**148**	3112
Organic peroxide type C, liquid	**146**	3103
Organic peroxide type C, liquid, temperature controlled	**148**	3113
Organic peroxide type C, solid	**146**	3104
Organic peroxide type C, solid, temperature controlled	**148**	3114
Organic peroxide type D, liquid	**145**	3105
Organic peroxide type D, liquid, temperature controlled	**148**	3115
Organic peroxide type D, solid	**145**	3106
Organic peroxide type D, solid, temperature controlled	**148**	3116
Organic peroxide type E, liquid	**145**	3107
Organic peroxide type E, liquid, temperature controlled	**148**	3117
Organic peroxide type E, solid	**145**	3108
Organic peroxide type E, solid, temperature controlled	**148**	3118
Organic peroxide type F, liquid	**145**	3109
Organic peroxide type F, liquid, temperature controlled	**148**	3119
Organic peroxide type F, solid	**145**	3110
Organic peroxide type F, solid, temperature controlled	**148**	3120
Organic phosphate compound mixed with compressed gas	**123**	1955
Organic phosphate mixed with compressed gas	**123**	1955
Organic phosphorus compound mixed with compressed gas	**123**	1955
Organic pigments, self-heating	**135**	3313
Organoarsenic compound, liquid, n.o.s.	**151**	3280
Organoarsenic compound, solid, n.o.s.	**151**	3465
Organochlorine pesticide, liquid, flammable, poisonous	**131**	2762
Organochlorine pesticide, liquid, flammable, toxic	**131**	2762
Organochlorine pesticide, liquid, poisonous	**151**	2996
Organochlorine pesticide, liquid, poisonous, flammable	**131**	2995
Organochlorine pesticide, liquid, toxic	**151**	2996
Organochlorine pesticide, liquid, toxic, flammable	**131**	2995
Organochlorine pesticide, solid, poisonous	**151**	2761
Organochlorine pesticide, solid, toxic	**151**	2761
Organometallic compound, liquid, poisonous, n.o.s.	**151**	3282
Organometallic compound, liquid, toxic, n.o.s.	**151**	3282
Organometallic compound, poisonous, liquid, n.o.s.	**151**	3282
Organometallic compound, poisonous, solid, n.o.s.	**151**	3467
Organometallic compound, solid, poisonous, n.o.s.	**151**	3467
Organometallic compound, solid, toxic, n.o.s.	**151**	3467
Organometallic compound, toxic, liquid, n.o.s.	**151**	3282

Name of Material	Guide No.	ID No.
Organometallic compound, toxic, solid, n.o.s.	**151**	3467
Organometallic substance, liquid, pyrophoric	**135**	3392
Organometallic substance, liquid, pyrophoric, water-reactive	**135**	3394
Organometallic substance, liquid, water-reactive	**135**	3398
Organometallic substance, liquid, water-reactive, flammable	**138**	3399
Organometallic substance, solid, pyrophoric	**135**	3391
Organometallic substance, solid, pyrophoric, water-reactive	**135**	3393
Organometallic substance, solid, self-heating	**138**	3400
Organometallic substance, solid, water-reactive	**135**	3395
Organometallic substance, solid, water-reactive, flammable	**138**	3396
Organometallic substance, solid, water-reactive, self-heating	**138**	3397
Organophosphorus compound, liquid, poisonous, n.o.s.	**151**	3278
Organophosphorus compound, liquid, toxic, n.o.s.	**151**	3278
Organophosphorus compound, poisonous, flammable, n.o.s.	**131**	3279
Organophosphorus compound, poisonous, liquid, n.o.s.	**151**	3278
Organophosphorus compound, poisonous, solid, n.o.s.	**151**	3464
Organophosphorus compound, solid, poisonous, n.o.s.	**151**	3464
Organophosphorus compound, solid, toxic, n.o.s.	**151**	3464
Organophosphorus compound, toxic, flammable, n.o.s.	**131**	3279
Organophosphorus compound, toxic, liquid, n.o.s.	**151**	3278
Organophosphorus compound, toxic, solid, n.o.s.	**151**	3464
Organophosphorus pesticide, liquid, flammable, poisonous	**131**	2784
Organophosphorus pesticide, liquid, flammable, toxic	**131**	2784
Organophosphorus pesticide, liquid, poisonous	**152**	3018
Organophosphorus pesticide, liquid, poisonous, flammable	**131**	3017
Organophosphorus pesticide, liquid, toxic	**152**	3018
Organophosphorus pesticide, liquid, toxic, flammable	**131**	3017
Organophosphorus pesticide, solid, poisonous	**152**	2783
Organophosphorus pesticide, solid, toxic	**152**	2783
Organotin compound, liquid, n.o.s.	**153**	2788
Organotin compound, solid, n.o.s.	**153**	3146
Organotin pesticide, liquid, flammable, poisonous	**131**	2787
Organotin pesticide, liquid, flammable, toxic	**131**	2787
Organotin pesticide, liquid, poisonous	**153**	3020
Organotin pesticide, liquid, poisonous, flammable	**131**	3019
Organotin pesticide, liquid, toxic	**153**	3020
Organotin pesticide, liquid, toxic, flammable	**131**	3019
Organotin pesticide, solid, poisonous	**153**	2786

Name of Material	Guide No.	ID No.
Organotin pesticide, solid, toxic	**153**	2786
Osmium tetroxide	**154**	2471
Other regulated substances, liquid, n.o.s.	**171**	3082
Other regulated substances, solid, n.o.s.	**171**	3077
Oxidizing liquid, corrosive, n.o.s.	**140**	3098
Oxidizing liquid, n.o.s.	**140**	3139
Oxidizing liquid, poisonous, n.o.s.	**142**	3099
Oxidizing liquid, toxic, n.o.s.	**142**	3099
Oxidizing solid, corrosive, n.o.s.	**140**	3085
Oxidizing solid, flammable, n.o.s.	**140**	3137
Oxidizing solid, n.o.s.	**140**	1479
Oxidizing solid, poisonous, n.o.s.	**141**	3087
Oxidizing solid, self-heating, n.o.s.	**135**	3100
Oxidizing solid, toxic, n.o.s.	**141**	3087
Oxidizing solid, water-reactive, n.o.s.	**144**	3121
Oxygen	**122**	1072
Oxygen, compressed	**122**	1072
Oxygen, refrigerated liquid (cryogenic liquid)	**122**	1073
Oxygen and Carbon dioxide mixture, compressed	**122**	1014
Oxygen difluoride	**124**	2190
Oxygen difluoride, compressed	**124**	2190
Oxygen generator, chemical	**140**	3356
Oxygen generator, chemical, spent	**140**	3356
Packagings discarded, empty, uncleaned	**171**	3509
Paint (corrosive)	**153**	3066
Paint, corrosive, flammable	**132**	3470
Paint (flammable)	**128**	1263
Paint, flammable, corrosive	**132**	3469
Paint related material (corrosive)	**153**	3066
Paint related material, corrosive, flammable	**132**	3470
Paint related material (flammable)	**128**	1263
Paint related material, flammable, corrosive	**132**	3469
Paper, unsaturated oil treated	**133**	1379
Paraformaldehyde	**133**	2213
Paraldehyde	**129**	1264
Parathion and compressed gas mixture	**123**	1967
PCB	**171**	2315
PD	**152**	—
Pentaborane	**135**	1380
Pentachloroethane	**151**	1669
Pentachlorophenol	**154**	3155
Pentaerythrite tetranitrate mixture, desensitized, solid, n.o.s., with more than 10% but not more than 20% PETN	**113**	3344
Pentaerythritol tetranitrate mixture, desensitized, solid, n.o.s., with more than 10% but not more than 20% PETN	**113**	3344
Pentafluoroethane	**126**	3220
Pentafluoroethane and Ethylene oxide mixture, with not more than 7.9% Ethylene oxide	**126**	3298
Pentamethylheptane	**128**	2286

Name of Material	Guide No.	ID No.
Pentane-2,4-dione	**131**	2310
Pentanes	**128**	1265
Pentanols	**129**	1105
1-Pentene	**128**	1108
1-Pentol	**153P**	2705
Perchlorates, inorganic, aqueous solution, n.o.s.	**140**	3211
Perchlorates, inorganic, n.o.s.	**140**	1481
Perchloric acid, with more than 50% but not more than 72% acid	**143**	1873
Perchloric acid, with not more than 50% acid	**157**	1802
Perchloroethylene	**160**	1897
Perchloromethyl mercaptan	**157**	1670
Perchloryl fluoride	**124**	3083
Perfluoro(ethyl vinyl ether)	**115**	3154
Perfluoro(methyl vinyl ether)	**115**	3153
Perfumery products, with flammable solvents	**127**	1266
Permanganates, inorganic, aqueous solution, n.o.s.	**140**	3214
Permanganates, inorganic, n.o.s.	**140**	1482
Peroxides, inorganic, n.o.s.	**140**	1483
Peroxyacetic acid and hydrogen peroxide mixture, with acid(s), water and not more than 5% Peroxyacetic acid, stabilized	**140**	3149
Persulfates, inorganic, aqueous solution, n.o.s.	**140**	3216
Persulfates, inorganic, n.o.s.	**140**	3215
Persulphates, inorganic, aqueous solution, n.o.s.	**140**	3216
Persulphates, inorganic, n.o.s.	**140**	3215
Pesticide, liquid, flammable, poisonous, n.o.s.	**131**	3021
Pesticide, liquid, flammable, toxic, n.o.s.	**131**	3021
Pesticide, liquid, poisonous, flammable, n.o.s.	**131**	2903
Pesticide, liquid, poisonous, n.o.s.	**151**	2902
Pesticide, liquid, toxic, flammable, n.o.s.	**131**	2903
Pesticide, liquid, toxic, n.o.s.	**151**	2902
Pesticide, solid, poisonous, n.o.s.	**151**	2588
Pesticide, solid, toxic, n.o.s.	**151**	2588
PETN mixture, desensitized, solid, n.o.s., with more than 10% but not more than 20% PETN	**113**	3344
Petrol	**128**	1203
Petrol and ethanol mixture, with more than 10% ethanol	**127**	3475
Petroleum crude oil	**128**	1267
Petroleum distillates, n.o.s.	**128**	1268
Petroleum gases, liquefied	**115**	1075
Petroleum oil	**128**	1270
Petroleum products, n.o.s.	**128**	1268
Petroleum sour crude oil, flammable, poisonous	**131**	3494
Petroleum sour crude oil, flammable, toxic	**131**	3494
Phenacyl bromide	**153**	2645
Phenetidines	**153**	2311
Phenol, molten	**153**	2312
Phenol, solid	**153**	1671
Phenol solution	**153**	2821
Phenolates, liquid	**154**	2904
Phenolates, solid	**154**	2905

Name of Material	Guide No.	ID No.
Phenolsulfonic acid, liquid	**153**	1803
Phenolsulphonic acid, liquid	**153**	1803
Phenoxyacetic acid derivative pesticide, liquid, flammable, poisonous	**131**	3346
Phenoxyacetic acid derivative pesticide, liquid, flammable, toxic	**131**	3346
Phenoxyacetic acid derivative pesticide, liquid, poisonous	**153**	3348
Phenoxyacetic acid derivative pesticide, liquid, poisonous, flammable	**131**	3347
Phenoxyacetic acid derivative pesticide, liquid, toxic	**153**	3348
Phenoxyacetic acid derivative pesticide, liquid, toxic, flammable	**131**	3347
Phenoxyacetic acid derivative pesticide, solid, poisonous	**153**	3345
Phenoxyacetic acid derivative pesticide, solid, toxic	**153**	3345
Phenylacetonitrile, liquid	**152**	2470
Phenylacetyl chloride	**156**	2577
Phenylcarbylamine chloride	**151**	1672
Phenyl chloroformate	**156**	2746
Phenylenediamines	**153**	1673
Phenylhydrazine	**153**	2572
Phenyl isocyanate	**155**	2487
Phenyl mercaptan	**131**	2337
Phenylmercuric acetate	**151**	1674
Phenylmercuric compound, n.o.s.	**151**	2026
Phenylmercuric hydroxide	**151**	1894
Phenylmercuric nitrate	**151**	1895
Phenylphosphorus dichloride	**137**	2798
Phenylphosphorus thiodichloride	**137**	2799
Phenyltrichlorosilane	**156**	1804
Phenyl urea pesticide, liquid, poisonous	**151**	3002
Phenyl urea pesticide, liquid, toxic	**151**	3002
Phosgene	**125**	1076
9-Phosphabicyclononanes	**135**	2940
Phosphine	**119**	2199
Phosphine, adsorbed	**173**	3525
Phosphoric acid, solid	**154**	3453
Phosphoric acid, solution	**154**	1805
Phosphorous acid	**154**	2834
Phosphorus, amorphous	**133**	1338
Phosphorus, white, dry or under water or in solution	**136**	1381
Phosphorus, white, molten	**136**	2447
Phosphorus, yellow, dry or under water or in solution	**136**	1381
Phosphorus heptasulfide, free from yellow and white Phosphorus	**139**	1339
Phosphorus heptasulphide, free from yellow and white Phosphorus	**139**	1339
Phosphorus oxybromide, molten	**137**	2576
Phosphorus oxybromide, solid	**137**	1939
Phosphorus oxychloride	**137**	1810
Phosphorus pentabromide	**137**	2691
Phosphorus pentachloride	**137**	1806
Phosphorus pentafluoride	**125**	2198
Phosphorus pentafluoride, adsorbed	**173**	3524
Phosphorus pentafluoride, compressed	**125**	2198

Name of Material	Guide No.	ID No.
Phosphorus pentasulfide, free from yellow and white Phosphorus	**139**	1340
Phosphorus pentasulphide, free from yellow and white Phosphorus	**139**	1340
Phosphorus pentoxide	**137**	1807
Phosphorus sesquisulfide, free from yellow and white Phosphorus	**139**	1341
Phosphorus sesquisulphide, free from yellow and white Phosphorus	**139**	1341
Phosphorus tribromide	**137**	1808
Phosphorus trichloride	**137**	1809
Phosphorus trioxide	**157**	2578
Phosphorus trisulfide, free from yellow and white Phosphorus	**139**	1343
Phosphorus trisulphide, free from yellow and white Phosphorus	**139**	1343
Phthalic anhydride	**156**	2214
Picolines	**129**	2313
Picric acid, wetted with not less than 10% water	**113**	3364
Picric acid, wetted with not less than 30% water	**113**	1344
Picrite, wetted with not less than 20% water	**113**	1336
Picryl chloride, wetted with not less than 10% water	**113**	3365
Pinene (alpha)	**128**	2368
Pine oil	**129**	1272
Piperazine	**153**	2579
Piperidine	**132**	2401
Plastic molding compound	**171**	3314
Plastics moulding compound	**171**	3314

Name of Material	Guide No.	ID No.
Plastics, nitrocellulose-based, self-heating, n.o.s.	**135**	2006
Poisonous by inhalation liquid, corrosive, flammable, n.o.s. (Inhalation Hazard Zone A)	**131**	3492
Poisonous by inhalation liquid, corrosive, flammable, n.o.s. (Inhalation Hazard Zone B)	**131**	3493
Poisonous by inhalation liquid, corrosive, n.o.s. (Inhalation Hazard Zone A)	**154**	3389
Poisonous by inhalation liquid, corrosive, n.o.s. (Inhalation Hazard Zone B)	**154**	3390
Poisonous by inhalation liquid, flammable, corrosive, n.o.s. (Inhalation Hazard Zone A)	**131**	3488
Poisonous by inhalation liquid, flammable, corrosive, n.o.s. (Inhalation Hazard Zone B)	**131**	3489
Poisonous by inhalation liquid, flammable, n.o.s. (Inhalation Hazard Zone A)	**131**	3383
Poisonous by inhalation liquid, flammable, n.o.s. (Inhalation Hazard Zone B)	**131**	3384
Poisonous by inhalation liquid, n.o.s. (Inhalation Hazard Zone A)	**151**	3381
Poisonous by inhalation liquid, n.o.s. (Inhalation Hazard Zone B)	**151**	3382
Poisonous by inhalation liquid, oxidizing, n.o.s. (Inhalation Hazard Zone A)	**142**	3387
Poisonous by inhalation liquid, oxidizing, n.o.s. (Inhalation Hazard Zone B)	**142**	3388
Poisonous by inhalation liquid, water-reactive, flammable, n.o.s. (Inhalation Hazard Zone A)	**155**	3490

Name of Material	Guide No.	ID No.
Poisonous by inhalation liquid, water-reactive, flammable, n.o.s. (Inhalation Hazard Zone B)	155	3491
Poisonous by inhalation liquid, water-reactive, n.o.s. (Inhalation Hazard Zone A)	139	3385
Poisonous by inhalation liquid, water-reactive, n.o.s. (Inhalation Hazard Zone B)	139	3386
Poisonous liquid, corrosive, inorganic, n.o.s.	154	3289
Poisonous liquid, corrosive, organic, n.o.s.	154	2927
Poisonous liquid, flammable, organic, n.o.s.	131	2929
Poisonous liquid, inorganic, n.o.s.	151	3287
Poisonous liquid, organic, n.o.s.	153	2810
Poisonous liquid, oxidizing, n.o.s.	142	3122
Poisonous liquid, water-reactive, n.o.s.	139	3123
Poisonous solid, corrosive, inorganic, n.o.s.	154	3290
Poisonous solid, corrosive, organic, n.o.s.	154	2928
Poisonous solid, flammable, organic, n.o.s.	134	2930
Poisonous solid, inorganic, n.o.s.	151	3288
Poisonous solid, organic, n.o.s.	154	2811
Poisonous solid, oxidizing, n.o.s.	141	3086
Poisonous solid, self-heating, n.o.s.	136	3124
Poisonous solid, water-reactive, n.o.s.	139	3125
Polyamines, flammable, corrosive, n.o.s.	132	2733

Name of Material	Guide No.	ID No.
Polyamines, liquid, corrosive, flammable, n.o.s.	132	2734
Polyamines, liquid, corrosive, n.o.s.	153	2735
Polyamines, solid, corrosive, n.o.s.	154	3259
Polychlorinated biphenyls, liquid	171	2315
Polychlorinated biphenyls, solid	171	3432
Polyester resin kit, liquid base material	128	3269
Polyester resin kit, solid base material	128P	3527
Polyhalogenated biphenyls, liquid	171	3151
Polyhalogenated biphenyls, solid	171	3152
Polyhalogenated terphenyls, liquid	171	3151
Polyhalogenated terphenyls, solid	171	3152
Polymeric beads, expandable	171	2211
Polymerizing substance, liquid, stabilized, n.o.s.	149P	3532
Polymerizing substance, liquid, temperature controlled, n.o.s.	150P	3534
Polymerizing substance, solid, stabilized, n.o.s.	149P	3531
Polymerizing substance, solid, temperature controlled, n.o.s.	150P	3533
Potassium	138	2257
Potassium, metal alloys, liquid	138	1420
Potassium, metal alloys, solid	138	3403
Potassium arsenate	151	1677
Potassium arsenite	154	1678
Potassium borohydride	138	1870

Name of Material	Guide No.	ID No.
Potassium bromate	**140**	1484
Potassium chlorate	**140**	1485
Potassium chlorate, aqueous solution	**140**	2427
Potassium cuprocyanide	**157**	1679
Potassium cyanide, solid	**157**	1680
Potassium cyanide, solution	**157**	3413
Potassium dithionite	**135**	1929
Potassium fluoride, solid	**154**	1812
Potassium fluoride, solution	**154**	3422
Potassium fluoroacetate	**151**	2628
Potassium fluorosilicate	**151**	2655
Potassium hydrogen difluoride, solid	**154**	1811
Potassium hydrogen difluoride, solution	**154**	3421
Potassium hydrogen sulfate	**154**	2509
Potassium hydrogen sulphate	**154**	2509
Potassium hydrosulfite	**135**	1929
Potassium hydrosulphite	**135**	1929
Potassium hydroxide, solid	**154**	1813
Potassium hydroxide, solution	**154**	1814
Potassium metavanadate	**151**	2864
Potassium monoxide	**154**	2033
Potassium nitrate	**140**	1486
Potassium nitrate and Sodium nitrate mixture	**140**	1499
Potassium nitrate and Sodium nitrite mixture	**140**	1487
Potassium nitrite	**140**	1488
Potassium perchlorate	**140**	1489
Potassium permanganate	**140**	1490
Potassium peroxide	**144**	1491
Potassium persulfate	**140**	1492
Potassium persulphate	**140**	1492
Potassium phosphide	**139**	2012
Potassium sodium alloys, liquid	**138**	1422
Potassium sodium alloys, solid	**138**	3404
Potassium sulfide, anhydrous	**135**	1382
Potassium sulfide, hydrated, with not less than 30% water of crystallization	**153**	1847
Potassium sulfide, with less than 30% water of crystallization	**135**	1382
Potassium sulphide, anhydrous	**135**	1382
Potassium sulphide, hydrated, with not less than 30% water of crystallization	**153**	1847
Potassium sulphide, with less than 30% water of crystallization	**135**	1382
Potassium superoxide	**143**	2466
Printing ink, flammable	**129**	1210
Printing ink related material, flammable	**129**	1210
Propadiene, stabilized	**116P**	2200
Propadiene and Methylacetylene mixture, stabilized	**116P**	1060
Propane	**115**	1075
Propane	**115**	1978
Propane-Ethane mixture, refrigerated liquid	**115**	1961
Propanethiols	**130**	2402
n-Propanol	**129**	1274
Propionaldehyde	**129P**	1275
Propionic acid	**153**	1848
Propionic acid, with not less than 10% and less than 90% acid	**153**	1848

Name of Material	Guide No.	ID No.
Propionic acid, with not less than 90% acid	**153**	3463
Propionic anhydride	**156**	2496
Propionitrile	**131**	2404
Propionyl chloride	**132**	1815
n-Propyl acetate	**129**	1276
Propyl alcohol, normal	**129**	1274
Propylamine	**132**	1277
n-Propyl benzene	**128**	2364
Propyl chloride	**129**	1278
n-Propyl chloroformate	**155**	2740
Propylene	**115**	1075
Propylene	**115**	1077
Propylene, Ethylene and Acetylene in mixture, refrigerated liquid containing at least 71.5% Ethylene with not more than 22.5% Acetylene and not more than 6% Propylene	**115**	3138
Propylene chlorohydrin	**131**	2611
1,2-Propylenediamine	**132**	2258
Propyleneimine, stabilized	**131P**	1921
Propylene oxide	**127P**	1280
Propylene oxide and Ethylene oxide mixture, with not more than 30% Ethylene oxide	**131P**	2983
Propylene tetramer	**128**	2850
Propyl formates	**129**	1281
n-Propyl isocyanate	**155P**	2482
n-Propyl nitrate	**128**	1865
Propyltrichlorosilane	**155**	1816
Pyrethroid pesticide, liquid, flammable, poisonous	**131**	3350
Pyrethroid pesticide, liquid, flammable, toxic	**131**	3350

Name of Material	Guide No.	ID No.
Pyrethroid pesticide, liquid, poisonous	**151**	3352
Pyrethroid pesticide, liquid, poisonous, flammable	**131**	3351
Pyrethroid pesticide, liquid, toxic	**151**	3352
Pyrethroid pesticide, liquid, toxic, flammable	**131**	3351
Pyrethroid pesticide, solid, poisonous	**151**	3349
Pyrethroid pesticide, solid, toxic	**151**	3349
Pyridine	**129**	1282
Pyrophoric alloy, n.o.s.	**135**	1383
Pyrophoric liquid, inorganic, n.o.s.	**135**	3194
Pyrophoric liquid, organic, n.o.s.	**135**	2845
Pyrophoric metal, n.o.s.	**135**	1383
Pyrophoric solid, inorganic, n.o.s.	**135**	3200
Pyrophoric solid, organic, n.o.s.	**135**	2846
Pyrosulfuryl chloride	**137**	1817
Pyrosulphuryl chloride	**137**	1817
Pyrrolidine	**132**	1922
Quinoline	**154**	2656
Radioactive material, excepted package, articles	**161**	2911
Radioactive material, excepted package, articles manufactured from depleted Uranium	**161**	2909
Radioactive material, excepted package, articles manufactured from natural Thorium	**161**	2909

Name of Material	Guide No.	ID No.
Radioactive material, excepted package, articles manufactured from natural Uranium	**161**	2909
Radioactive material, excepted package, empty packaging	**161**	2908
Radioactive material, excepted package, instruments	**161**	2911
Radioactive material, excepted package, limited quantity of material	**161**	2910
Radioactive material, low specific activity (LSA-I), non fissile or fissile-excepted	**162**	2912
Radioactive material, low specific activity (LSA-II), fissile	**165**	3324
Radioactive material, low specific activity (LSA-II), non fissile or fissile-excepted	**162**	3321
Radioactive material, low specific activity (LSA-III), fissile	**165**	3325
Radioactive material, low specific activity (LSA-III), non fissile or fissile-excepted	**162**	3322
Radioactive material, surface contaminated objects (SCO-I), fissile	**165**	3326
Radioactive material, surface contaminated objects (SCO-I), non fissile or fissile-excepted	**162**	2913
Radioactive material, surface contaminated objects (SCO-II), fissile	**165**	3326
Radioactive material, surface contaminated objects (SCO-II), non fissile or fissile-excepted	**162**	2913
Radioactive material, transported under special arrangement, fissile	**165**	3331
Radioactive material, transported under special arrangement, non fissile or fissile-excepted	**163**	2919
Radioactive material, Type A package, fissile, non-special form	**165**	3327
Radioactive material, Type A package, non-special form, non fissile or fissile-excepted	**163**	2915
Radioactive material, Type A package, special form, fissile	**165**	3333
Radioactive material, Type A package, special form, non fissile or fissile-excepted	**164**	3332
Radioactive material, Type B(M) package, fissile	**165**	3329
Radioactive material, Type B(M) package, non fissile or fissile-excepted	**163**	2917
Radioactive material, Type B(U) package, fissile	**165**	3328
Radioactive material, Type B(U) package, non fissile or fissile-excepted	**163**	2916
Radioactive material, Type C package, fissile	**165**	3330
Radioactive material, Type C package, non fissile or fissile excepted	**163**	3323
Radioactive material, Uranium hexafluoride, fissile	**166**	2977
Radioactive material, Uranium hexafluoride, non fissile or fissile-excepted	**166**	2978
Rags, oily	**133**	1856

Name of Material	Guide No.	ID No.
Receptacles, small, containing gas	**115**	2037
Red phosphorus	**133**	1338
Refrigerant gas, n.o.s.	**126**	1078
Refrigerant gases, n.o.s. (flammable)	**115**	1954
Refrigerant gas R-12	**126**	1028
Refrigerant gas R-12B1	**126**	1974
Refrigerant gas R-12B2	**171**	1941
Refrigerant gas R-13	**126**	1022
Refrigerant gas R-13B1	**126**	1009
Refrigerant gas R-14	**126**	1982
Refrigerant gas R-14, compressed	**126**	1982
Refrigerant gas R-21	**126**	1029
Refrigerant gas R-22	**126**	1018
Refrigerant gas R-23	**126**	1984
Refrigerant gas R-32	**115**	3252
Refrigerant gas R-40	**115**	1063
Refrigerant gas R-41	**115**	2454
Refrigerant gas R-114	**126**	1958
Refrigerant gas R-115	**126**	1020
Refrigerant gas R-116	**126**	2193
Refrigerant gas R-116, compressed	**126**	2193
Refrigerant gas R-124	**126**	1021
Refrigerant gas R-125	**126**	3220
Refrigerant gas R-133a	**126**	1983
Refrigerant gas R-134a	**126**	3159
Refrigerant gas R-142b	**115**	2517
Refrigerant gas R-143a	**115**	2035
Refrigerant gas R-152a	**115**	1030
Refrigerant gas R-161	**115**	2453

Name of Material	Guide No.	ID No.
Refrigerant gas R-218	**126**	2424
Refrigerant gas R-227	**126**	3296
Refrigerant gas R-404A	**126**	3337
Refrigerant gas R-407A	**126**	3338
Refrigerant gas R-407B	**126**	3339
Refrigerant gas R-407C	**126**	3340
Refrigerant gas R-500	**126**	2602
Refrigerant gas R-502	**126**	1973
Refrigerant gas R-503	**126**	2599
Refrigerant gas R-1113	**119P**	1082
Refrigerant gas R-1132a	**116P**	1959
Refrigerant gas R-1216	**126**	1858
Refrigerant gas R-1318	**126**	2422
Refrigerant gas RC-318	**126**	1976
Refrigerating machines, containing Ammonia solutions (UN2672)	**126**	2857
Refrigerating machines, containing flammable, non-poisonous, liquefied gas	**115**	3358
Refrigerating machines, containing flammable, non-toxic, liquefied gas	**115**	3358
Refrigerating machines, containing non-flammable, non-poisonous gases	**126**	2857
Refrigerating machines, containing non-flammable, non-toxic gases	**126**	2857
Regulated medical waste, n.o.s.	**158**	3291
Resin solution	**127**	1866
Resorcinol	**153**	2876
Rosin oil	**127**	1286
Rubber scrap, powdered or granulated	**133**	1345

Name of Material	Guide No.	ID No.
Rubber shoddy, powdered or granulated	**133**	1345
Rubber solution	**127**	1287
Rubidium	**138**	1423
Rubidium hydroxide, solid	**154**	2678
Rubidium hydroxide, solution	**154**	2677
SA	**119**	—
Safety devices	**171**	3268
Sarin	**153**	—
Seat-belt pre-tensioners	**171**	3268
Seed cake, with more than 1.5% oil and not more than 11% moisture	**135**	1386
Seed cake, with not more than 1.5% oil and not more than 11% moisture	**135**	2217
Selenates	**151**	2630
Selenic acid	**154**	1905
Selenites	**151**	2630
Selenium compound, liquid, n.o.s.	**151**	3440
Selenium compound, solid, n.o.s.	**151**	3283
Selenium disulfide	**153**	2657
Selenium disulphide	**153**	2657
Selenium hexafluoride	**125**	2194
Selenium oxychloride	**157**	2879
Self-defense spray, non-pressurized	**171**	3334
Self-heating liquid, corrosive, inorganic, n.o.s.	**136**	3188
Self-heating liquid, corrosive, organic, n.o.s.	**136**	3185
Self-heating liquid, inorganic, n.o.s.	**135**	3186
Self-heating liquid, organic, n.o.s.	**135**	3183
Self-heating liquid, poisonous, inorganic, n.o.s.	**136**	3187
Self-heating liquid, poisonous, organic, n.o.s.	**136**	3184
Self-heating liquid, toxic, inorganic, n.o.s.	**136**	3187
Self-heating liquid, toxic, organic, n.o.s.	**136**	3184
Self-heating solid, corrosive, inorganic, n.o.s.	**136**	3192
Self-heating solid, corrosive, organic, n.o.s.	**136**	3126
Self-heating solid, inorganic, n.o.s.	**135**	3190
Self-heating solid, organic, n.o.s.	**135**	3088
Self-heating solid, oxidizing, n.o.s.	**135**	3127
Self-heating solid, poisonous, inorganic, n.o.s.	**136**	3191
Self-heating solid, poisonous, organic, n.o.s.	**136**	3128
Self-heating solid, toxic, inorganic, n.o.s.	**136**	3191
Self-heating solid, toxic, organic, n.o.s.	**136**	3128
Self-reactive liquid type B	**149**	3221
Self-reactive liquid type B, temperature controlled	**150**	3231
Self-reactive liquid type C	**149**	3223
Self-reactive liquid type C, temperature controlled	**150**	3233
Self-reactive liquid type D	**149**	3225
Self-reactive liquid type D, temperature controlled	**150**	3235
Self-reactive liquid type E	**149**	3227
Self-reactive liquid type E, temperature controlled	**150**	3237
Self-reactive liquid type F	**149**	3229

Name of Material	Guide No.	ID No.
Self-reactive liquid type F, temperature controlled	**150**	3239
Self-reactive solid type B	**149**	3222
Self-reactive solid type B, temperature controlled	**150**	3232
Self-reactive solid type C	**149**	3224
Self-reactive solid type C, temperature controlled	**150**	3234
Self-reactive solid type D	**149**	3226
Self-reactive solid type D, temperature controlled	**150**	3236
Self-reactive solid type E	**149**	3228
Self-reactive solid type E, temperature controlled	**150**	3238
Self-reactive solid type F	**149**	3230
Self-reactive solid type F, temperature controlled	**150**	3240
Shale oil	**128**	1288
Silane	**116**	2203
Silane, compressed	**116**	2203
Silicon powder, amorphous	**170**	1346
Silicon tetrachloride	**157**	1818
Silicon tetrafluoride	**125**	1859
Silicon tetrafluoride, adsorbed	**173**	3521
Silicon tetrafluoride, compressed	**125**	1859
Silver arsenite	**151**	1683
Silver cyanide	**151**	1684
Silver nitrate	**140**	1493
Silver picrate, wetted with not less than 30% water	**113**	1347
Sludge acid	**153**	1906
Smokeless powder for small arms	**133**	3178
Soda lime, with more than 4% Sodium hydroxide	**154**	1907

Name of Material	Guide No.	ID No.
Sodium	**138**	1428
Sodium aluminate, solid	**154**	2812
Sodium aluminate, solution	**154**	1819
Sodium aluminum hydride	**138**	2835
Sodium ammonium vanadate	**154**	2863
Sodium arsanilate	**154**	2473
Sodium arsenate	**151**	1685
Sodium arsenite, aqueous solution	**154**	1686
Sodium arsenite, solid	**151**	2027
Sodium azide	**153**	1687
Sodium, batteries containing	**138**	3292
Sodium bisulfate, solution	**154**	2837
Sodium bisulphate, solution	**154**	2837
Sodium borohydride	**138**	1426
Sodium borohydride and Sodium hydroxide solution, with not more than 12% Sodium borohydride and not more than 40% Sodium hydroxide	**157**	3320
Sodium bromate	**140**	1494
Sodium cacodylate	**152**	1688
Sodium carbonate peroxyhydrate	**140**	3378
Sodium chlorate	**140**	1495
Sodium chlorate, aqueous solution	**140**	2428
Sodium chlorite	**143**	1496
Sodium chloroacetate	**151**	2659
Sodium cuprocyanide, solid	**157**	2316
Sodium cuprocyanide, solution	**157**	2317
Sodium cyanide, solid	**157**	1689
Sodium cyanide, solution	**157**	3414
Sodium dichloroisocyanurate	**140**	2465

Name of Material	Guide No.	ID No.
Sodium dichloro-s-triazinetrione	**140**	2465
Sodium dinitro-o-cresolate, wetted with not less than 10% water	**113**	3369
Sodium dinitro-o-cresolate, wetted with not less than 15% water	**113**	1348
Sodium dithionite	**135**	1384
Sodium fluoride, solid	**154**	1690
Sodium fluoride, solution	**154**	3415
Sodium fluoroacetate	**151**	2629
Sodium fluorosilicate	**154**	2674
Sodium hydride	**138**	1427
Sodium hydrogendifluoride	**154**	2439
Sodium hydrosulfide, hydrated, with not less than 25% water of crystallization	**154**	2949
Sodium hydrosulfide, with less than 25% water of crystallization	**135**	2318
Sodium hydrosulfide, with not less than 25% water of crystallization	**154**	2949
Sodium hydrosulfite	**135**	1384
Sodium hydrosulphide, hydrated, with not less than 25% water of crystallization	**154**	2949
Sodium hydrosulphide, with less than 25% water of crystallization	**135**	2318
Sodium hydrosulphide, with not less than 25% water of crystallization	**154**	2949
Sodium hydrosulphite	**135**	1384
Sodium hydroxide, solid	**154**	1823
Sodium hydroxide, solution	**154**	1824
Sodium hypochlorite	**154**	1791
Sodium methylate, dry	**138**	1431
Sodium methylate, solution in alcohol	**132**	1289
Sodium monoxide	**157**	1825
Sodium nitrate	**140**	1498
Sodium nitrate and Potassium nitrate mixture	**140**	1499
Sodium nitrite	**141**	1500
Sodium nitrite and Potassium nitrate mixture	**140**	1487
Sodium pentachlorophenate	**154**	2567
Sodium perborate monohydrate	**140**	3377
Sodium perchlorate	**140**	1502
Sodium permanganate	**140**	1503
Sodium peroxide	**144**	1504
Sodium peroxoborate, anhydrous	**140**	3247
Sodium persulfate	**140**	1505
Sodium persulphate	**140**	1505
Sodium phosphide	**139**	1432
Sodium picramate, wetted with not less than 20% water	**113**	1349
Sodium potassium alloys, liquid	**138**	1422
Sodium potassium alloys, solid	**138**	3404
Sodium sulfide, anhydrous	**135**	1385
Sodium sulfide, hydrated, with not less than 30% water	**153**	1849
Sodium sulfide, with less than 30% water of crystallization	**135**	1385
Sodium sulphide, anhydrous	**135**	1385
Sodium sulphide, hydrated, with not less than 30% water	**153**	1849
Sodium sulphide, with less than 30% water of crystallization	**135**	1385
Sodium superoxide	**143**	2547

Name of Material	Guide No.	ID No.
Solids containing corrosive liquid, n.o.s.	154	3244
Solids containing flammable liquid, n.o.s.	133	3175
Solids containing poisonous liquid, n.o.s.	151	3243
Solids containing toxic liquid, n.o.s.	151	3243
Soman	153	—
Stannic chloride, anhydrous	137	1827
Stannic chloride, pentahydrate	154	2440
Stannic phosphides	139	1433
Stibine	119	2676
Straw, wet, damp or contaminated with oil	133	1327
Strontium arsenite	151	1691
Strontium chlorate	143	1506
Strontium nitrate	140	1507
Strontium perchlorate	140	1508
Strontium peroxide	143	1509
Strontium phosphide	139	2013
Strychnine	151	1692
Strychnine salts	151	1692
Styrene monomer, stabilized	128P	2055
Substituted nitrophenol pesticide, liquid, flammable, poisonous	131	2780
Substituted nitrophenol pesticide, liquid, flammable, toxic	131	2780
Substituted nitrophenol pesticide, liquid, poisonous	153	3014
Substituted nitrophenol pesticide, liquid, poisonous, flammable	131	3013
Substituted nitrophenol pesticide, liquid, toxic	153	3014

Name of Material	Guide No.	ID No.
Substituted nitrophenol pesticide, liquid, toxic, flammable	131	3013
Substituted nitrophenol pesticide, solid, poisonous	153	2779
Substituted nitrophenol pesticide, solid, toxic	153	2779
Sulfamic acid	154	2967
Sulfur	133	1350
Sulfur, molten	133	2448
Sulfur chlorides	137	1828
Sulfur dioxide	125	1079
Sulfur hexafluoride	126	1080
Sulfuric acid	137	1830
Sulfuric acid, fuming	137	1831
Sulfuric acid, spent	137	1832
Sulfuric acid, with more than 51% acid	137	1830
Sulfuric acid, with not more than 51% acid	157	2796
Sulfuric acid and Hydrofluoric acid mixture	157	1786
Sulfurous acid	154	1833
Sulfur tetrafluoride	125	2418
Sulfur trioxide, stabilized	137	1829
Sulfuryl chloride	137	1834
Sulfuryl fluoride	123	2191
Sulphamic acid	154	2967
Sulphur	133	1350
Sulphur, molten	133	2448
Sulphur chlorides	137	1828
Sulphur dioxide	125	1079
Sulphur hexafluoride	126	1080
Sulphuric acid	137	1830
Sulphuric acid, fuming	137	1831

Name of Material	Guide No.	ID No.
Sulphuric acid, spent	**137**	1832
Sulphuric acid, with more than 51% acid	**137**	1830
Sulphuric acid, with not more than 51% acid	**157**	2796
Sulphuric acid and Hydrofluoric acid mixture	**157**	1786
Sulphurous acid	**154**	1833
Sulphur tetrafluoride	**125**	2418
Sulphur trioxide, stabilized	**137**	1829
Sulphuryl chloride	**137**	1834
Sulphuryl fluoride	**123**	2191
Tabun	**153**	—
Tars, liquid	**130**	1999
Tear gas candles	**159**	1700
Tear gas devices	**159**	1693
Tear gas grenades	**159**	1700
Tear gas substance, liquid, n.o.s.	**159**	1693
Tear gas substance, solid, n.o.s.	**159**	3448
Tellurium compound, n.o.s.	**151**	3284
Tellurium hexafluoride	**125**	2195
Terpene hydrocarbons, n.o.s.	**128**	2319
Terpinolene	**128**	2541
Tetrabromoethane	**159**	2504
1,1,2,2-Tetrachloroethane	**151**	1702
Tetrachloroethylene	**160**	1897
Tetraethyl dithiopyrophosphate	**153**	1704
Tetraethylenepentamine	**153**	2320
Tetraethyl silicate	**129**	1292
1,1,1,2-Tetrafluoroethane	**126**	3159
Tetrafluoroethane and Ethylene oxide mixture, with not more than 5.6% Ethylene oxide	**126**	3299

Name of Material	Guide No.	ID No.
Tetrafluoroethylene, stabilized	**116P**	1081
Tetrafluoromethane	**126**	1982
Tetrafluoromethane, compressed	**126**	1982
1,2,3,6-Tetrahydrobenzaldehyde	**129**	2498
Tetrahydrofuran	**127**	2056
Tetrahydrofurfurylamine	**129**	2943
Tetrahydrophthalic anhydrides	**156**	2698
1,2,3,6-Tetrahydropyridine	**129**	2410
Tetrahydrothiophene	**130**	2412
Tetramethylammonium hydroxide, solid	**153**	3423
Tetramethylammonium hydroxide, solution	**153**	1835
Tetramethylsilane	**130**	2749
Tetranitromethane	**143**	1510
Tetrapropyl orthotitanate	**128**	2413
Textile waste, wet	**133**	1857
Thallium chlorate	**141**	2573
Thallium compound, n.o.s.	**151**	1707
Thallium nitrate	**141**	2727
4-Thiapentanal	**152**	2785
Thickened GD	**153**	—
Thioacetic acid	**129**	2436
Thiocarbamate pesticide, liquid, flammable, poisonous	**131**	2772
Thiocarbamate pesticide, liquid, flammable, toxic	**131**	2772
Thiocarbamate pesticide, liquid, poisonous	**151**	3006
Thiocarbamate pesticide, liquid, poisonous, flammable	**131**	3005
Thiocarbamate pesticide, liquid, toxic	**151**	3006

Name of Material	Guide No.	ID No.
Thiocarbamate pesticide, liquid, toxic, flammable	**131**	3005
Thiocarbamate pesticide, solid, poisonous	**151**	2771
Thiocarbamate pesticide, solid, toxic	**151**	2771
Thioglycol	**153**	2966
Thioglycolic acid	**153**	1940
Thiolactic acid	**153**	2936
Thionyl chloride	**137**	1836
Thiophene	**130**	2414
Thiophosgene	**157**	2474
Thiophosphoryl chloride	**157**	1837
Thiourea dioxide	**135**	3341
Tinctures, medicinal	**127**	1293
Tin tetrachloride	**137**	1827
Titanium disulfide	**135**	3174
Titanium disulphide	**135**	3174
Titanium hydride	**170**	1871
Titanium powder, dry	**135**	2546
Titanium powder, wetted with not less than 25% water	**170**	1352
Titanium sponge granules	**170**	2878
Titanium sponge powders	**170**	2878
Titanium tetrachloride	**137**	1838
Titanium trichloride, pyrophoric	**135**	2441
Titanium trichloride mixture	**157**	2869
Titanium trichloride mixture, pyrophoric	**135**	2441
TNT, wetted with not less than 10% water	**113**	3366
TNT, wetted with not less than 30% water	**113**	1356
Toluene	**130**	1294
2,4-Toluenediamine, solid	**151**	1709

Name of Material	Guide No.	ID No.
2,4-Toluenediamine, solution	**151**	3418
Toluene diisocyanate	**156**	2078
Toluidines, liquid	**153**	1708
Toluidines, solid	**153**	3451
2,4-Toluylenediamine, solid	**151**	1709
2,4-Toluylenediamine, solution	**151**	3418
Toxic by inhalation liquid, corrosive, flammable, n.o.s. (Inhalation Hazard Zone A)	**131**	3492
Toxic by inhalation liquid, corrosive, flammable, n.o.s. (Inhalation Hazard Zone B)	**131**	3493
Toxic by inhalation liquid, corrosive, n.o.s. (Inhalation Hazard Zone A)	**154**	3389
Toxic by inhalation liquid, corrosive, n.o.s. (Inhalation Hazard Zone B)	**154**	3390
Toxic by inhalation liquid, flammable, corrosive, n.o.s. (Inhalation Hazard Zone A)	**131**	3488
Toxic by inhalation liquid, flammable, corrosive, n.o.s. (Inhalation Hazard Zone B)	**131**	3489
Toxic by inhalation liquid, flammable, n.o.s. (Inhalation Hazard Zone A)	**131**	3383
Toxic by inhalation liquid, flammable, n.o.s. (Inhalation Hazard Zone B)	**131**	3384
Toxic by inhalation liquid, n.o.s. (Inhalation Hazard Zone A)	**151**	3381
Toxic by inhalation liquid, n.o.s. (Inhalation Hazard Zone B)	**151**	3382
Toxic by inhalation liquid, oxidizing, n.o.s. (Inhalation Hazard Zone A)	**142**	3387
Toxic by inhalation liquid, oxidizing, n.o.s. (Inhalation Hazard Zone B)	**142**	3388

Name of Material	Guide No.	ID No.
Toxic by inhalation liquid, water-reactive, flammable, n.o.s. (Inhalation Hazard Zone A)	**155**	3490
Toxic by inhalation liquid, water-reactive, flammable, n.o.s. (Inhalation Hazard Zone B)	**155**	3491
Toxic by inhalation liquid, water-reactive, n.o.s. (Inhalation Hazard Zone A)	**139**	3385
Toxic by inhalation liquid, water-reactive, n.o.s. (Inhalation Hazard Zone B)	**139**	3386
Toxic liquid, corrosive, inorganic, n.o.s.	**154**	3289
Toxic liquid, corrosive, organic, n.o.s.	**154**	2927
Toxic liquid, flammable, organic, n.o.s.	**131**	2929
Toxic liquid, inorganic, n.o.s.	**151**	3287
Toxic liquid, organic, n.o.s.	**153**	2810
Toxic liquid, oxidizing, n.o.s.	**142**	3122
Toxic liquid, water-reactive, n.o.s.	**139**	3123
Toxic solid, corrosive, inorganic, n.o.s.	**154**	3290
Toxic solid, corrosive, organic, n.o.s.	**154**	2928
Toxic solid, flammable, inorganic, n.o.s.	**134**	3535
Toxic solid, flammable, organic, n.o.s.	**134**	2930
Toxic solid, inorganic, n.o.s.	**151**	3288
Toxic solid, organic, n.o.s.	**154**	2811
Toxic solid, oxidizing, n.o.s.	**141**	3086
Toxic solid, self-heating, n.o.s.	**136**	3124
Toxic solid, water-reactive, n.o.s.	**139**	3125

Name of Material	Guide No.	ID No.
Toxins	**153**	——
Toxins, extracted from living sources, liquid, n.o.s.	**153**	3172
Toxins, extracted from living sources, solid, n.o.s.	**153**	3462
Triallylamine	**132**	2610
Triallyl borate	**156**	2609
Triazine pesticide, liquid, flammable, poisonous	**131**	2764
Triazine pesticide, liquid, flammable, toxic	**131**	2764
Triazine pesticide, liquid, poisonous	**151**	2998
Triazine pesticide, liquid, poisonous, flammable	**131**	2997
Triazine pesticide, liquid, toxic	**151**	2998
Triazine pesticide, liquid, toxic, flammable	**131**	2997
Triazine pesticide, solid, poisonous	**151**	2763
Triazine pesticide, solid, toxic	**151**	2763
Tributylamine	**153**	2542
Tributylphosphane	**135**	3254
Trichloroacetic acid	**153**	1839
Trichloroacetic acid, solution	**153**	2564
Trichloroacetyl chloride	**156**	2442
Trichlorobenzenes, liquid	**153**	2321
Trichlorobutene	**152**	2322
1,1,1-Trichloroethane	**160**	2831
Trichloroethylene	**160**	1710
Trichloroisocyanuric acid, dry	**140**	2468
Trichlorosilane	**139**	1295
Tricresyl phosphate	**151**	2574
Triethylamine	**132**	1296
Triethylenetetramine	**153**	2259

Name of Material	Guide No.	ID No.
Triethyl phosphite	**130**	2323
Trifluoroacetic acid	**154**	2699
Trifluoroacetyl chloride	**125**	3057
Trifluorochloroethylene, stabilized	**119P**	1082
1,1,1-Trifluoroethane	**115**	2035
Trifluoromethane	**126**	1984
Trifluoromethane, refrigerated liquid	**120**	3136
Trifluoromethane and Chlorotrifluoromethane azeotropic mixture with approximately 60% Chlorotrifluoromethane	**126**	2599
2-Trifluoromethylaniline	**153**	2942
3-Trifluoromethylaniline	**153**	2948
Triisobutylene	**128**	2324
Triisopropyl borate	**129**	2616
Trimethoxysilane	**132**	9269
Trimethylacetyl chloride	**131**	2438
Trimethylamine, anhydrous	**118**	1083
Trimethylamine, aqueous solution	**132**	1297
1,3,5-Trimethylbenzene	**129**	2325
Trimethyl borate	**129**	2416
Trimethylchlorosilane	**155**	1298
Trimethylcyclohexylamine	**153**	2326
Trimethylhexamethylenediamines	**153**	2327
Trimethylhexamethylene diisocyanate	**156**	2328
Trimethyl phosphite	**130**	2329
Trinitrobenzene, wetted with not less than 10% water	**113**	3367
Trinitrobenzene, wetted with not less than 30% water	**113**	1354
Trinitrobenzoic acid, wetted with not less than 10% water	**113**	3368
Trinitrobenzoic acid, wetted with not less than 30% water	**113**	1355
Trinitrochlorobenzene, wetted with not less than 10% water	**113**	3365
Trinitrophenol, wetted with not less than 10% water	**113**	3364
Trinitrophenol, wetted with not less than 30% water	**113**	1344
Trinitrotoluene, wetted with not less than 10% water	**113**	3366
Trinitrotoluene, wetted with not less than 30% water	**113**	1356
Tripropylamine	**132**	2260
Tripropylene	**128**	2057
Tris-(1-aziridinyl)phosphine oxide, solution	**152**	2501
Tungsten hexafluoride	**125**	2196
Turpentine	**128**	1299
Turpentine substitute	**128**	1300
Undecane	**128**	2330
Uranium hexafluoride, radioactive material, excepted package, less than 0.1 kg per package, non-fissile or fissile-excepted	**166**	3507
Uranium hexafluoride, radioactive material, fissile	**166**	2977
Uranium hexafluoride, radioactive material, non fissile or fissile-excepted	**166**	2978
Urea hydrogen peroxide	**140**	1511
Urea nitrate, wetted with not less than 10% water	**113**	3370
Urea nitrate, wetted with not less than 20% water	**113**	1357
Valeraldehyde	**129**	2058
Valeryl chloride	**132**	2502

Name of Material	Guide No.	ID No.
Vanadium compound, n.o.s.	**151**	3285
Vanadium oxytrichloride	**137**	2443
Vanadium pentoxide	**151**	2862
Vanadium tetrachloride	**137**	2444
Vanadium trichloride	**157**	2475
Vanadyl sulfate	**151**	2931
Vanadyl sulphate	**151**	2931
Vehicle, flammable gas powered	**115**	3166
Vehicle, flammable liquid powered	**128**	3166
Vehicle, fuel cell, flammable gas powered	**115**	3166
Vehicle, fuel cell, flammable liquid powered	**128**	3166
Vinyl acetate, stabilized	**129P**	1301
Vinyl bromide, stabilized	**116P**	1085
Vinyl butyrate, stabilized	**129P**	2838
Vinyl chloride, stabilized	**116P**	1086
Vinyl chloroacetate	**155**	2589
Vinyl ethyl ether, stabilized	**127P**	1302
Vinyl fluoride, stabilized	**116P**	1860
Vinylidene chloride, stabilized	**130P**	1303
Vinyl isobutyl ether, stabilized	**127P**	1304
Vinyl methyl ether, stabilized	**116P**	1087
Vinylpyridines, stabilized	**131P**	3073
Vinyltoluenes, stabilized	**130P**	2618
Vinyltrichlorosilane	**155P**	1305
Vinyltrichlorosilane, stabilized	**155P**	1305
VX	**153**	—
Water-reactive liquid, corrosive, n.o.s.	**138**	3129
Water-reactive liquid, n.o.s.	**138**	3148

Name of Material	Guide No.	ID No.
Water-reactive liquid, poisonous, n.o.s.	**139**	3130
Water-reactive liquid, toxic, n.o.s.	**139**	3130
Water-reactive solid, corrosive, n.o.s.	**138**	3131
Water-reactive solid, flammable, n.o.s.	**138**	3132
Water-reactive solid, n.o.s.	**138**	2813
Water-reactive solid, oxidizing, n.o.s.	**138**	3133
Water-reactive solid, poisonous, n.o.s.	**139**	3134
Water-reactive solid, self-heating, n.o.s.	**138**	3135
Water-reactive solid, toxic, n.o.s.	**139**	3134
Wheelchair, electric, with batteries	**154**	3171
White asbestos	**171**	2590
White phosphorus, dry or under water or in solution	**136**	1381
White phosphorus, molten	**136**	2447
Wood preservatives, liquid	**129**	1306
Wool waste, wet	**133**	1387
Xanthates	**135**	3342
Xenon	**120**	2036
Xenon, compressed	**120**	2036
Xenon, refrigerated liquid (cryogenic liquid)	**120**	2591
Xylenes	**130**	1307
Xylenols, liquid	**153**	3430
Xylenols, solid	**153**	2261
Xylidines, liquid	**153**	1711
Xylidines, solid	**153**	3452
Xylyl bromide, liquid	**152**	1701

Name of Material	Guide No.	ID No.
Xylyl bromide, solid	**152**	3417
Yellow phosphorus, dry or under water or in solution	**136**	1381
Zinc ammonium nitrite	**140**	1512
Zinc arsenate	**151**	1712
Zinc arsenate and Zinc arsenite mixture	**151**	1712
Zinc arsenite	**151**	1712
Zinc arsenite and Zinc arsenate mixture	**151**	1712
Zinc ashes	**138**	1435
Zinc bromate	**140**	2469
Zinc chlorate	**140**	1513
Zinc chloride, anhydrous	**154**	2331
Zinc chloride, solution	**154**	1840
Zinc cyanide	**151**	1713
Zinc dithionite	**171**	1931
Zinc dross	**138**	1435
Zinc dust	**138**	1436
Zinc fluorosilicate	**151**	2855
Zinc hydrosulfite	**171**	1931
Zinc hydrosulphite	**171**	1931
Zinc nitrate	**140**	1514
Zinc permanganate	**140**	1515
Zinc peroxide	**143**	1516
Zinc phosphide	**139**	1714
Zinc powder	**138**	1436
Zinc residue	**138**	1435
Zinc resinate	**133**	2714
Zinc silicofluoride	**151**	2855
Zinc skimmings	**138**	1435
Zirconium, dry, coiled wire, finished metal sheets or strip	**170**	2858

Name of Material	Guide No.	ID No.
Zirconium, dry, finished sheets, strips or coiled wire	**135**	2009
Zirconium hydride	**138**	1437
Zirconium nitrate	**140**	2728
Zirconium picramate, wetted with not less than 20% water	**113**	1517
Zirconium powder, dry	**135**	2008
Zirconium powder, wetted with not less than 25% water	**170**	1358
Zirconium scrap	**135**	1932
Zirconium suspended in a flammable liquid	**170**	1308
Zirconium suspended in a liquid (flammable)	**170**	1308
Zirconium tetrachloride	**137**	2503

NOTES

SUGGESTED OPERATIONS SHOULD ONLY BE PERFORMED BY ADEQUATELY TRAINED AND EQUIPPED PERSONNEL

HOW TO USE THE ORANGE GUIDES

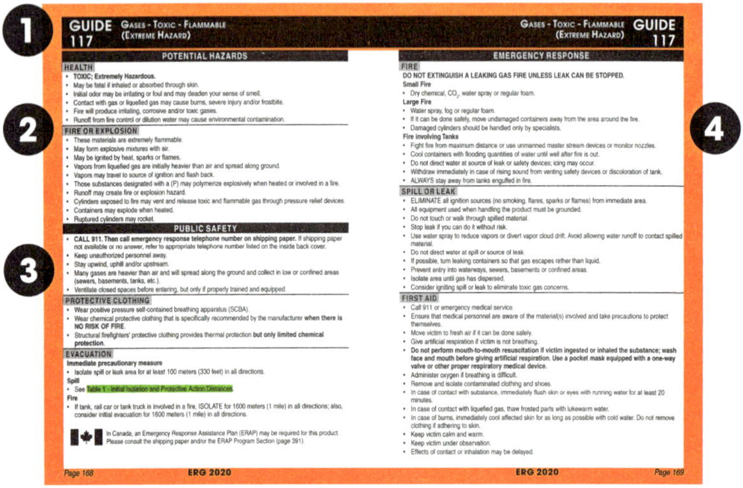

1

2

3

4

GUIDE 117 GASES - TOXIC - FLAMMABLE (EXTREME HAZARD)

POTENTIAL HAZARDS

HEALTH

- **TOXIC; Extremely Hazardous.**
- May be fatal if inhaled or absorbed through skin.
- Initial odor may be irritating or foul and may deaden your sense of smell.
- Contact with gas or liquefied gas may cause burns, severe injury and/or frostbite.
- Fire will produce irritating, corrosive and/or toxic gases.
- Runoff from fire control or dilution water may cause environmental contamination.

FIRE OR EXPLOSION

- These materials are extremely flammable.
- May form explosive mixtures with air.
- May be ignited by heat, sparks or flames.
- Vapors from liquefied gas are initially heavier than air and spread along ground.
- Vapors may travel to source of ignition and flash back.
- Those substances designated with a (P) may polymerize explosively when heated or involved in a fire.
- Runoff may create fire or explosion hazard.
- Cylinders exposed to fire may vent and release toxic and flammable gas through pressure relief devices.
- Containers may explode when heated.
- Ruptured cylinders may rocket.

PUBLIC SAFETY

- **CALL 911. Then call emergency response telephone number on shipping paper.** If shipping paper not available or no answer, refer to appropriate telephone number listed on the inside back cover.
- Keep unauthorized personnel away.
- Stay upwind, uphill and/or upstream.
- Many gases are heavier than air and will spread along the ground and collect in low or confined areas (sewers, basements, tanks, etc.).
- Ventilate closed spaces before entering, but only if properly trained and equipped.

PROTECTIVE CLOTHING

- Wear positive pressure self-contained breathing apparatus (SCBA).
- Wear chemical protective clothing that is specifically recommended by the manufacturer **when there is NO RISK OF FIRE.**
- Structural firefighters' protective clothing provides thermal protection **but only limited chemical protection.**

EVACUATION

Immediate precautionary measure

- Isolate spill or leak area for at least 100 meters (330 feet) in all directions.

Spill

- See Table 1 - Initial Isolation and Protective Action Distances.

Fire

- If tank, rail car or tank truck is involved in a fire, ISOLATE for 1600 meters (1 mile) in all directions; also, consider initial evacuation for 1600 meters (1 mile) in all directions.

In Canada, an Emergency Response Assistance Plan (ERAP) may be required for this product. Please consult the shipping paper and/or the ERAP Program Section (page 391).

Page 168 ERG 2020

GASES - TOXIC - FLAMMABLE (EXTREME HAZARD) **GUIDE 117**

EMERGENCY RESPONSE

FIRE

DO NOT EXTINGUISH A LEAKING GAS FIRE UNLESS LEAK CAN BE STOPPED.

Small Fire

- Dry chemical, CO_2, water spray or regular foam.

Large Fire

- Water spray, fog or regular foam.
- If it can be done safely, move undamaged containers away from the area around the fire.
- Damaged cylinders should be handled only by specialists.

Fire involving Tanks

- Fight fire from maximum distance or use unmanned master stream devices or monitor nozzles.
- Cool containers with flooding quantities of water until well after fire is out.
- Do not direct water at source of leak or safety devices; icing may occur.
- Withdraw immediately in case of rising sound from venting safety devices or discoloration of tank.
- ALWAYS stay away from tanks engulfed in fire.

SPILL OR LEAK

- ELIMINATE all ignition sources (no smoking, flares, sparks or flames) from immediate area.
- All equipment used when handling the product must be grounded.
- Do not touch or walk through spilled material.
- Stop leak if you can do it without risk.
- Use water spray to reduce vapors or divert vapor cloud drift. Avoid allowing water runoff to contact spilled material.
- Do not direct water at spill or source of leak.
- If possible, turn leaking containers so that gas escapes rather than liquid.
- Prevent entry into waterways, sewers, basements or confined areas.
- Isolate area until gas has dispersed.
- Consider igniting spill or leak to eliminate toxic gas concerns.

FIRST AID

- Call 911 or emergency medical service.
- Ensure that medical personnel are aware of the material(s) involved and take precautions to protect themselves.
- Move victim to fresh air if it can be done safely.
- Give artificial respiration if victim is not breathing.
- **Do not perform mouth-to-mouth resuscitation if victim ingested or inhaled the substance; wash face and mouth before giving artificial respiration. Use a pocket mask equipped with a one-way valve or other proper respiratory medical device.**
- Administer oxygen if breathing is difficult.
- Remove and isolate contaminated clothing and shoes.
- In case of contact with substance, immediately flush skin or eyes with running water for at least 20 minutes.
- In case of contact with liquefied gas, thaw frosted parts with lukewarm water.
- In case of burns, immediately cool affected skin for as long as possible with cold water. Do not remove clothing if adhering to skin.
- Keep victim calm and warm.
- Keep victim under observation.
- Effects of contact or inhalation may be delayed.

ERG 2020 Page 169

1 GUIDE NUMBER AND TITLE

- The guide title identifies the general hazards associated with the materials in this Guide.

2 POTENTIAL HAZARDS

- Emergency responders should consult this section first!
- Describes the material hazard in terms of **FIRE OR EXPLOSION** and **HEALTH** effects upon exposure.
- The primary potential hazard is listed first.
- Allows the responders to make decisions to protect the emergency response team, and the surrounding population.

3 PUBLIC SAFETY

- This section is divided into three subsections:
  - **General Information:** describes initial precautionary measures to be taken by those first on the scene.
  - **PROTECTIVE CLOTHING:** provides general guidance on personal protective equipment requirements including respiratory protection. The protective clothing information is general and correct selection is situation dependent, after considering the physical and chemical properties of the material, weather conditions, spill versus fire, topography, etc.
  - **EVACUATION:** suggests protective distances for immediate precautionary measures defined for small and large spills, including suggested guidance for conditions where fire is present or likely (potential fragmentation hazard).
    - The term "isolate" indicates a zone of no entry that applies to the public and first responders who are not equipped, trained, and prepared to mitigate the incident.
    - The term "evacuate" indicates people should be removed from inside this zone, if it can be done safely. If removal is too risky, sheltering-in-place can also be considered in this zone. Evacuation aims to protect as many people as possible, and applies mainly to the public.
- Materials highlighted in green in the yellow-bordered and blue-bordered pages direct the reader to consult Table 1, detailing specific response distances for toxic inhalation hazard materials, water-reactive materials and chemical warfare agents (green-bordered pages).

  If a Canadian flag appears in this section, and the incident is located in Canada, an Emergency Response Assistance Plan (ERAP) may be required for this product.

4 EMERGENCY RESPONSE

- This section is divided into three subsections:
  - **FIRE:** provides extinguishing procedures for **Small Fire**, **Large Fire**, and/or **Fire Involving Tanks or Car/Trailer Loads**
  - **SPILL OR LEAK:** includes general recommendations, and may describe the response procedure for **Small Spill** and **Large Spill**
  - **FIRST AID:** provides general guidance prior to seeking expert medical care.

GUIDE 111 MIXED LOAD/UNIDENTIFIED CARGO

POTENTIAL HAZARDS

FIRE OR EXPLOSION

- May explode from heat, shock, friction or contamination.
- May react violently or explosively on contact with air, water or foam.
- May be ignited by heat, sparks or flames.
- Vapors may travel to source of ignition and flash back.
- Containers may explode when heated.
- Ruptured cylinders may rocket.

HEALTH

- Inhalation, ingestion or contact with substance may cause severe injury, infection, disease or death.
- High concentration of gas may cause asphyxiation without warning.
- Contact may cause burns to skin and eyes.
- Fire or contact with water may produce irritating, toxic and/or corrosive gases.
- Runoff from fire control or dilution water may cause environmental contamination.

PUBLIC SAFETY

- **CALL 911. Then call emergency response telephone number on shipping paper**. If shipping paper not available or no answer, refer to appropriate telephone number listed on the inside back cover.
- Keep unauthorized personnel away.
- Stay upwind, uphill and/or upstream.

PROTECTIVE CLOTHING

- Wear positive pressure self-contained breathing apparatus (SCBA).
- Structural firefighters' protective clothing provides thermal protection **but only limited chemical protection**.

EVACUATION

Immediate precautionary measure

- Isolate spill or leak area for at least 100 meters (330 feet) in all directions.

Fire

- If tank, rail car or tank truck is involved in a fire, ISOLATE for 800 meters (1/2 mile) in all directions; also, consider initial evacuation for 800 meters (1/2 mile) in all directions.

EMERGENCY RESPONSE

FIRE

CAUTION: Material may react with extinguishing agent.

Small Fire

- Dry chemical, CO_2, water spray or regular foam.

Large Fire

- Water spray, fog or regular foam.
- If it can be done safely, move undamaged containers away from the area around the fire.

Fire Involving Tanks

- Cool containers with flooding quantities of water until well after fire is out.
- Do not get water inside containers.
- Withdraw immediately in case of rising sound from venting safety devices or discoloration of tank.
- ALWAYS stay away from tanks engulfed in fire.

SPILL OR LEAK

- Do not touch or walk through spilled material.
- ELIMINATE all ignition sources (no smoking, flares, sparks or flames) from immediate area.
- All equipment used when handling the product must be grounded.
- Keep combustibles (wood, paper, oil, etc.) away from spilled material.
- Use water spray to reduce vapors or divert vapor cloud drift. Avoid allowing water runoff to contact spilled material.
- Prevent entry into waterways, sewers, basements or confined areas.

Small Spill

- Pick up with sand or other non-combustible absorbent material and place into containers for later disposal.

Large Spill

- Dike far ahead of liquid spill for later disposal.

FIRST AID

- Call 911 or emergency medical service.
- Ensure that medical personnel are aware of the material(s) involved and take precautions to protect themselves.
- Move victim to fresh air if it can be done safely.
- Give artificial respiration if victim is not breathing.
- **Do not perform mouth-to-mouth resuscitation if victim ingested or inhaled the substance; wash face and mouth before giving artificial respiration. Use a pocket mask equipped with a one-way valve or other proper respiratory medical device.**
- Administer oxygen if breathing is difficult.
- Remove and isolate contaminated clothing and shoes.
- In case of contact with substance, immediately flush skin or eyes with running water for at least 20 minutes.
- Shower and wash with soap and water.
- Keep victim calm and warm.
- Effects of exposure (inhalation, ingestion or skin contact) to substance may be delayed.

GUIDE 112 EXPLOSIVES* - DIVISION 1.1, 1.2, 1.3 OR 1.5

POTENTIAL HAZARDS

FIRE OR EXPLOSION

- **MAY EXPLODE AND THROW FRAGMENTS 1600 METERS (1 MILE) OR MORE IF FIRE REACHES CARGO.**
- **For information on "Compatibility Group" letters, refer to Glossary section.**

HEALTH

- Fire may produce irritating, corrosive and/or toxic gases.

PUBLIC SAFETY

- **CALL 911. Then call emergency response telephone number on shipping paper.** If shipping paper not available or no answer, refer to appropriate telephone number listed on the inside back cover.
- Move people out of line of sight of the scene and away from windows.
- Keep unauthorized personnel away.
- Stay upwind, uphill and/or upstream.
- Ventilate closed spaces before entering, but only if properly trained and equipped.

PROTECTIVE CLOTHING

- Wear positive pressure self-contained breathing apparatus (SCBA).
- Structural firefighters' protective clothing provides thermal protection **but only limited chemical protection.**

EVACUATION

Immediate precautionary measure

- Isolate spill or leak area immediately for at least 500 meters (1/3 mile) in all directions.

Large Spill

- **Consider initial evacuation for 800 meters (1/2 mile) in all directions.**

Fire

- If rail car or trailer is involved in a fire, ISOLATE for 1600 meters (1 mile) in all directions; also, initiate evacuation including emergency responders for 1600 meters (1 mile) in all directions.

In Canada, an Emergency Response Assistance Plan (ERAP) may be required for this product. Please consult the shipping paper and/or the ERAP Program Section (page 390).

*** FOR INFORMATION ON "COMPATIBILITY GROUP" LETTERS, REFER TO THE GLOSSARY SECTION.**

EMERGENCY RESPONSE

FIRE

CARGO Fire

- **DO NOT fight fire when fire reaches cargo! Cargo may EXPLODE!**
- Stop all traffic and clear the area for at least 1600 meters (1 mile) in all directions and let burn.
- **Do not move cargo or vehicle if cargo has been exposed to heat.**

TIRE or VEHICLE Fire

- **Use plenty of water - FLOOD it! If water is not available, use CO_2, dry chemical or dirt.**
- If possible, and WITHOUT RISK, use unmanned master stream devices or monitor nozzles from maximum distance to prevent fire from spreading to cargo area.
- Pay special attention to tire fires as re-ignition may occur. Stand by, at a safe distance, with extinguisher ready for possible re-ignition.

SPILL OR LEAK

- ELIMINATE all ignition sources (no smoking, flares, sparks or flames) from immediate area.
- All equipment used when handling the product must be grounded.
- Do not touch or walk through spilled material.
- DO NOT OPERATE RADIO TRANSMITTERS WITHIN 100 METERS (330 FEET) OF ELECTRIC DETONATORS.
- **DO NOT CLEAN-UP OR DISPOSE OF, EXCEPT UNDER SUPERVISION OF A SPECIALIST.**

FIRST AID

- Call 911 or emergency medical service.
- Ensure that medical personnel are aware of the material(s) involved and take precautions to protect themselves.
- Move victim to fresh air if it can be done safely.
- Give artificial respiration if victim is not breathing.
- Administer oxygen if breathing is difficult.
- Remove and isolate contaminated clothing and shoes.
- In case of contact with substance, immediately flush skin or eyes with running water for at least 20 minutes.

*** FOR INFORMATION ON "COMPATIBILITY GROUP" LETTERS, REFER TO THE GLOSSARY SECTION.**

GUIDE 113 FLAMMABLE MATERIALS (WET/DESENSITIZED EXPLOSIVE)

POTENTIAL HAZARDS

FIRE OR EXPLOSION

- Flammable/combustible material.
- May be ignited by heat, sparks or flames.
- **DRIED OUT material may explode if exposed to heat, flame, friction or shock; treat as an explosive (GUIDE 112).**
- **Keep material wet with water or treat as an explosive (GUIDE 112).**
- Runoff to sewer may create fire or explosion hazard.

HEALTH

- **Some are toxic** and may be fatal if inhaled, ingested or absorbed through skin. Specifically, Dinitrophenol, wetted (UN1320); Dinitrophenolates, wetted (UN1321), Sodium dinitro-o-cresolate, wetted (UN1348); and Barium azide, wetted (UN1571) are known to be toxic.
- Contact may cause burns to skin and eyes.
- Fire may produce irritating, corrosive and/or toxic gases.
- Runoff from fire control or dilution water may cause environmental contamination.

PUBLIC SAFETY

- **CALL 911. Then call emergency response telephone number on shipping paper.** If shipping paper not available or no answer, refer to appropriate telephone number listed on the inside back cover.
- Keep unauthorized personnel away.
- Stay upwind, uphill and/or upstream.
- Ventilate closed spaces before entering, but only if properly trained and equipped.

PROTECTIVE CLOTHING

- Wear positive pressure self-contained breathing apparatus (SCBA).
- Structural firefighters' protective clothing provides thermal protection **but only limited chemical protection**.

EVACUATION

Immediate precautionary measure

- Isolate spill or leak area immediately for at least 100 meters (330 feet) in all directions.

Large Spill

- **Consider initial evacuation for 500 meters (1/3 mile) in all directions.**

Fire

- If tank, rail car or tank truck is involved in a fire, ISOLATE for 800 meters (1/2 mile) in all directions; also, consider initial evacuation for 800 meters (1/2 mile) in all directions.

In Canada, an Emergency Response Assistance Plan (ERAP) may be required for this product. Please consult the shipping paper and/or the ERAP Program Section (page 390).

EMERGENCY RESPONSE

FIRE

CARGO Fire

- **DO NOT fight fire when fire reaches cargo! Cargo may EXPLODE!**
- Stop all traffic and clear the area for at least 1600 meters (1 mile) in all directions and let burn.
- **Do not move cargo or vehicle if cargo has been exposed to heat.**

TIRE or VEHICLE Fire

- **Use plenty of water - FLOOD it! If water is not available, use CO_2, dry chemical or dirt.**
- If possible, and WITHOUT RISK, use unmanned master stream devices or monitor nozzles from maximum distance to prevent fire from spreading to cargo area.
- Pay special attention to tire fires as re-ignition may occur. Stand by, at a safe distance, with extinguisher ready for possible re-ignition.

SPILL OR LEAK

- ELIMINATE all ignition sources (no smoking, flares, sparks or flames) from immediate area.
- All equipment used when handling the product must be grounded.
- Do not touch or walk through spilled material.

Small Spill

- Flush area with large amounts of water.

Large Spill

- Wet down with water and dike for later disposal.
- KEEP "WETTED" PRODUCT WET BY SLOWLY ADDING FLOODING QUANTITIES OF WATER.

FIRST AID

- Call 911 or emergency medical service.
- Ensure that medical personnel are aware of the material(s) involved and take precautions to protect themselves.
- Move victim to fresh air if it can be done safely.
- Give artificial respiration if victim is not breathing.
- Administer oxygen if breathing is difficult.
- Remove and isolate contaminated clothing and shoes.
- In case of contact with substance, immediately flush skin or eyes with running water for at least 20 minutes.

GUIDE 114 EXPLOSIVES* - DIVISION 1.4 OR 1.6

POTENTIAL HAZARDS

FIRE OR EXPLOSION

- **MAY EXPLODE AND THROW FRAGMENTS 800 METERS (1/2 MILE) OR MORE IF FIRE REACHES CARGO.**
- **For information on "Compatibility Group" letters, refer to Glossary section.**

HEALTH

- Fire may produce irritating, corrosive and/or toxic gases.

PUBLIC SAFETY

- **CALL 911. Then call emergency response telephone number on shipping paper.** If shipping paper not available or no answer, refer to appropriate telephone number listed on the inside back cover.
- Move people out of line of sight of the scene and away from windows.
- Keep unauthorized personnel away.
- Stay upwind, uphill and/or upstream.
- Ventilate closed spaces before entering, but only if properly trained and equipped.

PROTECTIVE CLOTHING

- Wear positive pressure self-contained breathing apparatus (SCBA).
- Structural firefighters' protective clothing provides thermal protection **but only limited chemical protection.**

EVACUATION

Immediate precautionary measure

- Isolate spill or leak area immediately for at least 100 meters (330 feet) in all directions.

Large Spill

- **Consider initial evacuation for 250 meters (800 feet) in all directions.**

Fire

- If rail car or trailer is involved in a fire, ISOLATE for 800 meters (1/2 mile) in all directions; also initiate evacuation including emergency responders for 800 meters (1/2 mile) in all directions.
- If fire threatens cargo area containing packages bearing the 1.4S label or packages containing material classified as 1.4S, consider isolating at least 15 meters (50 feet) in all directions.

In Canada, an Emergency Response Assistance Plan (ERAP) may be required for this product. Please consult the shipping paper and/or the ERAP Program Section (page 390).

* FOR INFORMATION ON "COMPATIBILITY GROUP" LETTERS, REFER TO THE GLOSSARY SECTION.

EMERGENCY RESPONSE

FIRE

CARGO Fire

- **DO NOT fight fire when fire reaches cargo! Cargo may EXPLODE!**
- Stop all traffic and clear the area for at least 800 meters (1/2 mile) in all directions and let burn.
- **Do not move cargo or vehicle if cargo has been exposed to heat.**

TIRE or VEHICLE Fire

- **Use plenty of water - FLOOD it! If water is not available, use CO_2, dry chemical or dirt.**
- If possible, and WITHOUT RISK, use unmanned master stream devices or monitor nozzles from maximum distance to prevent fire from spreading to cargo area.
- Pay special attention to tire fires as re-ignition may occur. Stand by, at a safe distance, with extinguisher ready for possible re-ignition.

CLASS 1.4S Fire

- Packages bearing the 1.4S label or packages containing material classified as 1.4S are designed or packaged in such a manner that when involved in a fire, they may burn vigorously with localized detonations and projection of fragments.
- Effects are usually confined to immediate vicinity of packages.
- Fight fire with normal precautions from a reasonable distance.

SPILL OR LEAK

- ELIMINATE all ignition sources (no smoking, flares, sparks or flames) from immediate area.
- All equipment used when handling the product must be grounded.
- Do not touch or walk through spilled material.
- DO NOT OPERATE RADIO TRANSMITTERS WITHIN 100 METERS (330 FEET) OF ELECTRIC DETONATORS.
- **DO NOT CLEAN-UP OR DISPOSE OF, EXCEPT UNDER SUPERVISION OF A SPECIALIST.**

FIRST AID

- Call 911 or emergency medical service.
- Ensure that medical personnel are aware of the material(s) involved and take precautions to protect themselves.
- Move victim to fresh air if it can be done safely.
- Give artificial respiration if victim is not breathing.
- Administer oxygen if breathing is difficult.
- Remove and isolate contaminated clothing and shoes.
- In case of contact with substance, immediately flush skin or eyes with running water for at least 20 minutes.

*** FOR INFORMATION ON "COMPATIBILITY GROUP" LETTERS, REFER TO THE GLOSSARY SECTION.**

GUIDE 115 GASES - FLAMMABLE (INCLUDING REFRIGERATED LIQUIDS)

POTENTIAL HAZARDS

FIRE OR EXPLOSION

- **EXTREMELY FLAMMABLE.**
- Will be easily ignited by heat, sparks or flames.
- Will form explosive mixtures with air.
- Vapors from liquefied gas are initially heavier than air and spread along ground.

CAUTION: Hydrogen (UN1049), Deuterium (UN1957), Hydrogen, refrigerated liquid (UN1966), Methane (UN1971) and Hydrogen and Methane mixture, compressed (UN2034) are lighter than air and will rise. Hydrogen and Deuterium fires are difficult to detect since they burn with an invisible flame. Use an alternate method of detection (thermal camera, broom handle, etc.)

- Vapors may travel to source of ignition and flash back.
- Cylinders exposed to fire may vent and release flammable gas through pressure relief devices.
- Containers may explode when heated.
- Ruptured cylinders may rocket.

HEALTH

- Vapors may cause dizziness or asphyxiation without warning.
- Some may be irritating if inhaled at high concentrations.
- Contact with gas or liquefied gas may cause burns, severe injury and/or frostbite.
- Fire may produce irritating and/or toxic gases.

PUBLIC SAFETY

- **CALL 911. Then call emergency response telephone number on shipping paper.** If shipping paper not available or no answer, refer to appropriate telephone number listed on the inside back cover.
- Keep unauthorized personnel away.
- Stay upwind, uphill and/or upstream.
- Many gases are heavier than air and will spread along the ground and collect in low or confined areas (sewers, basements, tanks, etc.).

PROTECTIVE CLOTHING

- Wear positive pressure self-contained breathing apparatus (SCBA).
- Structural firefighters' protective clothing provides thermal protection **but only limited chemical protection**.
- Always wear thermal protective clothing when handling refrigerated/cryogenic liquids.

EVACUATION

Immediate precautionary measure

- Isolate spill or leak area for at least 100 meters (330 feet) in all directions.

Large Spill

- Consider initial downwind evacuation for at least 800 meters (1/2 mile).

Fire

- If tank, rail car or tank truck is involved in a fire, ISOLATE for 1600 meters (1 mile) in all directions; also, consider initial evacuation for 1600 meters (1 mile) in all directions.
- In fires involving Liquefied Petroleum Gases (LPG) (UN1075), Butane (UN1011), Butylene (UN1012), Isobutylene (UN1055), Propylene (UN1077), Isobutane (UN1969), and Propane (UN1978), also refer to BLEVE – SAFETY PRECAUTIONS (Page 366).

In Canada, an Emergency Response Assistance Plan (ERAP) may be required for this product. Please consult the shipping paper and/or the ERAP Program Section (page 390).

EMERGENCY RESPONSE

FIRE

- **DO NOT EXTINGUISH A LEAKING GAS FIRE UNLESS LEAK CAN BE STOPPED.**

CAUTION: Hydrogen (UN1049), Deuterium (UN1957), Hydrogen, refrigerated liquid (UN1966) and Hydrogen and Methane mixture, compressed (UN2034) will burn with an invisible flame. Use an alternate method of detection (thermal camera, broom handle, etc.)

Small Fire

- Dry chemical or CO_2.

Large Fire

- Water spray or fog.
- If it can be done safely, move undamaged containers away from the area around the fire.

CAUTION: For **LNG - Liquefied natural gas (UN1972)** pool fires, DO NOT USE water. Use dry chemical or high-expansion foam.

Fire Involving Tanks

- Fight fire from maximum distance or use unmanned master stream devices or monitor nozzles.
- Cool containers with flooding quantities of water until well after fire is out.
- Do not direct water at source of leak or safety devices; icing may occur.
- Withdraw immediately in case of rising sound from venting safety devices or discoloration of tank.
- ALWAYS stay away from tanks engulfed in fire.
- For massive fire, use unmanned master stream devices or monitor nozzles; if this is impossible, withdraw from area and let fire burn.

SPILL OR LEAK

- ELIMINATE all ignition sources (no smoking, flares, sparks or flames) from immediate area.
- All equipment used when handling the product must be grounded.
- Do not touch or walk through spilled material.
- Stop leak if you can do it without risk.
- If possible, turn leaking containers so that gas escapes rather than liquid.
- Use water spray to reduce vapors or divert vapor cloud drift. Avoid allowing water runoff to contact spilled material.
- Do not direct water at spill or source of leak.

CAUTION: For **LNG - Liquefied natural gas (UN1972)**, DO NOT apply water, regular or alcohol-resistant foam directly on spill. Use a high-expansion foam if available to reduce vapors.

- Prevent spreading of vapors through sewers, ventilation systems and confined areas.
- Isolate area until gas has dispersed.

CAUTION: When in contact with refrigerated/cryogenic liquids, many materials become brittle and are likely to break without warning.

FIRST AID

- Call 911 or emergency medical service.
- Ensure that medical personnel are aware of the material(s) involved and take precautions to protect themselves.
- Move victim to fresh air if it can be done safely.
- Give artificial respiration if victim is not breathing.
- Administer oxygen if breathing is difficult.
- Remove and isolate contaminated clothing and shoes.
- Clothing frozen to the skin should be thawed before being removed.
- In case of contact with liquefied gas, thaw frosted parts with lukewarm water.
- In case of burns, immediately cool affected skin for as long as possible with cold water. Do not remove clothing if adhering to skin.
- Keep victim calm and warm.

GUIDE 116 GASES - FLAMMABLE (UNSTABLE)

POTENTIAL HAZARDS

FIRE OR EXPLOSION

- **EXTREMELY FLAMMABLE.**
- Will be easily ignited by heat, sparks or flames.
- Will form explosive mixtures with air. Acetylene (UN1001, UN3374) may react explosively even in the absence of air.
- Silane (UN2203) will ignite spontaneously in air.
- Those substances designated with a **(P)** may polymerize explosively when heated or involved in a fire.
- Vapors from liquefied gas are initially heavier than air and spread along ground.
- Vapors may travel to source of ignition and flash back.
- Cylinders exposed to fire may vent and release flammable gas through pressure relief devices.
- Containers may explode when heated.
- Ruptured cylinders may rocket.

HEALTH

- Vapors may cause dizziness or asphyxiation without warning.
- Some may be toxic if inhaled at high concentrations.
- Contact with gas or liquefied gas may cause burns, severe injury and/or frostbite.
- Fire may produce irritating and/or toxic gases.

PUBLIC SAFETY

- **CALL 911. Then call emergency response telephone number on shipping paper.** If shipping paper not available or no answer, refer to appropriate telephone number listed on the inside back cover.
- Keep unauthorized personnel away.
- Stay upwind, uphill and/or upstream.
- Many gases are heavier than air and will spread along the ground and collect in low or confined areas (sewers, basements, tanks, etc.).

PROTECTIVE CLOTHING

- Wear positive pressure self-contained breathing apparatus (SCBA).
- Structural firefighters' protective clothing provides thermal protection **but only limited chemical protection**.

EVACUATION

Immediate precautionary measure

- Isolate spill or leak area for at least 100 meters (330 feet) in all directions.

Large Spill

- Consider initial downwind evacuation for at least 800 meters (1/2 mile).

Fire

- If tank, rail car or tank truck is involved in a fire, ISOLATE for 1600 meters (1 mile) in all directions; also, consider initial evacuation for 1600 meters (1 mile) in all directions.

In Canada, an Emergency Response Assistance Plan (ERAP) may be required for this product. Please consult the shipping paper and/or the ERAP Program Section (page 390).

EMERGENCY RESPONSE

FIRE

- **DO NOT EXTINGUISH A LEAKING GAS FIRE UNLESS LEAK CAN BE STOPPED.**

Small Fire

- Dry chemical or CO_2.

Large Fire

- Water spray or fog.
- If it can be done safely, move undamaged containers away from the area around the fire.

Fire Involving Tanks

- Fight fire from maximum distance or use unmanned master stream devices or monitor nozzles.
- Cool containers with flooding quantities of water until well after fire is out.
- Do not direct water at source of leak or safety devices; icing may occur.
- Withdraw immediately in case of rising sound from venting safety devices or discoloration of tank.
- ALWAYS stay away from tanks engulfed in fire.
- For massive fire, use unmanned master stream devices or monitor nozzles; if this is impossible, withdraw from area and let fire burn.

SPILL OR LEAK

- ELIMINATE all ignition sources (no smoking, flares, sparks or flames) from immediate area.
- All equipment used when handling the product must be grounded.
- Stop leak if you can do it without risk.
- Do not touch or walk through spilled material.
- Do not direct water at spill or source of leak.
- Use water spray to reduce vapors or divert vapor cloud drift. Avoid allowing water runoff to contact spilled material.
- If possible, turn leaking containers so that gas escapes rather than liquid.
- Prevent entry into waterways, sewers, basements or confined areas.
- Isolate area until gas has dispersed.

FIRST AID

- Call 911 or emergency medical service.
- Ensure that medical personnel are aware of the material(s) involved and take precautions to protect themselves.
- Move victim to fresh air if it can be done safely.
- Give artificial respiration if victim is not breathing.
- Administer oxygen if breathing is difficult.
- Remove and isolate contaminated clothing and shoes.
- In case of contact with liquefied gas, thaw frosted parts with lukewarm water.
- In case of burns, immediately cool affected skin for as long as possible with cold water. Do not remove clothing if adhering to skin.
- Keep victim calm and warm.

GUIDE 117 GASES - TOXIC - FLAMMABLE (EXTREME HAZARD)

POTENTIAL HAZARDS

HEALTH

- **TOXIC; Extremely Hazardous.**
- May be fatal if inhaled or absorbed through skin.
- Initial odor may be irritating or foul and may deaden your sense of smell.
- Contact with gas or liquefied gas may cause burns, severe injury and/or frostbite.
- Fire will produce irritating, corrosive and/or toxic gases.
- Runoff from fire control or dilution water may cause environmental contamination.

FIRE OR EXPLOSION

- These materials are extremely flammable.
- May form explosive mixtures with air.
- May be ignited by heat, sparks or flames.
- Vapors from liquefied gas are initially heavier than air and spread along ground.
- Vapors may travel to source of ignition and flash back.
- Those substances designated with a **(P)** may polymerize explosively when heated or involved in a fire.
- Runoff may create fire or explosion hazard.
- Cylinders exposed to fire may vent and release toxic and flammable gas through pressure relief devices.
- Containers may explode when heated.
- Ruptured cylinders may rocket.

PUBLIC SAFETY

- **CALL 911. Then call emergency response telephone number on shipping paper.** If shipping paper not available or no answer, refer to appropriate telephone number listed on the inside back cover.
- Keep unauthorized personnel away.
- Stay upwind, uphill and/or upstream.
- Many gases are heavier than air and will spread along the ground and collect in low or confined areas (sewers, basements, tanks, etc.).
- Ventilate closed spaces before entering, but only if properly trained and equipped.

PROTECTIVE CLOTHING

- Wear positive pressure self-contained breathing apparatus (SCBA).
- Wear chemical protective clothing that is specifically recommended by the manufacturer **when there is NO RISK OF FIRE**.
- Structural firefighters' protective clothing provides thermal protection **but only limited chemical protection**.

EVACUATION

Immediate precautionary measure

- Isolate spill or leak area for at least 100 meters (330 feet) in all directions.

Spill

- See Table 1 - Initial Isolation and Protective Action Distances.

Fire

- If tank, rail car or tank truck is involved in a fire, ISOLATE for 1600 meters (1 mile) in all directions; also, consider initial evacuation for 1600 meters (1 mile) in all directions.

In Canada, an Emergency Response Assistance Plan (ERAP) may be required for this product. Please consult the shipping paper and/or the ERAP Program Section (page 390).

EMERGENCY RESPONSE

FIRE

- **DO NOT EXTINGUISH A LEAKING GAS FIRE UNLESS LEAK CAN BE STOPPED.**

Small Fire

- Dry chemical, CO_2, water spray or regular foam.

Large Fire

- Water spray, fog or regular foam.
- If it can be done safely, move undamaged containers away from the area around the fire.
- Damaged cylinders should be handled only by specialists.

Fire Involving Tanks

- Fight fire from maximum distance or use unmanned master stream devices or monitor nozzles.
- Cool containers with flooding quantities of water until well after fire is out.
- Do not direct water at source of leak or safety devices; icing may occur.
- Withdraw immediately in case of rising sound from venting safety devices or discoloration of tank.
- ALWAYS stay away from tanks engulfed in fire.

SPILL OR LEAK

- ELIMINATE all ignition sources (no smoking, flares, sparks or flames) from immediate area.
- All equipment used when handling the product must be grounded.
- Do not touch or walk through spilled material.
- Stop leak if you can do it without risk.
- Use water spray to reduce vapors or divert vapor cloud drift. Avoid allowing water runoff to contact spilled material.
- Do not direct water at spill or source of leak.
- If possible, turn leaking containers so that gas escapes rather than liquid.
- Prevent entry into waterways, sewers, basements or confined areas.
- Isolate area until gas has dispersed.
- Consider igniting spill or leak to eliminate toxic gas concerns.

FIRST AID

- Call 911 or emergency medical service.
- Ensure that medical personnel are aware of the material(s) involved and take precautions to protect themselves.
- Move victim to fresh air if it can be done safely.
- Give artificial respiration if victim is not breathing.
- **Do not perform mouth-to-mouth resuscitation if victim ingested or inhaled the substance; wash face and mouth before giving artificial respiration. Use a pocket mask equipped with a one-way valve or other proper respiratory medical device.**
- Administer oxygen if breathing is difficult.
- Remove and isolate contaminated clothing and shoes.
- In case of contact with substance, immediately flush skin or eyes with running water for at least 20 minutes.
- In case of contact with liquefied gas, thaw frosted parts with lukewarm water.
- In case of burns, immediately cool affected skin for as long as possible with cold water. Do not remove clothing if adhering to skin.
- Keep victim calm and warm.
- Keep victim under observation.
- Effects of contact or inhalation may be delayed.

GUIDE 118 Gases - Flammable - Corrosive

POTENTIAL HAZARDS

FIRE OR EXPLOSION

- **EXTREMELY FLAMMABLE.**
- May be ignited by heat, sparks or flames.
- May form explosive mixtures with air.
- Vapors from liquefied gas are initially heavier than air and spread along ground.
- Vapors may travel to source of ignition and flash back.
- Some of these materials may react violently with water.
- Cylinders exposed to fire may vent and release flammable gas through pressure relief devices.
- Containers may explode when heated.
- Ruptured cylinders may rocket.

HEALTH

- May cause toxic effects if inhaled.
- Vapors are extremely irritating.
- Contact with gas or liquefied gas may cause burns, severe injury and/or frostbite.
- Fire will produce irritating, corrosive and/or toxic gases.
- Runoff from fire control or dilution water may cause environmental contamination.

PUBLIC SAFETY

- **CALL 911. Then call emergency response telephone number on shipping paper.** If shipping paper not available or no answer, refer to appropriate telephone number listed on the inside back cover.
- Keep unauthorized personnel away.
- Stay upwind, uphill and/or upstream.
- Many gases are heavier than air and will spread along the ground and collect in low or confined areas (sewers, basements, tanks, etc.).
- Ventilate closed spaces before entering, but only if properly trained and equipped.

PROTECTIVE CLOTHING

- Wear positive pressure self-contained breathing apparatus (SCBA).
- Wear chemical protective clothing that is specifically recommended by the manufacturer **when there is NO RISK OF FIRE**.
- Structural firefighters' protective clothing provides thermal protection **but only limited chemical protection**.

EVACUATION

Immediate precautionary measure

- Isolate spill or leak area for at least 100 meters (330 feet) in all directions.

Large Spill

- Consider initial downwind evacuation for at least 800 meters (1/2 mile).

Fire

- If tank, rail car or tank truck is involved in a fire, ISOLATE for 1600 meters (1 mile) in all directions; also, consider initial evacuation for 1600 meters (1 mile) in all directions.

In Canada, an Emergency Response Assistance Plan (ERAP) may be required for this product. Please consult the shipping paper and/or the ERAP Program Section (page 390).

EMERGENCY RESPONSE

FIRE

- **DO NOT EXTINGUISH A LEAKING GAS FIRE UNLESS LEAK CAN BE STOPPED.**

Small Fire

- Dry chemical or CO_2.

Large Fire

- Water spray, fog or regular foam.
- If it can be done safely, move undamaged containers away from the area around the fire.
- Damaged cylinders should be handled only by specialists.

Fire Involving Tanks

- Fight fire from maximum distance or use unmanned master stream devices or monitor nozzles.
- Cool containers with flooding quantities of water until well after fire is out.
- Do not direct water at source of leak or safety devices; icing may occur.
- Withdraw immediately in case of rising sound from venting safety devices or discoloration of tank.
- ALWAYS stay away from tanks engulfed in fire.

SPILL OR LEAK

- ELIMINATE all ignition sources (no smoking, flares, sparks or flames) from immediate area.
- All equipment used when handling the product must be grounded.
- Do not touch or walk through spilled material.
- Stop leak if you can do it without risk.
- If possible, turn leaking containers so that gas escapes rather than liquid.
- Use water spray to reduce vapors or divert vapor cloud drift. Avoid allowing water runoff to contact spilled material.
- Do not direct water at spill or source of leak.
- Isolate area until gas has dispersed.

FIRST AID

- Call 911 or emergency medical service.
- Ensure that medical personnel are aware of the material(s) involved and take precautions to protect themselves.
- Move victim to fresh air if it can be done safely.
- Give artificial respiration if victim is not breathing.
- **Do not perform mouth-to-mouth resuscitation if victim ingested or inhaled the substance; wash face and mouth before giving artificial respiration. Use a pocket mask equipped with a one-way valve or other proper respiratory medical device.**
- Administer oxygen if breathing is difficult.
- Remove and isolate contaminated clothing and shoes.
- In case of contact with liquefied gas, thaw frosted parts with lukewarm water.
- In case of burns, immediately cool affected skin for as long as possible with cold water. Do not remove clothing if adhering to skin.
- Keep victim calm and warm.
- Keep victim under observation.
- Effects of contact or inhalation may be delayed.

GUIDE 119 GASES - TOXIC - FLAMMABLE

POTENTIAL HAZARDS

HEALTH

- **TOXIC; may be fatal if inhaled or absorbed through skin. Some may cause severe skin burns and eye damage.**
- Contact with gas or liquefied gas may cause burns, severe injury and/or frostbite.
- Fire will produce irritating, corrosive and/or toxic gases.
- Runoff from fire control or dilution water may cause environmental contamination.

FIRE OR EXPLOSION

- Flammable; may be ignited by heat, sparks or flames.
- May form explosive mixtures with air. Ethylene oxide (UN1040) may react explosively even in the absence of air.
- Those substances designated with a **(P)** may polymerize explosively when heated or involved in a fire.
- Vapors from liquefied gas are initially heavier than air and spread along ground.
- Vapors may travel to source of ignition and flash back.
- Some of these materials may react violently with water.
- Cylinders exposed to fire may vent and release toxic and flammable gas through pressure relief devices.
- Containers may explode when heated.
- Ruptured cylinders may rocket.
- Runoff may create fire or explosion hazard.

PUBLIC SAFETY

- **CALL 911. Then call emergency response telephone number on shipping paper.** If shipping paper not available or no answer, refer to appropriate telephone number listed on the inside back cover.
- Keep unauthorized personnel away.
- Stay upwind, uphill and/or upstream.
- Many gases are heavier than air and will spread along the ground and collect in low or confined areas (sewers, basements, tanks, etc.).
- Ventilate closed spaces before entering, but only if properly trained and equipped.

PROTECTIVE CLOTHING

- Wear positive pressure self-contained breathing apparatus (SCBA).
- Wear chemical protective clothing that is specifically recommended by the manufacturer **when there is NO RISK OF FIRE**.
- Structural firefighters' protective clothing provides thermal protection **but only limited chemical protection**.

EVACUATION

Immediate precautionary measure

- Isolate spill or leak area for at least 100 meters (330 feet) in all directions.

Spill

- For highlighted materials: see Table 1 - Initial Isolation and Protective Action Distances.
- For non-highlighted materials: increase the immediate precautionary measure distance, in the downwind direction, as necessary.

Fire

- If tank, rail car or tank truck is involved in a fire, ISOLATE for 1600 meters (1 mile) in all directions; also, consider initial evacuation for 1600 meters (1 mile) in all directions.

In Canada, an Emergency Response Assistance Plan (ERAP) may be required for this product. Please consult the shipping paper and/or the ERAP Program Section (page 390).

EMERGENCY RESPONSE

FIRE

- **DO NOT EXTINGUISH A LEAKING GAS FIRE UNLESS LEAK CAN BE STOPPED.**

Small Fire

- Dry chemical, CO_2, water spray or alcohol-resistant foam.

Large Fire

- Water spray, fog or alcohol-resistant foam.
- **FOR CHLOROSILANES, DO NOT USE WATER;** use AFFF alcohol-resistant medium-expansion foam.
- If it can be done safely, move undamaged containers away from the area around the fire.
- Damaged cylinders should be handled only by specialists.

Fire Involving Tanks

- Fight fire from maximum distance or use unmanned master stream devices or monitor nozzles.
- Cool containers with flooding quantities of water until well after fire is out.
- Do not direct water at source of leak or safety devices; icing may occur.
- Withdraw immediately in case of rising sound from venting safety devices or discoloration of tank.
- ALWAYS stay away from tanks engulfed in fire.

SPILL OR LEAK

- ELIMINATE all ignition sources (no smoking, flares, sparks or flames) from immediate area.
- All equipment used when handling the product must be grounded.
- Do not touch or walk through spilled material.
- Stop leak if you can do it without risk.
- Do not direct water at spill or source of leak.
- Use water spray to reduce vapors or divert vapor cloud drift. Avoid allowing water runoff to contact spilled material.
- **FOR CHLOROSILANES**, use AFFF alcohol-resistant medium-expansion foam to reduce vapors.
- If possible, turn leaking containers so that gas escapes rather than liquid.
- Prevent entry into waterways, sewers, basements or confined areas.
- Isolate area until gas has dispersed.

FIRST AID

- Call 911 or emergency medical service.
- Ensure that medical personnel are aware of the material(s) involved and take precautions to protect themselves.
- Move victim to fresh air if it can be done safely.
- Give artificial respiration if victim is not breathing.
- **Do not perform mouth-to-mouth resuscitation if victim ingested or inhaled the substance; wash face and mouth before giving artificial respiration. Use a pocket mask equipped with a one-way valve or other proper respiratory medical device.**
- Administer oxygen if breathing is difficult.
- Remove and isolate contaminated clothing and shoes.
- In case of contact with substance, immediately flush skin or eyes with running water for at least 20 minutes.
- In case of contact with liquefied gas, thaw frosted parts with lukewarm water.
- In case of burns, immediately cool affected skin for as long as possible with cold water. Do not remove clothing if adhering to skin.
- Keep victim calm and warm.
- Keep victim under observation.
- Effects of contact or inhalation may be delayed.

GUIDE 120 GASES - INERT (INCLUDING REFRIGERATED LIQUIDS)

POTENTIAL HAZARDS

HEALTH

- Vapors may cause dizziness or asphyxiation without warning.
- Vapors from liquefied gas are initially heavier than air and spread along ground.
- Contact with gas or liquefied gas may cause burns, severe injury and/or frostbite.

FIRE OR EXPLOSION

- **Non-flammable gases.**
- Containers may explode when heated.
- Ruptured cylinders may rocket.

PUBLIC SAFETY

- **CALL 911. Then call emergency response telephone number on shipping paper.** If shipping paper not available or no answer, refer to appropriate telephone number listed on the inside back cover.
- Keep unauthorized personnel away.
- Stay upwind, uphill and/or upstream.
- Many gases are heavier than air and will spread along the ground and collect in low or confined areas (sewers, basements, tanks, etc.).
- Ventilate closed spaces before entering, but only if properly trained and equipped.

PROTECTIVE CLOTHING

- Wear positive pressure self-contained breathing apparatus (SCBA).
- Structural firefighters' protective clothing provides thermal protection **but only limited chemical protection**.
- Always wear thermal protective clothing when handling refrigerated/cryogenic liquids or solids.

EVACUATION

Immediate precautionary measure

- Isolate spill or leak area for at least 100 meters (330 feet) in all directions.

Large Spill

- Consider initial downwind evacuation for at least 100 meters (330 feet).

Fire

- If tank, rail car or tank truck is involved in a fire, ISOLATE for 800 meters (1/2 mile) in all directions; also, consider initial evacuation for 800 meters (1/2 mile) in all directions.

EMERGENCY RESPONSE

FIRE

- Use extinguishing agent suitable for type of surrounding fire.
- If it can be done safely, move undamaged containers away from the area around the fire.
- Damaged cylinders should be handled only by specialists.

Fire Involving Tanks

- Fight fire from maximum distance or use unmanned master stream devices or monitor nozzles.
- Cool containers with flooding quantities of water until well after fire is out.
- Do not direct water at source of leak or safety devices; icing may occur.
- Withdraw immediately in case of rising sound from venting safety devices or discoloration of tank.
- ALWAYS stay away from tanks engulfed in fire.

SPILL OR LEAK

- Do not touch or walk through spilled material.
- Stop leak if you can do it without risk.
- Use water spray to reduce vapors or divert vapor cloud drift. Avoid allowing water runoff to contact spilled material.
- Do not direct water at spill or source of leak.
- If possible, turn leaking containers so that gas escapes rather than liquid.
- Prevent entry into waterways, sewers, basements or confined areas.
- Allow substance to evaporate.
- Ventilate the area.

CAUTION: When in contact with refrigerated/cryogenic liquids, many materials become brittle and are likely to break without warning.

FIRST AID

- Call 911 or emergency medical service.
- Ensure that medical personnel are aware of the material(s) involved and take precautions to protect themselves.
- Move victim to fresh air if it can be done safely.
- Give artificial respiration if victim is not breathing.
- Administer oxygen if breathing is difficult.
- Clothing frozen to the skin should be thawed before being removed.
- In case of contact with liquefied gas, thaw frosted parts with lukewarm water.
- Keep victim calm and warm.

Page intentionally left blank

There are no materials that refer to this guide.

Page intentionally left blank

There are no materials that refer to this guide.

GUIDE 122 GASES - OXIDIZING (INCLUDING REFRIGERATED LIQUIDS)

POTENTIAL HAZARDS

FIRE OR EXPLOSION

- Substance does not burn but will support combustion.
- Some may react explosively with fuels.
- May ignite combustibles (wood, paper, oil, clothing, etc.).
- Vapors from liquefied gas are initially heavier than air and spread along ground.
- Runoff may create fire or explosion hazard.
- Containers may explode when heated.
- Ruptured cylinders may rocket.

HEALTH

- Vapors may cause dizziness or asphyxiation without warning.
- Contact with gas or liquefied gas may cause burns, severe injury and/or frostbite.
- Fire may produce irritating and/or toxic gases.

PUBLIC SAFETY

- **CALL 911. Then call emergency response telephone number on shipping paper.** If shipping paper not available or no answer, refer to appropriate telephone number listed on the inside back cover.
- Keep unauthorized personnel away.
- Stay upwind, uphill and/or upstream.
- Many gases are heavier than air and will spread along the ground and collect in low or confined areas (sewers, basements, tanks, etc.).
- Ventilate closed spaces before entering, but only if properly trained and equipped.

PROTECTIVE CLOTHING

- Wear positive pressure self-contained breathing apparatus (SCBA).
- Wear chemical protective clothing that is specifically recommended by the manufacturer **when there is NO RISK OF FIRE**.
- Structural firefighters' protective clothing provides thermal protection **but only limited chemical protection**.
- Always wear thermal protective clothing when handling refrigerated/cryogenic liquids.

EVACUATION

Immediate precautionary measure

- Isolate spill or leak area for at least 100 meters (330 feet) in all directions.

Large Spill

- Consider initial downwind evacuation for at least 500 meters (1/3 mile).

Fire

- If tank, rail car or tank truck is involved in a fire, ISOLATE for 800 meters (1/2 mile) in all directions; also, consider initial evacuation for 800 meters (1/2 mile) in all directions.

In Canada, an Emergency Response Assistance Plan (ERAP) may be required for this product. Please consult the shipping paper and/or the ERAP Program Section (page 390).

EMERGENCY RESPONSE

FIRE

- Use extinguishing agent suitable for type of surrounding fire.

Small Fire

- Dry chemical or CO_2.

Large Fire

- Water spray, fog or regular foam.
- If it can be done safely, move undamaged containers away from the area around the fire.
- Damaged cylinders should be handled only by specialists.

Fire Involving Tanks

- Fight fire from maximum distance or use unmanned master stream devices or monitor nozzles.
- Cool containers with flooding quantities of water until well after fire is out.
- Do not direct water at source of leak or safety devices; icing may occur.
- Withdraw immediately in case of rising sound from venting safety devices or discoloration of tank.
- ALWAYS stay away from tanks engulfed in fire.
- For massive fire, use unmanned master stream devices or monitor nozzles; if this is impossible, withdraw from area and let fire burn.

SPILL OR LEAK

- Keep combustibles (wood, paper, oil, etc.) away from spilled material.
- Do not touch or walk through spilled material.
- Stop leak if you can do it without risk.
- If possible, turn leaking containers so that gas escapes rather than liquid.
- Do not direct water at spill or source of leak.
- Use water spray to reduce vapors or divert vapor cloud drift. Avoid allowing water runoff to contact spilled material.
- Prevent entry into waterways, sewers, basements or confined areas.
- Allow substance to evaporate.
- Isolate area until gas has dispersed.

CAUTION: When in contact with refrigerated/cryogenic liquids, many materials become brittle and are likely to break without warning.

FIRST AID

- Call 911 or emergency medical service.
- Ensure that medical personnel are aware of the material(s) involved and take precautions to protect themselves.
- Move victim to fresh air if it can be done safely.
- Give artificial respiration if victim is not breathing.
- Administer oxygen if breathing is difficult.
- Remove and isolate contaminated clothing and shoes.
- Clothing frozen to the skin should be thawed before being removed.
- In case of contact with liquefied gas, thaw frosted parts with lukewarm water.
- Keep victim calm and warm.

GUIDE 123 GASES - TOXIC

POTENTIAL HAZARDS

HEALTH

- **TOXIC; may be fatal if inhaled or absorbed through skin.**
- Vapors may be irritating and/or corrosive.
- Contact with gas or liquefied gas may cause burns, severe injury and/or frostbite.
- Fire will produce irritating, corrosive and/or toxic gases.
- Runoff from fire control or dilution water may cause environmental contamination.

FIRE OR EXPLOSION

- Some may burn but none ignite readily.
- Vapors from liquefied gas are initially heavier than air and spread along ground.
- Cylinders exposed to fire may vent and release toxic and/or corrosive gas through pressure relief devices.
- Containers may explode when heated.
- Ruptured cylinders may rocket.

PUBLIC SAFETY

- **CALL 911. Then call emergency response telephone number on shipping paper.** If shipping paper not available or no answer, refer to appropriate telephone number listed on the inside back cover.
- Keep unauthorized personnel away.
- Stay upwind, uphill and/or upstream.
- Many gases are heavier than air and will spread along the ground and collect in low or confined areas (sewers, basements, tanks, etc.).
- Ventilate closed spaces before entering, but only if properly trained and equipped.

PROTECTIVE CLOTHING

- Wear positive pressure self-contained breathing apparatus (SCBA).
- Wear chemical protective clothing that is specifically recommended by the manufacturer **when there is NO RISK OF FIRE**.
- Structural firefighters' protective clothing provides thermal protection **but only limited chemical protection**.

EVACUATION

Immediate precautionary measure

- Isolate spill or leak area for at least 100 meters (330 feet) in all directions.

Spill

- For highlighted materials: see Table 1 - Initial Isolation and Protective Action Distances.
- For non-highlighted materials: increase the immediate precautionary measure distance, in the downwind direction, as necessary.

Fire

- If tank, rail car or tank truck is involved in a fire, ISOLATE for 800 meters (1/2 mile) in all directions; also, consider initial evacuation for 800 meters (1/2 mile) in all directions.

In Canada, an Emergency Response Assistance Plan (ERAP) may be required for this product. Please consult the shipping paper and/or the ERAP Program Section (page 390).

EMERGENCY RESPONSE

FIRE

Small Fire

- Dry chemical or CO_2.

Large Fire

- Water spray, fog or regular foam.
- Do not get water inside containers.
- If it can be done safely, move undamaged containers away from the area around the fire.
- Damaged cylinders should be handled only by specialists.

Fire Involving Tanks

- Fight fire from maximum distance or use unmanned master stream devices or monitor nozzles.
- Cool containers with flooding quantities of water until well after fire is out.
- Do not direct water at source of leak or safety devices; icing may occur.
- Withdraw immediately in case of rising sound from venting safety devices or discoloration of tank.
- ALWAYS stay away from tanks engulfed in fire.

SPILL OR LEAK

- Do not touch or walk through spilled material.
- Stop leak if you can do it without risk.
- If possible, turn leaking containers so that gas escapes rather than liquid.
- Prevent entry into waterways, sewers, basements or confined areas.
- Use water spray to reduce vapors or divert vapor cloud drift. Avoid allowing water runoff to contact spilled material.
- Do not direct water at spill or source of leak.
- Isolate area until gas has dispersed.

FIRST AID

- Call 911 or emergency medical service.
- Ensure that medical personnel are aware of the material(s) involved and take precautions to protect themselves.
- Move victim to fresh air if it can be done safely.
- Give artificial respiration if victim is not breathing.
- **Do not perform mouth-to-mouth resuscitation if victim ingested or inhaled the substance; wash face and mouth before giving artificial respiration. Use a pocket mask equipped with a one-way valve or other proper respiratory medical device.**
- Administer oxygen if breathing is difficult.
- Remove and isolate contaminated clothing and shoes.
- In case of contact with liquefied gas, thaw frosted parts with lukewarm water.
- In case of contact with substance, immediately flush skin or eyes with running water for at least 20 minutes.
- Keep victim calm and warm.
- Keep victim under observation.
- Effects of contact or inhalation may be delayed.

GUIDE 124 GASES - TOXIC AND/OR CORROSIVE - OXIDIZING

POTENTIAL HAZARDS

HEALTH

- **TOXIC; may be fatal if inhaled or absorbed through skin.**
- Fire will produce irritating, corrosive and/or toxic gases.
- Contact with gas or liquefied gas may cause burns, severe injury and/or frostbite.
- Runoff from fire control or dilution water may cause environmental contamination.

FIRE OR EXPLOSION

- Substance does not burn but will support combustion.
- Vapors from liquefied gas are initially heavier than air and spread along ground.
- These are strong oxidizers and will react vigorously or explosively with many materials including fuels.
- May ignite combustibles (wood, paper, oil, clothing, etc.).
- Some will react violently with air, moist air and/or water.
- Cylinders exposed to fire may vent and release toxic and/or corrosive gas through pressure relief devices.
- Containers may explode when heated.
- Ruptured cylinders may rocket.

PUBLIC SAFETY

- **CALL 911. Then call emergency response telephone number on shipping paper.** If shipping paper not available or no answer, refer to appropriate telephone number listed on the inside back cover.
- Keep unauthorized personnel away.
- Stay upwind, uphill and/or upstream.
- Many gases are heavier than air and will spread along the ground and collect in low or confined areas (sewers, basements, tanks, etc.).
- Ventilate closed spaces before entering, but only if properly trained and equipped.

PROTECTIVE CLOTHING

- Wear positive pressure self-contained breathing apparatus (SCBA).
- Wear chemical protective clothing that is specifically recommended by the manufacturer **when there is NO RISK OF FIRE**.
- Structural firefighters' protective clothing provides thermal protection **but only limited chemical protection**.

EVACUATION

Immediate precautionary measure

- Isolate spill or leak area for at least 100 meters (330 feet) in all directions.

Spill

- See Table 1 - Initial Isolation and Protective Action Distances.

Fire

- If tank, rail car or tank truck is involved in a fire, ISOLATE for 800 meters (1/2 mile) in all directions; also, consider initial evacuation for 800 meters (1/2 mile) in all directions.

In Canada, an Emergency Response Assistance Plan (ERAP) may be required for this product. Please consult the shipping paper and/or the ERAP Program Section (page 390).

EMERGENCY RESPONSE

FIRE

Small Fire

CAUTION: These materials do not burn but will support combustion. Some will react violently with water.

- Contain fire and let burn. If fire must be fought, water spray or fog is recommended.
- **Water only; no dry chemical, CO_2 or Halon®**.
- Do not get water inside containers.
- If it can be done safely, move undamaged containers away from the area around the fire.
- Damaged cylinders should be handled only by specialists.

Fire Involving Tanks

- Fight fire from maximum distance or use unmanned master stream devices or monitor nozzles.
- Cool containers with flooding quantities of water until well after fire is out.
- Do not direct water at source of leak or safety devices; icing may occur.
- Withdraw immediately in case of rising sound from venting safety devices or discoloration of tank.
- ALWAYS stay away from tanks engulfed in fire.
- For massive fire, use unmanned master stream devices or monitor nozzles; if this is impossible, withdraw from area and let fire burn.

SPILL OR LEAK

- Do not touch or walk through spilled material.
- Keep combustibles (wood, paper, oil, etc.) away from spilled material.
- Stop leak if you can do it without risk.
- Use water spray to reduce vapors or divert vapor cloud drift. Avoid allowing water runoff to contact spilled material.
- Do not direct water at spill or source of leak.
- If possible, turn leaking containers so that gas escapes rather than liquid.
- Prevent entry into waterways, sewers, basements or confined areas.
- Isolate area until gas has dispersed.
- Ventilate the area.

FIRST AID

- Call 911 or emergency medical service.
- Ensure that medical personnel are aware of the material(s) involved and take precautions to protect themselves.
- Move victim to fresh air if it can be done safely.
- Give artificial respiration if victim is not breathing.
- **Do not perform mouth-to-mouth resuscitation if victim ingested or inhaled the substance; wash face and mouth before giving artificial respiration. Use a pocket mask equipped with a one-way valve or other proper respiratory medical device.**
- Administer oxygen if breathing is difficult.
- Clothing frozen to the skin should be thawed before being removed.
- Remove and isolate contaminated clothing and shoes.
- In case of contact with substance, immediately flush skin or eyes with running water for at least 20 minutes.
- Keep victim calm and warm.
- Keep victim under observation.
- Effects of contact or inhalation may be delayed.

GUIDE 125 Gases - Toxic and/or Corrosive

POTENTIAL HAZARDS

HEALTH

- **TOXIC; may be fatal if inhaled, ingested or absorbed through skin.**
- Vapors are extremely irritating and corrosive.
- Contact with gas or liquefied gas may cause burns, severe injury and/or frostbite.
- Fire will produce irritating, corrosive and/or toxic gases.
- Runoff from fire control or dilution water may cause environmental contamination.

FIRE OR EXPLOSION

- Some may burn but none ignite readily.
- Vapors from liquefied gas are initially heavier than air and spread along ground.
- Some of these materials may react violently with water.
- Cylinders exposed to fire may vent and release toxic and/or corrosive gas through pressure relief devices.
- Containers may explode when heated.
- Ruptured cylinders may rocket.
- For UN1005: Anhydrous ammonia, at high concentrations in confined spaces, presents a flammability risk if a source of ignition is introduced.

PUBLIC SAFETY

- **CALL 911. Then call emergency response telephone number on shipping paper.** If shipping paper not available or no answer, refer to appropriate telephone number listed on the inside back cover.
- Keep unauthorized personnel away.
- Stay upwind, uphill and/or upstream.
- Many gases are heavier than air and will spread along the ground and collect in low or confined areas (sewers, basements, tanks, etc.).
- Ventilate closed spaces before entering, but only if properly trained and equipped.

PROTECTIVE CLOTHING

- Wear positive pressure self-contained breathing apparatus (SCBA).
- Wear chemical protective clothing that is specifically recommended by the manufacturer **when there is NO RISK OF FIRE.**
- Structural firefighters' protective clothing provides thermal protection **but only limited chemical protection**.

EVACUATION

Immediate precautionary measure

- Isolate spill or leak area for at least 100 meters (330 feet) in all directions.

Spill

- For highlighted materials: see Table 1 - Initial Isolation and Protective Action Distances.
- For non-highlighted materials: increase the immediate precautionary measure distance, in the downwind direction, as necessary.

Fire

- If tank, rail car or tank truck is involved in a fire, ISOLATE for 1600 meters (1 mile) in all directions; also, consider initial evacuation for 1600 meters (1 mile) in all directions.

In Canada, an Emergency Response Assistance Plan (ERAP) may be required for this product. Please consult the shipping paper and/or the ERAP Program Section (page 390).

EMERGENCY RESPONSE

FIRE

Small Fire

- Dry chemical or CO_2.

Large Fire

- Water spray, fog or regular foam.
- If it can be done safely, move undamaged containers away from the area around the fire.
- Do not get water inside containers.
- Damaged cylinders should be handled only by specialists.

Fire Involving Tanks

- Fight fire from maximum distance or use unmanned master stream devices or monitor nozzles.
- Cool containers with flooding quantities of water until well after fire is out.
- Do not direct water at source of leak or safety devices; icing may occur.
- Withdraw immediately in case of rising sound from venting safety devices or discoloration of tank.
- ALWAYS stay away from tanks engulfed in fire.

SPILL OR LEAK

- Do not touch or walk through spilled material.
- Stop leak if you can do it without risk.
- If possible, turn leaking containers so that gas escapes rather than liquid.
- Prevent entry into waterways, sewers, basements or confined areas.
- Do not direct water at spill or source of leak.
- Use water spray to reduce vapors or divert vapor cloud drift. Avoid allowing water runoff to contact spilled material.
- Isolate area until gas has dispersed.

FIRST AID

- Call 911 or emergency medical service.
- Ensure that medical personnel are aware of the material(s) involved and take precautions to protect themselves.
- Move victim to fresh air if it can be done safely.
- Give artificial respiration if victim is not breathing.
- **Do not perform mouth-to-mouth resuscitation if victim ingested or inhaled the substance; wash face and mouth before giving artificial respiration. Use a pocket mask equipped with a one-way valve or other proper respiratory medical device.**
- Administer oxygen if breathing is difficult.
- Remove and isolate contaminated clothing and shoes.
- In case of contact with liquefied gas, thaw frosted parts with lukewarm water.
- In case of contact with substance, immediately flush skin or eyes with running water for at least 20 minutes.
- **In case of skin contact with hydrogen fluoride, anhydrous (UN1052)**, if calcium gluconate gel is available, rinse 5 minutes, then apply gel. Otherwise, continue rinsing until medical treatment is available.
- Keep victim calm and warm.
- Keep victim under observation.
- Effects of contact or inhalation may be delayed.

GUIDE 126 Gases - Compressed or Liquefied (Including Refrigerant Gases)

POTENTIAL HAZARDS

FIRE OR EXPLOSION

- Some may burn but none ignite readily.
- Containers may explode when heated.
- Ruptured cylinders may rocket.

CAUTION: Aerosols (UN1950) may contain a flammable propellant.

HEALTH

- Vapors may cause dizziness or asphyxiation without warning.
- Vapors from liquefied gas are initially heavier than air and spread along ground.
- Contact with gas or liquefied gas may cause burns, severe injury and/or frostbite.
- Fire may produce irritating, corrosive and/or toxic gases.

PUBLIC SAFETY

- **CALL 911. Then call emergency response telephone number on shipping paper**. If shipping paper not available or no answer, refer to appropriate telephone number listed on the inside back cover.
- Keep unauthorized personnel away.
- Stay upwind, uphill and/or upstream.
- Many gases are heavier than air and will spread along the ground and collect in low or confined areas (sewers, basements, tanks, etc.).
- Ventilate closed spaces before entering, but only if properly trained and equipped.

PROTECTIVE CLOTHING

- Wear positive pressure self-contained breathing apparatus (SCBA).
- Wear chemical protective clothing that is specifically recommended by the manufacturer **when there is NO RISK OF FIRE**.
- Structural firefighters' protective clothing provides thermal protection **but only limited chemical protection**.

EVACUATION

Immediate precautionary measure

- Isolate spill or leak area for at least 100 meters (330 feet) in all directions.

Large Spill

- Consider initial downwind evacuation for at least 500 meters (1/3 mile).

Fire

- If tank, rail car or tank truck is involved in a fire, ISOLATE for 800 meters (1/2 mile) in all directions; also, consider initial evacuation for 800 meters (1/2 mile) in all directions.

EMERGENCY RESPONSE

FIRE

- Use extinguishing agent suitable for type of surrounding fire.

Small Fire

- Dry chemical or CO_2.

Large Fire

- Water spray, fog or regular foam.
- If it can be done safely, move undamaged containers away from the area around the fire.
- Damaged cylinders should be handled only by specialists.

Fire Involving Tanks

- Fight fire from maximum distance or use unmanned master stream devices or monitor nozzles.
- Cool containers with flooding quantities of water until well after fire is out.
- Do not direct water at source of leak or safety devices; icing may occur.
- Withdraw immediately in case of rising sound from venting safety devices or discoloration of tank.
- ALWAYS stay away from tanks engulfed in fire.
- Some of these materials, if spilled, may evaporate leaving a flammable residue.

SPILL OR LEAK

- Do not touch or walk through spilled material.
- Stop leak if you can do it without risk.
- Do not direct water at spill or source of leak.
- Use water spray to reduce vapors or divert vapor cloud drift. Avoid allowing water runoff to contact spilled material.
- If possible, turn leaking containers so that gas escapes rather than liquid.
- Prevent entry into waterways, sewers, basements or confined areas.
- Allow substance to evaporate.
- Ventilate the area.

FIRST AID

- Call 911 or emergency medical service.
- Ensure that medical personnel are aware of the material(s) involved and take precautions to protect themselves.
- Move victim to fresh air if it can be done safely.
- Give artificial respiration if victim is not breathing.
- Administer oxygen if breathing is difficult.
- Remove and isolate contaminated clothing and shoes.
- In case of contact with liquefied gas, thaw frosted parts with lukewarm water.
- Keep victim calm and warm.

GUIDE 127 FLAMMABLE LIQUIDS (WATER-MISCIBLE)

POTENTIAL HAZARDS

FIRE OR EXPLOSION

- **HIGHLY FLAMMABLE: Will be easily ignited by heat, sparks or flames.**

CAUTION: Ethanol (UN1170) can burn with an invisible flame. Use an alternate method of detection (thermal camera, broom handle, etc.)

- Vapors may form explosive mixtures with air.
- Vapors may travel to source of ignition and flash back.
- Most vapors are heavier than air. They will spread along the ground and collect in low or confined areas (sewers, basements, tanks, etc.).
- Vapor explosion hazard indoors, outdoors or in sewers.
- Those substances designated with a **(P)** may polymerize explosively when heated or involved in a fire.
- Runoff to sewer may create fire or explosion hazard.
- Containers may explode when heated.
- Many liquids will float on water.

HEALTH

- Inhalation or contact with material may irritate or burn skin and eyes.
- Fire may produce irritating, corrosive and/or toxic gases.
- Vapors may cause dizziness or asphyxiation.
- Runoff from fire control or dilution water may cause environmental contamination.

PUBLIC SAFETY

- **CALL 911. Then call emergency response telephone number on shipping paper**. If shipping paper not available or no answer, refer to appropriate telephone number listed on the inside back cover.
- Keep unauthorized personnel away.
- Stay upwind, uphill and/or upstream.
- Ventilate closed spaces before entering, but only if properly trained and equipped.

PROTECTIVE CLOTHING

- Wear positive pressure self-contained breathing apparatus (SCBA).
- Structural firefighters' protective clothing provides thermal protection **but only limited chemical protection**.

EVACUATION

Immediate precautionary measure

- Isolate spill or leak area for at least 50 meters (150 feet) in all directions.

Large Spill

- Consider initial downwind evacuation for at least 300 meters (1000 feet).

Fire

- If tank, rail car or tank truck is involved in a fire, ISOLATE for 800 meters (1/2 mile) in all directions; also, consider initial evacuation for 800 meters (1/2 mile) in all directions.

In Canada, an Emergency Response Assistance Plan (ERAP) may be required for this product. Please consult the shipping paper and/or the ERAP Program Section (page 390).

EMERGENCY RESPONSE

FIRE

CAUTION: The majority of these products have a very low flash point. Use of water spray when fighting fire may be inefficient.

CAUTION: For fire involving UN1170, UN1987 or UN3475, alcohol-resistant foam should be used.

CAUTION: Ethanol (UN1170) can burn with an invisible flame. Use an alternate method of detection (thermal camera, broom handle, etc.)

Small Fire

- Dry chemical, CO_2, water spray or alcohol-resistant foam.

Large Fire

- Water spray, fog or alcohol-resistant foam.
- Avoid aiming straight or solid streams directly onto the product.
- If it can be done safely, move undamaged containers away from the area around the fire.

Fire Involving Tanks or Car/Trailer Loads

- Fight fire from maximum distance or use unmanned master stream devices or monitor nozzles.
- Cool containers with flooding quantities of water until well after fire is out.
- Withdraw immediately in case of rising sound from venting safety devices or discoloration of tank.
- ALWAYS stay away from tanks engulfed in fire.
- For massive fire, use unmanned master stream devices or monitor nozzles; if this is impossible, withdraw from area and let fire burn.

SPILL OR LEAK

- ELIMINATE all ignition sources (no smoking, flares, sparks or flames) from immediate area.
- All equipment used when handling the product must be grounded.
- Do not touch or walk through spilled material.
- Stop leak if you can do it without risk.
- Prevent entry into waterways, sewers, basements or confined areas.
- A vapor-suppressing foam may be used to reduce vapors.
- Absorb or cover with dry earth, sand or other non-combustible material and transfer to containers.
- Use clean, non-sparking tools to collect absorbed material.

Large Spill

- Dike far ahead of liquid spill for later disposal.
- Water spray may reduce vapor, but may not prevent ignition in closed spaces.

FIRST AID

- Call 911 or emergency medical service.
- Ensure that medical personnel are aware of the material(s) involved and take precautions to protect themselves.
- Move victim to fresh air if it can be done safely.
- Give artificial respiration if victim is not breathing.
- Administer oxygen if breathing is difficult.
- Remove and isolate contaminated clothing and shoes.
- In case of contact with substance, immediately flush skin or eyes with running water for at least 20 minutes.
- Wash skin with soap and water.
- In case of burns, immediately cool affected skin for as long as possible with cold water. Do not remove clothing if adhering to skin.
- Keep victim calm and warm.

GUIDE 128 FLAMMABLE LIQUIDS (WATER-IMMISCIBLE)

POTENTIAL HAZARDS

FIRE OR EXPLOSION

- **HIGHLY FLAMMABLE: Will be easily ignited by heat, sparks or flames.**
- Vapors may form explosive mixtures with air.
- Vapors may travel to source of ignition and flash back.
- Most vapors are heavier than air. They will spread along the ground and collect in low or confined areas (sewers, basements, tanks, etc.).
- Vapor explosion hazard indoors, outdoors or in sewers.
- Those substances designated with a **(P)** may polymerize explosively when heated or involved in a fire.
- Runoff to sewer may create fire or explosion hazard.
- Containers may explode when heated.
- Many liquids will float on water.
- Substance may be transported hot.
- For hybrid vehicles, GUIDE 147 (lithium ion batteries) or GUIDE 138 (sodium batteries) should also be consulted.
- **If molten aluminum is involved, refer to GUIDE 169.**

HEALTH

CAUTION: Petroleum crude oil (UN1267) may contain **TOXIC** hydrogen sulphide gas.

- Inhalation or contact with material may irritate or burn skin and eyes.
- Fire may produce irritating, corrosive and/or toxic gases.
- Vapors may cause dizziness or asphyxiation.
- Runoff from fire control or dilution water may cause environmental contamination.

PUBLIC SAFETY

- **CALL 911. Then call emergency response telephone number on shipping paper.** If shipping paper not available or no answer, refer to appropriate telephone number listed on the inside back cover.
- Keep unauthorized personnel away.
- Stay upwind, uphill and/or upstream.
- Ventilate closed spaces before entering, but only if properly trained and equipped.

PROTECTIVE CLOTHING

- Wear positive pressure self-contained breathing apparatus (SCBA).
- Structural firefighters' protective clothing provides thermal protection **but only limited chemical protection.**

EVACUATION

Immediate precautionary measure

- Isolate spill or leak area for at least 50 meters (150 feet) in all directions.

Large Spill

- Consider initial downwind evacuation for at least 300 meters (1000 feet).

Fire

- If tank, rail car or tank truck is involved in a fire, ISOLATE for 800 meters (1/2 mile) in all directions; also, consider initial evacuation for 800 meters (1/2 mile) in all directions.

In Canada, an Emergency Response Assistance Plan (ERAP) may be required for this product. Please consult the shipping paper and/or the ERAP Program Section (page 390).

EMERGENCY RESPONSE

FIRE

CAUTION: The majority of these products have a very low flash point. Use of water spray when fighting fire may be inefficient.

CAUTION: For mixtures containing alcohol or polar solvent, alcohol-resistant foam may be more effective.

Small Fire

- Dry chemical, CO_2, water spray or regular foam.

Large Fire

- Water spray, fog or regular foam.
- Avoid aiming straight or solid streams directly onto the product.
- If it can be done safely, move undamaged containers away from the area around the fire.

Fire Involving Tanks or Car/Trailer Loads

- Fight fire from maximum distance or use unmanned master stream devices or monitor nozzles.
- Cool containers with flooding quantities of water until well after fire is out.
- For petroleum crude oil, do not spray water directly into a breached tank car. This can lead to a dangerous boil over.
- Withdraw immediately in case of rising sound from venting safety devices or discoloration of tank.
- ALWAYS stay away from tanks engulfed in fire.
- For massive fire, use unmanned master stream devices or monitor nozzles; if this is impossible, withdraw from area and let fire burn.

SPILL OR LEAK

- ELIMINATE all ignition sources (no smoking, flares, sparks or flames) from immediate area.
- All equipment used when handling the product must be grounded.
- Do not touch or walk through spilled material.
- Stop leak if you can do it without risk.
- Prevent entry into waterways, sewers, basements or confined areas.
- A vapor-suppressing foam may be used to reduce vapors.
- Absorb or cover with dry earth, sand or other non-combustible material and transfer to containers.
- Use clean, non-sparking tools to collect absorbed material.

Large Spill

- Dike far ahead of liquid spill for later disposal.
- Water spray may reduce vapor, but may not prevent ignition in closed spaces.

FIRST AID

- Call 911 or emergency medical service.
- Ensure that medical personnel are aware of the material(s) involved and take precautions to protect themselves.
- Move victim to fresh air if it can be done safely.
- Give artificial respiration if victim is not breathing.
- Administer oxygen if breathing is difficult.
- Remove and isolate contaminated clothing and shoes.
- In case of contact with substance, immediately flush skin or eyes with running water for at least 20 minutes.
- Wash skin with soap and water.
- In case of burns, immediately cool affected skin for as long as possible with cold water. Do not remove clothing if adhering to skin.
- Keep victim calm and warm.

GUIDE 129 FLAMMABLE LIQUIDS (WATER-MISCIBLE/NOXIOUS)

POTENTIAL HAZARDS

FIRE OR EXPLOSION

- **HIGHLY FLAMMABLE: Will be easily ignited by heat, sparks or flames.**
- Vapors may form explosive mixtures with air.
- Vapors may travel to source of ignition and flash back.
- Most vapors are heavier than air. They will spread along the ground and collect in low or confined areas (sewers, basements, tanks, etc.).
- Vapor explosion hazard indoors, outdoors or in sewers.
- Those substances designated with a **(P)** may polymerize explosively when heated or involved in a fire.
- Runoff to sewer may create fire or explosion hazard.
- Containers may explode when heated.
- Many liquids will float on water.

HEALTH

- May cause toxic effects if inhaled or absorbed through skin.
- Inhalation or contact with material may irritate or burn skin and eyes.
- Fire will produce irritating, corrosive and/or toxic gases.
- Vapors may cause dizziness or asphyxiation.
- Runoff from fire control or dilution water may cause environmental contamination.

PUBLIC SAFETY

- **CALL 911. Then call emergency response telephone number on shipping paper.** If shipping paper not available or no answer, refer to appropriate telephone number listed on the inside back cover.
- Keep unauthorized personnel away.
- Stay upwind, uphill and/or upstream.
- Ventilate closed spaces before entering, but only if properly trained and equipped.

PROTECTIVE CLOTHING

- Wear positive pressure self-contained breathing apparatus (SCBA).
- Structural firefighters' protective clothing provides thermal protection **but only limited chemical protection.**

EVACUATION

Immediate precautionary measure

- Isolate spill or leak area for at least 50 meters (150 feet) in all directions.

Large Spill

- Consider initial downwind evacuation for at least 300 meters (1000 feet).

Fire

- If tank, rail car or tank truck is involved in a fire, ISOLATE for 800 meters (1/2 mile) in all directions; also, consider initial evacuation for 800 meters (1/2 mile) in all directions.

In Canada, an Emergency Response Assistance Plan (ERAP) may be required for this product. Please consult the shipping paper and/or the ERAP Program Section (page 390).

EMERGENCY RESPONSE

FIRE

CAUTION: The majority of these products have a very low flash point. Use of water spray when fighting fire may be inefficient.

Small Fire

- Dry chemical, CO_2, water spray or alcohol-resistant foam.
- **Do not use dry chemical extinguishers to control fires involving nitromethane (UN1261) or nitroethane (UN2842).**

Large Fire

- Water spray, fog or alcohol-resistant foam.
- Avoid aiming straight or solid streams directly onto the product.
- If it can be done safely, move undamaged containers away from the area around the fire.

Fire Involving Tanks or Car/Trailer Loads

- Fight fire from maximum distance or use unmanned master stream devices or monitor nozzles.
- Cool containers with flooding quantities of water until well after fire is out.
- Withdraw immediately in case of rising sound from venting safety devices or discoloration of tank.
- ALWAYS stay away from tanks engulfed in fire.
- For massive fire, use unmanned master stream devices or monitor nozzles; if this is impossible, withdraw from area and let fire burn.

SPILL OR LEAK

- ELIMINATE all ignition sources (no smoking, flares, sparks or flames) from immediate area.
- All equipment used when handling the product must be grounded.
- Do not touch or walk through spilled material.
- Stop leak if you can do it without risk.
- Prevent entry into waterways, sewers, basements or confined areas.
- A vapor-suppressing foam may be used to reduce vapors.
- Absorb or cover with dry earth, sand or other non-combustible material and transfer to containers.
- Use clean, non-sparking tools to collect absorbed material.

Large Spill

- Dike far ahead of liquid spill for later disposal.
- Water spray may reduce vapor, but may not prevent ignition in closed spaces.

FIRST AID

- Call 911 or emergency medical service.
- Ensure that medical personnel are aware of the material(s) involved and take precautions to protect themselves.
- Move victim to fresh air if it can be done safely.
- Give artificial respiration if victim is not breathing.
- Administer oxygen if breathing is difficult.
- Remove and isolate contaminated clothing and shoes.
- In case of contact with substance, immediately flush skin or eyes with running water for at least 20 minutes.
- Wash skin with soap and water.
- In case of burns, immediately cool affected skin for as long as possible with cold water. Do not remove clothing if adhering to skin.
- Keep victim calm and warm.
- Effects of exposure (inhalation, ingestion or skin contact) to substance may be delayed.

GUIDE 130 FLAMMABLE LIQUIDS (WATER-IMMISCIBLE/NOXIOUS)

POTENTIAL HAZARDS

FIRE OR EXPLOSION

- **HIGHLY FLAMMABLE: Will be easily ignited by heat, sparks or flames.**
- Vapors may form explosive mixtures with air.
- Vapors may travel to source of ignition and flash back.
- Most vapors are heavier than air. They will spread along the ground and collect in low or confined areas (sewers, basements, tanks, etc.).
- Vapor explosion hazard indoors, outdoors or in sewers.
- Those substances designated with a **(P)** may polymerize explosively when heated or involved in a fire.
- Runoff to sewer may create fire or explosion hazard.
- Containers may explode when heated.
- Many liquids will float on water.

HEALTH

- May cause toxic effects if inhaled or absorbed through skin.
- Inhalation or contact with material may irritate or burn skin and eyes.
- Fire will produce irritating, corrosive and/or toxic gases.
- Vapors may cause dizziness or asphyxiation.
- Runoff from fire control or dilution water may cause environmental contamination.

PUBLIC SAFETY

- **CALL 911. Then call emergency response telephone number on shipping paper.** If shipping paper not available or no answer, refer to appropriate telephone number listed on the inside back cover.
- Keep unauthorized personnel away.
- Stay upwind, uphill and/or upstream.
- Ventilate closed spaces before entering, but only if properly trained and equipped.

PROTECTIVE CLOTHING

- Wear positive pressure self-contained breathing apparatus (SCBA).
- Structural firefighters' protective clothing provides thermal protection **but only limited chemical protection**.

EVACUATION

Immediate precautionary measure

- Isolate spill or leak area for at least 50 meters (150 feet) in all directions.

Large Spill

- Consider initial downwind evacuation for at least 300 meters (1000 feet).

Fire

- If tank, rail car or tank truck is involved in a fire, ISOLATE for 800 meters (1/2 mile) in all directions; also, consider initial evacuation for 800 meters (1/2 mile) in all directions.

EMERGENCY RESPONSE

FIRE

CAUTION: The majority of these products have a very low flash point. Use of water spray when fighting fire may be inefficient.

Small Fire

- Dry chemical, CO_2, water spray or regular foam.

Large Fire

- Water spray, fog or regular foam.
- Avoid aiming straight or solid streams directly onto the product.
- If it can be done safely, move undamaged containers away from the area around the fire.

Fire Involving Tanks or Car/Trailer Loads

- Fight fire from maximum distance or use unmanned master stream devices or monitor nozzles.
- Cool containers with flooding quantities of water until well after fire is out.
- Withdraw immediately in case of rising sound from venting safety devices or discoloration of tank.
- ALWAYS stay away from tanks engulfed in fire.
- For massive fire, use unmanned master stream devices or monitor nozzles; if this is impossible, withdraw from area and let fire burn.

SPILL OR LEAK

- ELIMINATE all ignition sources (no smoking, flares, sparks or flames) from immediate area.
- All equipment used when handling the product must be grounded.
- Do not touch or walk through spilled material.
- Stop leak if you can do it without risk.
- Prevent entry into waterways, sewers, basements or confined areas.
- A vapor-suppressing foam may be used to reduce vapors.
- Absorb or cover with dry earth, sand or other non-combustible material and transfer to containers.
- Use clean, non-sparking tools to collect absorbed material.

Large Spill

- Dike far ahead of liquid spill for later disposal.
- Water spray may reduce vapor, but may not prevent ignition in closed spaces.

FIRST AID

- Call 911 or emergency medical service.
- Ensure that medical personnel are aware of the material(s) involved and take precautions to protect themselves.
- Move victim to fresh air if it can be done safely.
- Give artificial respiration if victim is not breathing.
- Administer oxygen if breathing is difficult.
- Remove and isolate contaminated clothing and shoes.
- In case of contact with substance, immediately flush skin or eyes with running water for at least 20 minutes.
- Wash skin with soap and water.
- In case of burns, immediately cool affected skin for as long as possible with cold water. Do not remove clothing if adhering to skin.
- Keep victim calm and warm.
- Effects of exposure (inhalation, ingestion or skin contact) to substance may be delayed.

GUIDE 131 FLAMMABLE LIQUIDS - TOXIC

POTENTIAL HAZARDS

HEALTH

- **TOXIC; may be fatal if inhaled, ingested or absorbed through skin.**
- Inhalation or contact with some of these materials will irritate or burn skin and eyes.
- Fire will produce irritating, corrosive and/or toxic gases.
- Vapors may cause dizziness or asphyxiation.
- Runoff from fire control or dilution water may cause environmental contamination.

FIRE OR EXPLOSION

- **HIGHLY FLAMMABLE: Will be easily ignited by heat, sparks or flames.**

CAUTION: Methanol (UN1230) will burn with an invisible flame. Use an alternate method of detection (thermal camera, broom handle, etc.)

- Vapors may form explosive mixtures with air.
- Vapors may travel to source of ignition and flash back.
- Most vapors are heavier than air. They will spread along the ground and collect in low or confined areas (sewers, basements, tanks, etc.).
- Vapor explosion and poison hazard indoors, outdoors or in sewers.
- Those substances designated with a **(P)** may polymerize explosively when heated or involved in a fire.
- Runoff to sewer may create fire or explosion hazard.
- Containers may explode when heated.
- Many liquids will float on water.

PUBLIC SAFETY

- **CALL 911. Then call emergency response telephone number on shipping paper.** If shipping paper not available or no answer, refer to appropriate telephone number listed on the inside back cover.
- Keep unauthorized personnel away.
- Stay upwind, uphill and/or upstream.
- Ventilate closed spaces before entering, but only if properly trained and equipped.

PROTECTIVE CLOTHING

- Wear positive pressure self-contained breathing apparatus (SCBA).
- Wear chemical protective clothing that is specifically recommended by the manufacturer **when there is NO RISK OF FIRE**.
- Structural firefighters' protective clothing provides thermal protection **but only limited chemical protection**.

EVACUATION

Immediate precautionary measure

- Isolate spill or leak area for at least 50 meters (150 feet) in all directions.

Spill

- For highlighted materials: see Table 1 - Initial Isolation and Protective Action Distances.
- For non-highlighted materials: increase the immediate precautionary measure distance, in the downwind direction, as necessary.

Fire

- If tank, rail car or tank truck is involved in a fire, ISOLATE for 800 meters (1/2 mile) in all directions; also, consider initial evacuation for 800 meters (1/2 mile) in all directions.

In Canada, an Emergency Response Assistance Plan (ERAP) may be required for this product. Please consult the shipping paper and/or the ERAP Program Section (page 390).

EMERGENCY RESPONSE

FIRE

CAUTION: The majority of these products have a very low flash point. Use of water spray when fighting fire may be inefficient.

CAUTION: Methanol (UN1230) will burn with an invisible flame. Use an alternate method of detection (thermal camera, broom handle, etc.)

Small Fire

- Dry chemical, CO_2, water spray or alcohol-resistant foam.

Large Fire

- Water spray, fog or alcohol-resistant foam.
- If it can be done safely, move undamaged containers away from the area around the fire.
- Dike runoff from fire control for later disposal.
- Avoid aiming straight or solid streams directly onto the product.

Fire Involving Tanks or Car/Trailer Loads

- Fight fire from maximum distance or use unmanned master stream devices or monitor nozzles.
- Cool containers with flooding quantities of water until well after fire is out.
- Withdraw immediately in case of rising sound from venting safety devices or discoloration of tank.
- ALWAYS stay away from tanks engulfed in fire.
- For massive fire, use unmanned master stream devices or monitor nozzles; if this is impossible, withdraw from area and let fire burn.

SPILL OR LEAK

- ELIMINATE all ignition sources (no smoking, flares, sparks or flames) from immediate area.
- All equipment used when handling the product must be grounded.
- Do not touch or walk through spilled material.
- Stop leak if you can do it without risk.
- Prevent entry into waterways, sewers, basements or confined areas.
- A vapor-suppressing foam may be used to reduce vapors.

Small Spill

- Absorb with earth, sand or other non-combustible material and transfer to containers for later disposal.
- Use clean, non-sparking tools to collect absorbed material.

Large Spill

- Dike far ahead of liquid spill for later disposal.
- Water spray may reduce vapor, but may not prevent ignition in closed spaces.

FIRST AID

- Call 911 or emergency medical service.
- Ensure that medical personnel are aware of the material(s) involved and take precautions to protect themselves.
- Move victim to fresh air if it can be done safely.
- Give artificial respiration if victim is not breathing.
- **Do not perform mouth-to-mouth resuscitation if victim ingested or inhaled the substance; wash face and mouth before giving artificial respiration. Use a pocket mask equipped with a one-way valve or other proper respiratory medical device.**
- Administer oxygen if breathing is difficult.
- Remove and isolate contaminated clothing and shoes.
- In case of contact with substance, immediately flush skin or eyes with running water for at least 20 minutes.
- Wash skin with soap and water.
- In case of burns, immediately cool affected skin for as long as possible with cold water. Do not remove clothing if adhering to skin.
- Keep victim calm and warm.
- Effects of exposure (inhalation, ingestion or skin contact) to substance may be delayed.

GUIDE 132 Flammable Liquids - Corrosive

POTENTIAL HAZARDS

FIRE OR EXPLOSION

- Flammable/combustible material.
- May be ignited by heat, sparks or flames.
- Vapors may form explosive mixtures with air.
- Vapors may travel to source of ignition and flash back.
- Most vapors are heavier than air. They will spread along the ground and collect in low or confined areas (sewers, basements, tanks, etc.).
- Vapor explosion hazard indoors, outdoors or in sewers.
- Those substances designated with a **(P)** may polymerize explosively when heated or involved in a fire.
- Runoff to sewer may create fire or explosion hazard.
- Containers may explode when heated.
- Many liquids will float on water.

HEALTH

- May cause toxic effects if inhaled or ingested.
- Contact with substance may cause severe burns to skin and eyes.
- Fire will produce irritating, corrosive and/or toxic gases.
- Vapors may cause dizziness or asphyxiation.
- Runoff from fire control or dilution water may cause environmental contamination.

PUBLIC SAFETY

- **CALL 911. Then call emergency response telephone number on shipping paper.** If shipping paper not available or no answer, refer to appropriate telephone number listed on the inside back cover.
- Keep unauthorized personnel away.
- Stay upwind, uphill and/or upstream.
- Ventilate closed spaces before entering, but only if properly trained and equipped.

PROTECTIVE CLOTHING

- Wear positive pressure self-contained breathing apparatus (SCBA).
- Wear chemical protective clothing that is specifically recommended by the manufacturer **when there is NO RISK OF FIRE**.
- Structural firefighters' protective clothing provides thermal protection **but only limited chemical protection**.

EVACUATION

Immediate precautionary measure

- Isolate spill or leak area for at least 50 meters (150 feet) in all directions.

Spill

- For highlighted materials: see Table 1 - Initial Isolation and Protective Action Distances.
- For non-highlighted materials: increase the immediate precautionary measure distance, in the downwind direction, as necessary.

Fire

- If tank, rail car or tank truck is involved in a fire, ISOLATE for 800 meters (1/2 mile) in all directions; also, consider initial evacuation for 800 meters (1/2 mile) in all directions.

In Canada, an Emergency Response Assistance Plan (ERAP) may be required for this product. Please consult the shipping paper and/or the ERAP Program Section (page 390).

EMERGENCY RESPONSE

FIRE

- **Some of these materials may react violently with water.**

Small Fire

- Dry chemical, CO_2, water spray or alcohol resistant foam.

Large Fire

- Water spray, fog or alcohol-resistant foam.
- If it can be done safely, move undamaged containers away from the area around the fire.
- Dike runoff from fire control for later disposal.
- Do not get water inside containers.

Fire Involving Tanks or Car/Trailer Loads

- Fight fire from maximum distance or use unmanned master stream devices or monitor nozzles.
- Cool containers with flooding quantities of water until well after fire is out.
- Withdraw immediately in case of rising sound from venting safety devices or discoloration of tank.
- ALWAYS stay away from tanks engulfed in fire.
- For massive fire, use unmanned master stream devices or monitor nozzles; if this is impossible, withdraw from area and let fire burn.

SPILL OR LEAK

- ELIMINATE all ignition sources (no smoking, flares, sparks or flames) from immediate area.
- All equipment used when handling the product must be grounded.
- Do not touch or walk through spilled material.
- Stop leak if you can do it without risk.
- Prevent entry into waterways, sewers, basements or confined areas.
- A vapor-suppressing foam may be used to reduce vapors.
- Absorb with earth, sand or other non-combustible material.
- For **hydrazine**, absorb with DRY sand or inert absorbent (vermiculite or absorbent pads).
- Use clean, non-sparking tools to collect absorbed material.

Large Spill

- Dike far ahead of liquid spill for later disposal.
- Water spray may reduce vapor, but may not prevent ignition in closed spaces.

FIRST AID

- Call 911 or emergency medical service.
- Ensure that medical personnel are aware of the material(s) involved and take precautions to protect themselves.
- Move victim to fresh air if it can be done safely.
- Give artificial respiration if victim is not breathing.
- **Do not perform mouth-to-mouth resuscitation if victim ingested or inhaled the substance; wash face and mouth before giving artificial respiration. Use a pocket mask equipped with a one-way valve or other proper respiratory medical device.**
- Administer oxygen if breathing is difficult.
- Remove and isolate contaminated clothing and shoes.
- In case of contact with substance, immediately flush skin or eyes with running water for at least 20 minutes.
- In case of burns, immediately cool affected skin for as long as possible with cold water. Do not remove clothing if adhering to skin.
- Keep victim calm and warm.
- Effects of exposure (inhalation, ingestion or skin contact) to substance may be delayed.

GUIDE 133 Flammable Solids

POTENTIAL HAZARDS

FIRE OR EXPLOSION

- Flammable/combustible material.
- May be ignited by friction, heat, sparks or flames.
- Some may burn rapidly with flare-burning effect.
- Powders, dusts, shavings, borings, turnings or cuttings may explode or burn with explosive violence.
- Substance may be transported in a molten form at a temperature that may be above its flash point.
- May re-ignite after fire is extinguished.

HEALTH

- Fire may produce irritating and/or toxic gases.
- Contact may cause burns to skin and eyes.
- Contact with molten substance may cause severe burns to skin and eyes.
- Runoff from fire control or dilution water may cause environmental contamination.

PUBLIC SAFETY

- **CALL 911. Then call emergency response telephone number on shipping paper.** If shipping paper not available or no answer, refer to appropriate telephone number listed on the inside back cover.
- Keep unauthorized personnel away.
- Stay upwind, uphill and/or upstream.

PROTECTIVE CLOTHING

- Wear positive pressure self-contained breathing apparatus (SCBA).
- Structural firefighters' protective clothing provides thermal protection **but only limited chemical protection**.

EVACUATION

Immediate precautionary measure

- Isolate spill or leak area for at least 25 meters (75 feet) in all directions.

Large Spill

- Consider initial downwind evacuation for at least 100 meters (330 feet).

Fire

- If tank, rail car or tank truck is involved in a fire, ISOLATE for 800 meters (1/2 mile) in all directions; also, consider initial evacuation for 800 meters (1/2 mile) in all directions.

In Canada, an Emergency Response Assistance Plan (ERAP) may be required for this product. Please consult the shipping paper and/or the ERAP Program Section (page 390).

EMERGENCY RESPONSE

FIRE

Small Fire

- Dry chemical, CO_2, sand, earth, water spray or regular foam.

Large Fire

- Water spray, fog or regular foam.
- If it can be done safely, move undamaged containers away from the area around the fire.

Fire Involving Metal Pigments or Pastes (e.g. "Aluminum Paste")

- Aluminum Paste fires should be treated as a combustible metal fire. Use DRY sand, graphite powder, dry sodium chloride-based extinguishers or class D extinguishers. Also, see GUIDE 170.

Fire Involving Tanks or Car/Trailer Loads

- Cool containers with flooding quantities of water until well after fire is out.
- For massive fire, use unmanned master stream devices or monitor nozzles; if this is impossible, withdraw from area and let fire burn.
- Withdraw immediately in case of rising sound from venting safety devices or discoloration of tank.
- ALWAYS stay away from tanks engulfed in fire.

SPILL OR LEAK

- ELIMINATE all ignition sources (no smoking, flares, sparks or flames) from immediate area.
- Do not touch or walk through spilled material.

Small Dry Spill

- With clean shovel, place material into clean, dry container and cover loosely; move containers from spill area.

Large Spill

- Wet down with water and dike for later disposal.
- Prevent entry into waterways, sewers, basements or confined areas.

FIRST AID

- Call 911 or emergency medical service.
- Ensure that medical personnel are aware of the material(s) involved and take precautions to protect themselves.
- Move victim to fresh air if it can be done safely.
- Give artificial respiration if victim is not breathing.
- Administer oxygen if breathing is difficult.
- Remove and isolate contaminated clothing and shoes.
- In case of contact with substance, immediately flush skin or eyes with running water for at least 20 minutes.
- Removal of solidified molten material from skin requires medical assistance.
- Keep victim calm and warm.

GUIDE 134 FLAMMABLE SOLIDS - TOXIC AND/OR CORROSIVE

POTENTIAL HAZARDS

FIRE OR EXPLOSION

- Flammable/combustible material.
- May be ignited by heat, sparks or flames.
- When heated, vapors may form explosive mixtures with air: indoors, outdoors and sewers explosion hazards.
- Contact with metals may evolve flammable hydrogen gas.
- Containers may explode when heated.

HEALTH

- **TOXIC;** inhalation, ingestion or skin contact with material may cause severe injury or death.
- Fire will produce irritating, corrosive and/or toxic gases.
- Runoff from fire control or dilution water may be corrosive and/or toxic and cause environmental contamination.

PUBLIC SAFETY

- **CALL 911. Then call emergency response telephone number on shipping paper**. If shipping paper not available or no answer, refer to appropriate telephone number listed on the inside back cover.
- Stay upwind, uphill and/or upstream.
- Keep unauthorized personnel away.
- Ventilate closed spaces before entering, but only if properly trained and equipped.

PROTECTIVE CLOTHING

- Wear positive pressure self-contained breathing apparatus (SCBA).
- Wear chemical protective clothing that is specifically recommended by the manufacturer **when there is NO RISK OF FIRE**.
- Structural firefighters' protective clothing provides thermal protection **but only limited chemical protection**.

EVACUATION

Immediate precautionary measure

- Isolate spill or leak area for at least 25 meters (75 feet) in all directions.

Large Spill

- Consider initial downwind evacuation for at least 100 meters (330 feet).

Fire

- If tank, rail car or tank truck is involved in a fire, ISOLATE for 800 meters (1/2 mile) in all directions; also, consider initial evacuation for 800 meters (1/2 mile) in all directions.

In Canada, an Emergency Response Assistance Plan (ERAP) may be required for this product. Please consult the shipping paper and/or the ERAP Program Section (page 390).

EMERGENCY RESPONSE

FIRE

Small Fire

- Dry chemical, CO_2, water spray or alcohol-resistant foam.

Large Fire

- Water spray, fog or alcohol-resistant foam.
- If it can be done safely, move undamaged containers away from the area around the fire.
- Avoid aiming straight or solid streams directly onto the product.
- Do not get water inside containers.
- Dike runoff from fire control for later disposal.

Fire Involving Tanks or Car/Trailer Loads

- Fight fire from maximum distance or use unmanned master stream devices or monitor nozzles.
- Cool containers with flooding quantities of water until well after fire is out.
- Withdraw immediately in case of rising sound from venting safety devices or discoloration of tank.
- ALWAYS stay away from tanks engulfed in fire.

SPILL OR LEAK

- ELIMINATE all ignition sources (no smoking, flares, sparks or flames) from immediate area.
- Stop leak if you can do it without risk.
- Do not touch damaged containers or spilled material unless wearing appropriate protective clothing.
- Prevent entry into waterways, sewers, basements or confined areas.
- Use clean, non-sparking tools to collect material and place it into loosely covered plastic containers for later disposal.

FIRST AID

- Call 911 or emergency medical service.
- Ensure that medical personnel are aware of the material(s) involved and take precautions to protect themselves.
- Move victim to fresh air if it can be done safely.
- Give artificial respiration if victim is not breathing.
- **Do not perform mouth-to-mouth resuscitation if victim ingested or inhaled the substance; wash face and mouth before giving artificial respiration. Use a pocket mask equipped with a one-way valve or other proper respiratory medical device.**
- Administer oxygen if breathing is difficult.
- Remove and isolate contaminated clothing and shoes.
- In case of contact with substance, immediately flush skin or eyes with running water for at least 20 minutes.
- For minor skin contact, avoid spreading material on unaffected skin.
- Keep victim calm and warm.
- Effects of exposure (inhalation, ingestion or skin contact) to substance may be delayed.

GUIDE 135 SUBSTANCES - SPONTANEOUSLY COMBUSTIBLE

POTENTIAL HAZARDS

FIRE OR EXPLOSION

- Flammable/combustible material.
- May ignite on contact with moist air or moisture.
- May burn rapidly with flare-burning effect.
- Some react vigorously or explosively on contact with water.
- Some may decompose explosively when heated or involved in a fire.
- May re-ignite after fire is extinguished.
- Runoff may create fire or explosion hazard.
- Containers may explode when heated.

HEALTH

- Fire will produce irritating, corrosive and/or toxic gases.
- Inhalation of decomposition products may cause severe injury or death.
- Contact with substance may cause severe burns to skin and eyes.
- Runoff from fire control or dilution water may cause environmental contamination.

CAUTION: Pentaborane (UN1380) is highly toxic and may be fatal if inhaled, ingested or absorbed through skin.

PUBLIC SAFETY

- **CALL 911. Then call emergency response telephone number on shipping paper.** If shipping paper not available or no answer, refer to appropriate telephone number listed on the inside back cover.
- Stay upwind, uphill and/or upstream.
- Keep unauthorized personnel away.

PROTECTIVE CLOTHING

- Wear positive pressure self-contained breathing apparatus (SCBA).
- Wear chemical protective clothing that is specifically recommended by the manufacturer **when there is NO RISK OF FIRE**.
- Structural firefighters' protective clothing provides thermal protection **but only limited chemical protection**.

EVACUATION

Immediate precautionary measure

- Isolate spill or leak area in all directions for at least 50 meters (150 feet) for liquids and at least 25 meters (75 feet) for solids.

Spill

- For highlighted materials: see Table 1 - Initial Isolation and Protective Action Distances.
- For non-highlighted materials: increase the immediate precautionary measure distance, in the downwind direction, as necessary.

Fire

- If tank, rail car or tank truck is involved in a fire, ISOLATE for 800 meters (1/2 mile) in all directions; also, consider initial evacuation for 800 meters (1/2 mile) in all directions.

In Canada, an Emergency Response Assistance Plan (ERAP) may be required for this product. Please consult the shipping paper and/or the ERAP Program Section (page 390).

EMERGENCY RESPONSE

FIRE

- **DO NOT USE WATER, CO_2 OR FOAM ON MATERIAL ITSELF.**
- Some of these materials may react violently with water.

CAUTION: For Xanthates, UN3342 and for Dithionite (Hydrosulfite/Hydrosulphite) UN1384, UN1923 and UN1929, USE FLOODING AMOUNTS OF WATER for SMALL AND LARGE fires to stop the reaction. Smothering will not work for these materials, they do not need air to burn.

Small Fire

- Dry chemical, soda ash, lime or DRY sand, **EXCEPT for UN1384, UN1923, UN1929 and UN3342**.

Large Fire

- DRY sand, dry chemical, soda ash or lime **EXCEPT for UN1384, UN1923, UN1929 and UN3342**, or withdraw from area and let fire burn.

CAUTION: UN3342 when flooded with water will continue to evolve flammable Carbon disulfide/Carbon disulphide vapors.

- If it can be done safely, move undamaged containers away from the area around the fire.

Fire Involving Tanks or Car/Trailer Loads

- Fight fire from maximum distance or use unmanned master stream devices or monitor nozzles.
- Do not get water inside containers or in contact with substance.
- Cool containers with flooding quantities of water until well after fire is out.
- Withdraw immediately in case of rising sound from venting safety devices or discoloration of tank.
- ALWAYS stay away from tanks engulfed in fire.

SPILL OR LEAK

- ELIMINATE all ignition sources (no smoking, flares, sparks or flames) from immediate area.
- Do not touch or walk through spilled material.
- Stop leak if you can do it without risk.

Small Spill

CAUTION: For spills of Xanthates, UN3342 and for Dithionite (Hydrosulfite/Hydrosulphite), UN1384, UN1923 and UN1929, dissolve in 5 parts water and collect for proper disposal.

CAUTION: UN3342 when flooded with water will continue to evolve flammable Carbon disulfide/Carbon disulphide vapors.

- Cover with DRY earth, DRY sand or other non-combustible material followed with plastic sheet to minimize spreading or contact with rain.
- Use clean, non-sparking tools to collect material and place it into loosely covered plastic containers for later disposal.
- Prevent entry into waterways, sewers, basements or confined areas.

FIRST AID

- Call 911 or emergency medical service.
- Ensure that medical personnel are aware of the material(s) involved and take precautions to protect themselves.
- Move victim to fresh air if it can be done safely.
- Give artificial respiration if victim is not breathing.
- Administer oxygen if breathing is difficult.
- Remove and isolate contaminated clothing and shoes.
- In case of contact with substance, immediately flush skin or eyes with running water for at least 20 minutes.
- Keep victim calm and warm.

GUIDE 136 SUBSTANCES - SPONTANEOUSLY COMBUSTIBLE - TOXIC AND/OR CORROSIVE (AIR-REACTIVE)

POTENTIAL HAZARDS

FIRE OR EXPLOSION

- Extremely flammable; will ignite itself if exposed to air.
- Burns rapidly, releasing dense, white, irritating fumes.
- Substance may be transported in a molten form.
- May re-ignite after fire is extinguished.
- Corrosive substances in contact with metals may produce flammable hydrogen gas.
- Containers may explode when heated.

HEALTH

- Fire will produce irritating, corrosive and/or toxic gases.
- **TOXIC**; ingestion of substance or inhalation of decomposition products will cause severe injury or death.
- Contact with substance may cause severe burns to skin and eyes.
- Some effects may be experienced due to skin absorption.
- Runoff from fire control or dilution water may be corrosive and/or toxic and cause environmental contamination.

PUBLIC SAFETY

- **CALL 911. Then call emergency response telephone number on shipping paper.** If shipping paper not available or no answer, refer to appropriate telephone number listed on the inside back cover.
- Stay upwind, uphill and/or upstream.
- Keep unauthorized personnel away.

PROTECTIVE CLOTHING

- Wear positive pressure self-contained breathing apparatus (SCBA).
- Wear chemical protective clothing that is specifically recommended by the manufacturer **when there is NO RISK OF FIRE**.
- Structural firefighters' protective clothing provides thermal protection **but only limited chemical protection**.
- **For Phosphorus (UN1381): Special aluminized protective clothing should be worn when direct contact with the substance is possible.**

EVACUATION

Immediate precautionary measure

- Isolate spill or leak area in all directions for at least 50 meters (150 feet) for liquids and at least 25 meters (75 feet) for solids.

Spill

- Consider initial downwind evacuation for at least 300 meters (1000 feet).

Fire

- If tank, rail car or tank truck is involved in a fire, ISOLATE for 800 meters (1/2 mile) in all directions; also, consider initial evacuation for 800 meters (1/2 mile) in all directions.

In Canada, an Emergency Response Assistance Plan (ERAP) may be required for this product. Please consult the shipping paper and/or the ERAP Program Section (page 390).

EMERGENCY RESPONSE

FIRE

Small Fire

- Water spray, wet sand or wet earth.

Large Fire

- Water spray or fog.
- **Do not scatter spilled material with high-pressure water streams.**
- If it can be done safely, move undamaged containers away from the area around the fire.

Fire Involving Tanks or Car/Trailer Loads

- Fight fire from maximum distance or use unmanned master stream devices or monitor nozzles.
- Cool containers with flooding quantities of water until well after fire is out.
- Withdraw immediately in case of rising sound from venting safety devices or discoloration of tank.
- ALWAYS stay away from tanks engulfed in fire.

SPILL OR LEAK

- ELIMINATE all ignition sources (no smoking, flares, sparks or flames) from immediate area.
- Do not touch or walk through spilled material.
- Do not touch damaged containers or spilled material unless wearing appropriate protective clothing.
- Stop leak if you can do it without risk.

Small Spill

- Cover with water, sand or earth. Shovel into metal container and keep material under water.

Large Spill

- Dike for later disposal and cover with wet sand or earth.
- Prevent entry into waterways, sewers, basements or confined areas.

FIRST AID

- Call 911 or emergency medical service.
- Ensure that medical personnel are aware of the material(s) involved and take precautions to protect themselves.
- Move victim to fresh air if it can be done safely.
- Give artificial respiration if victim is not breathing.
- Administer oxygen if breathing is difficult.
- In case of contact with substance, keep exposed skin areas immersed in water or covered with wet bandages until medical attention is received.
- Removal of solidified molten material from skin requires medical assistance.
- Remove and isolate contaminated clothing and shoes at the site and place in metal container filled with water. Fire hazard if allowed to dry.
- Effects of exposure (inhalation, ingestion or skin contact) to substance may be delayed.
- Keep victim calm and warm.

GUIDE 137 SUBSTANCES - WATER-REACTIVE - CORROSIVE

POTENTIAL HAZARDS

HEALTH

- CORROSIVE and/or TOXIC; inhalation, ingestion or contact (skin, eyes) with vapors, dusts or substance may cause severe injury, burns or death.
- Fire will produce irritating, corrosive and/or toxic gases.
- Reaction with water may generate much heat that will increase the concentration of fumes in the air.
- Contact with molten substance may cause severe burns to skin and eyes.
- Runoff from fire control or dilution water may cause environmental contamination.

FIRE OR EXPLOSION

- **EXCEPT FOR ACETIC ANHYDRIDE (UN1715), THAT IS FLAMMABLE,** some of these materials may burn, but none ignite readily.
- May ignite combustibles (wood, paper, oil, clothing, etc.).
- Substance will react with water (some violently), releasing corrosive and/or toxic gases and runoff.
- Flammable/toxic gases may accumulate in confined areas (basement, tanks, hopper/tank cars, etc.).
- Contact with metals may evolve flammable hydrogen gas.
- Containers may explode when heated or if contaminated with water.
- Substance may be transported in a molten form.

PUBLIC SAFETY

- **CALL 911. Then call emergency response telephone number on shipping paper.** If shipping paper not available or no answer, refer to appropriate telephone number listed on the inside back cover.
- Keep unauthorized personnel away.
- Stay upwind, uphill and/or upstream.
- Ventilate closed spaces before entering, but only if properly trained and equipped.

PROTECTIVE CLOTHING

- Wear positive pressure self-contained breathing apparatus (SCBA).
- Wear chemical protective clothing that is specifically recommended by the manufacturer **when there is NO RISK OF FIRE**.
- Structural firefighters' protective clothing provides thermal protection **but only limited chemical protection**.

EVACUATION

Immediate precautionary measure

- Isolate spill or leak area in all directions for at least 50 meters (150 feet) for liquids and at least 25 meters (75 feet) for solids.

Spill

- For highlighted materials: see Table 1 - Initial Isolation and Protective Action Distances.
- For non-highlighted materials: increase the immediate precautionary measure distance, in the downwind direction, as necessary.

Fire

- If tank, rail car or tank truck is involved in a fire, ISOLATE for 800 meters (1/2 mile) in all directions; also, consider initial evacuation for 800 meters (1/2 mile) in all directions.

In Canada, an Emergency Response Assistance Plan (ERAP) may be required for this product. Please consult the shipping paper and/or the ERAP Program Section (page 390).

EMERGENCY RESPONSE

FIRE

- **When material is not involved in fire, do not use water on material itself.**

Small Fire

- Dry chemical or CO_2.
- If it can be done safely, move undamaged containers away from the area around the fire.

Large Fire

- Flood fire area with large quantities of water, while knocking down vapors with water fog. If insufficient water supply, responders should withdraw.

Fire Involving Tanks or Car/Trailer Loads

- Cool containers with flooding quantities of water until well after fire is out.
- Do not get water inside containers.
- Withdraw immediately in case of rising sound from venting safety devices or discoloration of tank.
- ALWAYS stay away from tanks engulfed in fire.

SPILL OR LEAK

- Do not touch damaged containers or spilled material unless wearing appropriate protective clothing.
- Stop leak if you can do it without risk.
- Use water spray to reduce vapors; do not put water directly on leak, spill area or inside container.
- Keep combustibles (wood, paper, oil, etc.) away from spilled material.

Small Spill

- Cover with DRY earth, DRY sand or other non-combustible material followed with plastic sheet to minimize spreading or contact with rain.
- Use clean, non-sparking tools to collect material and place it into loosely covered plastic containers for later disposal.
- Prevent entry into waterways, sewers, basements or confined areas.

FIRST AID

- Call 911 or emergency medical service.
- Ensure that medical personnel are aware of the material(s) involved and take precautions to protect themselves.
- Move victim to fresh air if it can be done safely.
- Give artificial respiration if victim is not breathing.
- **Do not perform mouth-to-mouth resuscitation if victim ingested or inhaled the substance; wash face and mouth before giving artificial respiration. Use a pocket mask equipped with a one-way valve or other proper respiratory medical device.**
- Administer oxygen if breathing is difficult.
- Remove and isolate contaminated clothing and shoes.
- In case of contact with substance, immediately flush skin or eyes with running water for at least 20 minutes.
- For minor skin contact, avoid spreading material on unaffected skin.
- Removal of solidified molten material from skin requires medical assistance.
- Keep victim calm and warm.
- Effects of exposure (inhalation, ingestion or skin contact) to substance may be delayed.

GUIDE 138 SUBSTANCES - WATER-REACTIVE (EMITTING FLAMMABLE GASES)

POTENTIAL HAZARDS

FIRE OR EXPLOSION

- Produce flammable gases on contact with water.
- May ignite on contact with water or moist air.
- Some react vigorously or explosively on contact with water.
- May be ignited by heat, sparks or flames.
- May re-ignite after fire is extinguished.
- Some are transported in highly flammable liquids.
- Runoff may create fire or explosion hazard.

HEALTH

- Inhalation or contact with vapors, substance or decomposition products may cause severe injury or death.
- May produce corrosive solutions on contact with water.
- Fire will produce irritating, corrosive and/or toxic gases.
- Runoff from fire control or dilution water may cause environmental contamination.

PUBLIC SAFETY

- **CALL 911. Then call emergency response telephone number on shipping paper.** If shipping paper not available or no answer, refer to appropriate telephone number listed on the inside back cover.
- Keep unauthorized personnel away.
- Stay upwind, uphill and/or upstream.
- Ventilate closed spaces before entering, but only if properly trained and equipped.

PROTECTIVE CLOTHING

- Wear positive pressure self-contained breathing apparatus (SCBA).
- Wear chemical protective clothing that is specifically recommended by the manufacturer **when there is NO RISK OF FIRE**.
- Structural firefighters' protective clothing provides thermal protection **but only limited chemical protection.**

EVACUATION

Immediate precautionary measure

- Isolate spill or leak area in all directions for at least 50 meters (150 feet) for liquids and at least 25 meters (75 feet) for solids.

Spill

- For highlighted materials: see Table 1 - Initial Isolation and Protective Action Distances.
- For non-highlighted materials: increase the immediate precautionary measure distance, in the downwind direction, as necessary.

Fire

- If tank, rail car or tank truck is involved in a fire, ISOLATE for 800 meters (1/2 mile) in all directions; also, consider initial evacuation for 800 meters (1/2 mile) in all directions.

In Canada, an Emergency Response Assistance Plan (ERAP) may be required for this product. Please consult the shipping paper and/or the ERAP Program Section (page 390).

EMERGENCY RESPONSE

FIRE

- **DO NOT USE WATER OR FOAM.**

Small Fire

- Dry chemical, soda ash, lime or sand.

Large Fire

- DRY sand, dry chemical, soda ash or lime or withdraw from area and let fire burn.
- If it can be done safely, move undamaged containers away from the area around the fire.

Fire Involving Metals or Powders (Aluminum, Lithium, Magnesium, etc.)

- Use dry chemical, DRY sand, sodium chloride powder, graphite powder or class D extinguishers; in addition, for Lithium you may use Lith-X® powder or copper powder. Also, see GUIDE 170.

Fire Involving Tanks or Car/Trailer Loads

- Fight fire from maximum distance or use unmanned master stream devices or monitor nozzles.
- Do not get water inside containers.
- Cool containers with flooding quantities of water until well after fire is out.
- Withdraw immediately in case of rising sound from venting safety devices or discoloration of tank.
- ALWAYS stay away from tanks engulfed in fire.

SPILL OR LEAK

- ELIMINATE all ignition sources (no smoking, flares, sparks or flames) from immediate area.
- Do not touch or walk through spilled material.
- Stop leak if you can do it without risk.
- Use water spray to reduce vapors or divert vapor cloud drift. Avoid allowing water runoff to contact spilled material.
- **DO NOT GET WATER on spilled substance or inside containers.**

Small Spill

- Cover with DRY earth, DRY sand or other non-combustible material followed with plastic sheet to minimize spreading or contact with rain.
- Dike for later disposal; do not apply water unless directed to do so.

Powder Spill

- Cover powder spill with plastic sheet or tarp to minimize spreading and keep powder dry.
- **DO NOT CLEAN-UP OR DISPOSE OF, EXCEPT UNDER SUPERVISION OF A SPECIALIST.**

FIRST AID

- Call 911 or emergency medical service.
- Ensure that medical personnel are aware of the material(s) involved and take precautions to protect themselves.
- Move victim to fresh air if it can be done safely.
- Give artificial respiration if victim is not breathing.
- Administer oxygen if breathing is difficult.
- Remove and isolate contaminated clothing and shoes.
- In case of contact with substance, wipe from skin immediately; flush skin or eyes with running water for at least 20 minutes.
- Keep victim calm and warm.

GUIDE 139 SUBSTANCES - WATER-REACTIVE (EMITTING FLAMMABLE AND TOXIC GASES)

POTENTIAL HAZARDS

FIRE OR EXPLOSION

- Produce flammable and toxic gases on contact with water.
- May ignite on contact with water or moist air.
- Some react vigorously or explosively on contact with water.
- May be ignited by heat, sparks or flames.
- May re-ignite after fire is extinguished.
- Some are transported in highly flammable liquids.
- Containers may explode when heated.
- Runoff may create fire or explosion hazard.

HEALTH

- Highly toxic: contact with water produces toxic gas, may be fatal if inhaled.
- Inhalation or contact with vapors, substance or decomposition products may cause severe injury or death.
- May produce corrosive solutions on contact with water.
- Fire will produce irritating, corrosive and/or toxic gases.
- Runoff from fire control or dilution water may cause environmental contamination.

PUBLIC SAFETY

- **CALL 911. Then call emergency response telephone number on shipping paper.** If shipping paper not available or no answer, refer to appropriate telephone number listed on the inside back cover.
- Keep unauthorized personnel away.
- Stay upwind, uphill and/or upstream.
- Ventilate closed spaces before entering, but only if properly trained and equipped.

PROTECTIVE CLOTHING

- Wear positive pressure self-contained breathing apparatus (SCBA).
- Wear chemical protective clothing that is specifically recommended by the manufacturer **when there is NO RISK OF FIRE.**
- Structural firefighters' protective clothing provides thermal protection **but only limited chemical protection.**

EVACUATION

Immediate precautionary measure

- Isolate spill or leak area in all directions for at least 50 meters (150 feet) for liquids and at least 25 meters (75 feet) for solids.

Spill

- For highlighted materials: see Table 1 - Initial Isolation and Protective Action Distances.
- For non-highlighted materials: increase the immediate precautionary measure distance, in the downwind direction, as necessary.

Fire

- If tank, rail car or tank truck is involved in a fire, ISOLATE for 800 meters (1/2 mile) in all directions; also, consider initial evacuation for 800 meters (1/2 mile) in all directions.

In Canada, an Emergency Response Assistance Plan (ERAP) may be required for this product. Please consult the shipping paper and/or the ERAP Program Section (page 390).

EMERGENCY RESPONSE

FIRE

- **DO NOT USE WATER OR FOAM. (FOAM MAY BE USED FOR CHLOROSILANES, SEE BELOW)**

Small Fire

- Dry chemical, soda ash, lime or sand.

Large Fire

- DRY sand, dry chemical, soda ash or lime or withdraw from area and let fire burn.
- **FOR CHLOROSILANES, DO NOT USE WATER**; use AFFF alcohol-resistant medium-expansion foam; **DO NOT USE** dry chemicals, soda ash or lime on chlorosilane fires (large or small) as they may release large quantities of hydrogen gas that may explode.
- If it can be done safely, move undamaged containers away from the area around the fire.

Fire Involving Tanks or Car/Trailer Loads

- Fight fire from maximum distance or use unmanned master stream devices or monitor nozzles.
- Cool containers with flooding quantities of water until well after fire is out.
- Do not get water inside containers.
- Withdraw immediately in case of rising sound from venting safety devices or discoloration of tank.
- ALWAYS stay away from tanks engulfed in fire.

SPILL OR LEAK

- ELIMINATE all ignition sources (no smoking, flares, sparks or flames) from immediate area.
- Do not touch or walk through spilled material.
- Stop leak if you can do it without risk.
- **DO NOT GET WATER on spilled substance or inside containers.**
- Use water spray to reduce vapors or divert vapor cloud drift. Avoid allowing water runoff to contact spilled material.
- **FOR CHLOROSILANES**, use AFFF alcohol-resistant medium-expansion foam to reduce vapors.

Small Spill

- Cover with DRY earth, DRY sand or other non-combustible material followed with plastic sheet to minimize spreading or contact with rain.
- Dike for later disposal; do not apply water unless directed to do so.

Powder Spill

- Cover powder spill with plastic sheet or tarp to minimize spreading and keep powder dry.
- **DO NOT CLEAN-UP OR DISPOSE OF, EXCEPT UNDER SUPERVISION OF A SPECIALIST.**

FIRST AID

- Call 911 or emergency medical service.
- Ensure that medical personnel are aware of the material(s) involved and take precautions to protect themselves.
- Move victim to fresh air if it can be done safely.
- Give artificial respiration if victim is not breathing.
- **Do not perform mouth-to-mouth resuscitation if victim ingested or inhaled the substance; wash face and mouth before giving artificial respiration. Use a pocket mask equipped with a one-way valve or other proper respiratory medical device.**
- Administer oxygen if breathing is difficult.
- Remove and isolate contaminated clothing and shoes.
- In case of contact with substance, wipe from skin immediately; flush skin or eyes with running water for at least 20 minutes.
- Keep victim calm and warm.

GUIDE 140 OXIDIZERS

POTENTIAL HAZARDS

FIRE OR EXPLOSION

- These substances will accelerate burning when involved in a fire.
- Some may decompose explosively when heated or involved in a fire.
- May explode from heat or contamination.
- Some will react explosively with hydrocarbons (fuels).
- May ignite combustibles (wood, paper, oil, clothing, etc.).
- Containers may explode when heated.
- Runoff may create fire or explosion hazard.

HEALTH

- Inhalation, ingestion or contact (skin, eyes) with vapors or substance may cause severe injury, burns or death.
- Fire may produce irritating, corrosive and/or toxic gases.
- Runoff from fire control or dilution water may cause environmental contamination.

PUBLIC SAFETY

- **CALL 911. Then call emergency response telephone number on shipping paper.** If shipping paper not available or no answer, refer to appropriate telephone number listed on the inside back cover.
- Keep unauthorized personnel away.
- Stay upwind, uphill and/or upstream.
- Ventilate closed spaces before entering, but only if properly trained and equipped.

PROTECTIVE CLOTHING

- Wear positive pressure self-contained breathing apparatus (SCBA).
- Wear chemical protective clothing that is specifically recommended by the manufacturer **when there is NO RISK OF FIRE**.
- Structural firefighters' protective clothing provides thermal protection **but only limited chemical protection**.

EVACUATION

Immediate precautionary measure

- Isolate spill or leak area in all directions for at least 50 meters (150 feet) for liquids and at least 25 meters (75 feet) for solids.

Large Spill

- Consider initial downwind evacuation for at least 100 meters (330 feet).

Fire

- If tank, rail car or tank truck is involved in a fire, ISOLATE for 800 meters (1/2 mile) in all directions; also, consider initial evacuation for 800 meters (1/2 mile) in all directions.
- If **ammonium nitrate** is in a tank, rail car or tank truck and involved in a fire, ISOLATE for 1600 meters (1 mile) in all directions; also, initiate evacuation including emergency responders for 1600 meters (1 mile) in all directions.

In Canada, an Emergency Response Assistance Plan (ERAP) may be required for this product. Please consult the shipping paper and/or the ERAP Program Section (page 390).

EMERGENCY RESPONSE

FIRE

Small Fire

- Use water. Do not use dry chemicals or foams. CO_2 or Halon® may provide limited control.

Large Fire

- Flood fire area with water from a distance.
- Do not move cargo or vehicle if cargo has been exposed to heat.
- If it can be done safely, move undamaged containers away from the area around the fire.

Fire Involving Tanks or Car/Trailer Loads

- Fight fire from maximum distance or use unmanned master stream devices or monitor nozzles.
- Cool containers with flooding quantities of water until well after fire is out.
- ALWAYS stay away from tanks engulfed in fire.
- For massive fire, use unmanned master stream devices or monitor nozzles; if this is impossible, withdraw from area and let fire burn.

SPILL OR LEAK

- Keep combustibles (wood, paper, oil, etc.) away from spilled material.
- Do not touch damaged containers or spilled material unless wearing appropriate protective clothing.
- Stop leak if you can do it without risk.
- Do not get water inside containers.

Small Dry Spill

- With clean shovel, place material into clean, dry container and cover loosely; move containers from spill area.

Small Liquid Spill

- Use a non-combustible material like vermiculite or sand to soak up the product and place into a container for later disposal.

Large Spill

- Dike far ahead of liquid spill for later disposal.

FIRST AID

- Call 911 or emergency medical service.
- Ensure that medical personnel are aware of the material(s) involved and take precautions to protect themselves.
- Move victim to fresh air if it can be done safely.
- Give artificial respiration if victim is not breathing.
- Administer oxygen if breathing is difficult.
- Remove and isolate contaminated clothing and shoes.
- Contaminated clothing may be a fire risk when dry.
- In case of contact with substance, immediately flush skin or eyes with running water for at least 20 minutes.
- Keep victim calm and warm.

GUIDE 141 OXIDIZERS - TOXIC

POTENTIAL HAZARDS

FIRE OR EXPLOSION

- These substances will accelerate burning when involved in a fire.
- May explode from heat or contamination.
- Some may burn rapidly.
- Some will react explosively with hydrocarbons (fuels).
- May ignite combustibles (wood, paper, oil, clothing, etc.).
- Containers may explode when heated.
- Runoff may create fire or explosion hazard.

HEALTH

- Toxic by ingestion.
- Inhalation of dust is toxic.
- Fire may produce irritating, corrosive and/or toxic gases.
- Contact with substance may cause severe burns to skin and eyes.
- Runoff from fire control or dilution water may cause environmental contamination.

PUBLIC SAFETY

- **CALL 911. Then call emergency response telephone number on shipping paper**. If shipping paper not available or no answer, refer to appropriate telephone number listed on the inside back cover.
- Keep unauthorized personnel away.
- Stay upwind, uphill and/or upstream.
- Ventilate closed spaces before entering, but only if properly trained and equipped.

PROTECTIVE CLOTHING

- Wear positive pressure self-contained breathing apparatus (SCBA).
- Wear chemical protective clothing that is specifically recommended by the manufacturer **when there is NO RISK OF FIRE**.
- Structural firefighters' protective clothing provides thermal protection **but only limited chemical protection**.

EVACUATION

Immediate precautionary measure

- Isolate spill or leak area in all directions for at least 50 meters (150 feet) for liquids and at least 25 meters (75 feet) for solids.

Large Spill

- Consider initial downwind evacuation for at least 100 meters (330 feet).

Fire

- If tank, rail car or tank truck is involved in a fire, ISOLATE for 800 meters (1/2 mile) in all directions; also, consider initial evacuation for 800 meters (1/2 mile) in all directions.

In Canada, an Emergency Response Assistance Plan (ERAP) may be required for this product. Please consult the shipping paper and/or the ERAP Program Section (page 390).

EMERGENCY RESPONSE

FIRE

Small Fire

- Use water. Do not use dry chemicals or foams. CO_2 or Halon® may provide limited control.

Large Fire

- Flood fire area with water from a distance.
- Do not move cargo or vehicle if cargo has been exposed to heat.
- If it can be done safely, move undamaged containers away from the area around the fire.

Fire Involving Tanks or Car/Trailer Loads

- Fight fire from maximum distance or use unmanned master stream devices or monitor nozzles.
- Cool containers with flooding quantities of water until well after fire is out.
- ALWAYS stay away from tanks engulfed in fire.
- For massive fire, use unmanned master stream devices or monitor nozzles; if this is impossible, withdraw from area and let fire burn.

SPILL OR LEAK

- Keep combustibles (wood, paper, oil, etc.) away from spilled material.
- Do not touch damaged containers or spilled material unless wearing appropriate protective clothing.
- Stop leak if you can do it without risk.

Small Dry Spill

- With clean shovel, place material into clean, dry container and cover loosely; move containers from spill area.

Large Spill

- Dike far ahead of spill for later disposal.

FIRST AID

- Call 911 or emergency medical service.
- Ensure that medical personnel are aware of the material(s) involved and take precautions to protect themselves.
- Move victim to fresh air if it can be done safely.
- Give artificial respiration if victim is not breathing.
- Administer oxygen if breathing is difficult.
- Remove and isolate contaminated clothing and shoes.
- Contaminated clothing may be a fire risk when dry.
- In case of contact with substance, immediately flush skin or eyes with running water for at least 20 minutes.
- Keep victim calm and warm.

GUIDE 142 OXIDIZERS - TOXIC (LIQUID)

POTENTIAL HAZARDS

FIRE OR EXPLOSION

- These substances will accelerate burning when involved in a fire.
- May explode from heat or contamination.
- Some will react explosively with hydrocarbons (fuels).
- May ignite combustibles (wood, paper, oil, clothing, etc.).
- Containers may explode when heated.
- Runoff may create fire or explosion hazard.

HEALTH

- **TOXIC;** inhalation, ingestion or contact (skin, eyes) with vapors or substance may cause severe injury, burns or death.
- Fire may produce irritating, corrosive and/or toxic gases.
- Toxic/flammable fumes may accumulate in confined areas (basement, tanks, tank cars, etc.).
- Runoff from fire control or dilution water may cause environmental contamination.

PUBLIC SAFETY

- **CALL 911. Then call emergency response telephone number on shipping paper.** If shipping paper not available or no answer, refer to appropriate telephone number listed on the inside back cover.
- Keep unauthorized personnel away.
- Stay upwind, uphill and/or upstream.
- Ventilate closed spaces before entering, but only if properly trained and equipped.

PROTECTIVE CLOTHING

- Wear positive pressure self-contained breathing apparatus (SCBA).
- Wear chemical protective clothing that is specifically recommended by the manufacturer **when there is NO RISK OF FIRE**.
- Structural firefighters' protective clothing provides thermal protection **but only limited chemical protection**.

EVACUATION

Immediate precautionary measure

- Isolate spill or leak area for at least 50 meters (150 feet) in all directions.

Spill

- For highlighted materials: see Table 1 - Initial Isolation and Protective Action Distances.
- For non-highlighted materials: increase the immediate precautionary measure distance, in the downwind direction, as necessary.

Fire

- If tank, rail car or tank truck is involved in a fire, ISOLATE for 800 meters (1/2 mile) in all directions; also, consider initial evacuation for 800 meters (1/2 mile) in all directions.

In Canada, an Emergency Response Assistance Plan (ERAP) may be required for this product. Please consult the shipping paper and/or the ERAP Program Section (page 390).

EMERGENCY RESPONSE

FIRE

Small Fire

- Use water. Do not use dry chemicals or foams. CO_2 or Halon® may provide limited control.

Large Fire

- Flood fire area with water from a distance.
- Do not move cargo or vehicle if cargo has been exposed to heat.
- If it can be done safely, move undamaged containers away from the area around the fire.

Fire Involving Tanks or Car/Trailer Loads

- Fight fire from maximum distance or use unmanned master stream devices or monitor nozzles.
- Cool containers with flooding quantities of water until well after fire is out.
- ALWAYS stay away from tanks engulfed in fire.
- For massive fire, use unmanned master stream devices or monitor nozzles; if this is impossible, withdraw from area and let fire burn.

SPILL OR LEAK

- Keep combustibles (wood, paper, oil, etc.) away from spilled material.
- Do not touch damaged containers or spilled material unless wearing appropriate protective clothing.
- Stop leak if you can do it without risk.
- Use water spray to reduce vapors or divert vapor cloud drift.
- Do not get water inside containers.

Small Liquid Spill

- Use a non-combustible material like vermiculite or sand to soak up the product and place into a container for later disposal.

Large Spill

- Dike far ahead of liquid spill for later disposal.

FIRST AID

- Call 911 or emergency medical service.
- Ensure that medical personnel are aware of the material(s) involved and take precautions to protect themselves.
- Move victim to fresh air if it can be done safely.
- Give artificial respiration if victim is not breathing.
- **Do not perform mouth-to-mouth resuscitation if victim ingested or inhaled the substance; wash face and mouth before giving artificial respiration. Use a pocket mask equipped with a one-way valve or other proper respiratory medical device.**
- Administer oxygen if breathing is difficult.
- Remove and isolate contaminated clothing and shoes.
- Contaminated clothing may be a fire risk when dry.
- In case of contact with substance, immediately flush skin or eyes with running water for at least 20 minutes.
- Keep victim calm and warm.

GUIDE 143 OXIDIZERS (UNSTABLE)

POTENTIAL HAZARDS

FIRE OR EXPLOSION

- May explode from friction, heat or contamination.
- These substances will accelerate burning when involved in a fire.
- May ignite combustibles (wood, paper, oil, clothing, etc.).
- Some will react explosively with hydrocarbons (fuels).
- Containers may explode when heated.
- Runoff may create fire or explosion hazard.

HEALTH

- **TOXIC;** inhalation, ingestion or contact (skin, eyes) with vapors, dusts or substance may cause severe injury, burns or death.
- Fire may produce irritating and/or toxic gases.
- Toxic fumes or dust may accumulate in confined areas (basement, tanks, hopper/tank cars, etc.).
- Runoff from fire control or dilution water may cause environmental contamination.

PUBLIC SAFETY

- **CALL 911. Then call emergency response telephone number on shipping paper.** If shipping paper not available or no answer, refer to appropriate telephone number listed on the inside back cover.
- Keep unauthorized personnel away.
- Stay upwind, uphill and/or upstream.
- Ventilate closed spaces before entering, but only if properly trained and equipped.

PROTECTIVE CLOTHING

- Wear positive pressure self-contained breathing apparatus (SCBA).
- Wear chemical protective clothing that is specifically recommended by the manufacturer **when there is NO RISK OF FIRE**.
- Structural firefighters' protective clothing provides thermal protection **but only limited chemical protection**.

EVACUATION

Immediate precautionary measure

- Isolate spill or leak area in all directions for at least 50 meters (150 feet) for liquids and at least 25 meters (75 feet) for solids.

Spill

- For highlighted materials: see Table 1 - Initial Isolation and Protective Action Distances.
- For non-highlighted materials: increase the immediate precautionary measure distance, in the downwind direction, as necessary.

Fire

- If tank, rail car or tank truck is involved in a fire, ISOLATE for 800 meters (1/2 mile) in all directions; also, consider initial evacuation for 800 meters (1/2 mile) in all directions.

In Canada, an Emergency Response Assistance Plan (ERAP) may be required for this product. Please consult the shipping paper and/or the ERAP Program Section (page 390).

EMERGENCY RESPONSE

FIRE

Small Fire

- Use water. Do not use dry chemicals or foams. CO_2 or Halon® may provide limited control.

Large Fire

- Flood fire area with water from a distance.
- Do not move cargo or vehicle if cargo has been exposed to heat.
- If it can be done safely, move undamaged containers away from the area around the fire.
- Do not get water inside containers: a violent reaction may occur.

Fire Involving Tanks or Car/Trailer Loads

- Cool containers with flooding quantities of water until well after fire is out.
- Dike runoff from fire control for later disposal.
- ALWAYS stay away from tanks engulfed in fire.
- For massive fire, use unmanned master stream devices or monitor nozzles; if this is impossible, withdraw from area and let fire burn.

SPILL OR LEAK

- Keep combustibles (wood, paper, oil, etc.) away from spilled material.
- Do not touch damaged containers or spilled material unless wearing appropriate protective clothing.
- Use water spray to reduce vapors or divert vapor cloud drift.
- Prevent entry into waterways, sewers, basements or confined areas.

Small Spill

- Flush area with large amounts of water.

Large Spill

- **DO NOT CLEAN-UP OR DISPOSE OF, EXCEPT UNDER SUPERVISION OF A SPECIALIST.**

FIRST AID

- Call 911 or emergency medical service.
- Ensure that medical personnel are aware of the material(s) involved and take precautions to protect themselves.
- Move victim to fresh air if it can be done safely.
- Give artificial respiration if victim is not breathing.
- Administer oxygen if breathing is difficult.
- Remove and isolate contaminated clothing and shoes.
- Contaminated clothing may be a fire risk when dry.
- In case of contact with substance, immediately flush skin or eyes with running water for at least 20 minutes.
- Keep victim calm and warm.

GUIDE 144 OXIDIZERS (WATER-REACTIVE)

POTENTIAL HAZARDS

FIRE OR EXPLOSION

- May ignite combustibles (wood, paper, oil, clothing, etc.).
- React vigorously and/or explosively with water.
- Produce toxic and/or corrosive substances on contact with water.
- Flammable/toxic gases may accumulate in tanks and hopper cars.
- Some may produce flammable hydrogen gas upon contact with metals.
- Containers may explode when heated.
- Runoff may create fire or explosion hazard.

HEALTH

- **TOXIC;** inhalation or contact with vapor, substance, or decomposition products may cause severe injury or death.
- Fire will produce irritating, corrosive and/or toxic gases.
- Runoff from fire control or dilution water may cause environmental contamination.

PUBLIC SAFETY

- **CALL 911. Then call emergency response telephone number on shipping paper.** If shipping paper not available or no answer, refer to appropriate telephone number listed on the inside back cover.
- Keep unauthorized personnel away.
- Stay upwind, uphill and/or upstream.
- Ventilate closed spaces before entering, but only if properly trained and equipped.

PROTECTIVE CLOTHING

- Wear positive pressure self-contained breathing apparatus (SCBA).
- Wear chemical protective clothing that is specifically recommended by the manufacturer **when there is NO RISK OF FIRE**.
- Structural firefighters' protective clothing provides thermal protection **but only limited chemical protection**.

EVACUATION

Immediate precautionary measure

- Isolate spill or leak area in all directions for at least 50 meters (150 feet) for liquids and at least 25 meters (75 feet) for solids.

Spill

- For highlighted materials: see Table 1 - Initial Isolation and Protective Action Distances.
- For non-highlighted materials: increase the immediate precautionary measure distance, in the downwind direction, as necessary.

Fire

- If tank, rail car or tank truck is involved in a fire, ISOLATE for 800 meters (1/2 mile) in all directions; also, consider initial evacuation for 800 meters (1/2 mile) in all directions.

In Canada, an Emergency Response Assistance Plan (ERAP) may be required for this product. Please consult the shipping paper and/or the ERAP Program Section (page 390).

EMERGENCY RESPONSE

FIRE

- **DO NOT USE WATER OR FOAM.**

Small Fire

- Dry chemical, soda ash or lime.

Large Fire

- DRY sand, dry chemical, soda ash or lime or withdraw from area and let fire burn.
- Do not move cargo or vehicle if cargo has been exposed to heat.
- If it can be done safely, move undamaged containers away from the area around the fire.

Fire Involving Tanks or Car/Trailer Loads

- Fight fire from maximum distance or use unmanned master stream devices or monitor nozzles.
- Cool containers with flooding quantities of water until well after fire is out.
- Withdraw immediately in case of rising sound from venting safety devices or discoloration of tank.
- ALWAYS stay away from tanks engulfed in fire.

SPILL OR LEAK

- ELIMINATE all ignition sources (no smoking, flares, sparks or flames) from immediate area.
- Do not touch damaged containers or spilled material unless wearing appropriate protective clothing.
- Stop leak if you can do it without risk.
- Use water spray to reduce vapors or divert vapor cloud drift. Avoid allowing water runoff to contact spilled material.
- **DO NOT GET WATER on spilled substance or inside containers.**

Small Spill

- Cover with DRY earth, DRY sand or other non-combustible material followed with plastic sheet to minimize spreading or contact with rain.

Large Spill

- **DO NOT CLEAN-UP OR DISPOSE OF, EXCEPT UNDER SUPERVISION OF A SPECIALIST.**

FIRST AID

- Call 911 or emergency medical service.
- Ensure that medical personnel are aware of the material(s) involved and take precautions to protect themselves.
- Move victim to fresh air if it can be done safely.
- Give artificial respiration if victim is not breathing.
- **Do not perform mouth-to-mouth resuscitation if victim ingested or inhaled the substance; wash face and mouth before giving artificial respiration. Use a pocket mask equipped with a one-way valve or other proper respiratory medical device.**
- Administer oxygen if breathing is difficult.
- Remove and isolate contaminated clothing and shoes.
- Contaminated clothing may be a fire risk when dry.
- In case of contact with substance, immediately flush skin or eyes with running water for at least 20 minutes.
- Keep victim calm and warm.
- Keep victim under observation.
- Effects of contact or inhalation may be delayed.

GUIDE 145 ORGANIC PEROXIDES (HEAT AND CONTAMINATION SENSITIVE)

POTENTIAL HAZARDS

FIRE OR EXPLOSION

- May explode from heat or contamination.
- May ignite combustibles (wood, paper, oil, clothing, etc.).
- May be ignited by heat, sparks or flames.
- May burn rapidly with flare-burning effect.
- Containers may explode when heated.
- Runoff may create fire or explosion hazard.

HEALTH

- Fire may produce irritating, corrosive and/or toxic gases.
- Ingestion or contact (skin, eyes) with substance may cause severe injury or burns.
- Runoff from fire control or dilution water may cause environmental contamination.

PUBLIC SAFETY

- **CALL 911. Then call emergency response telephone number on shipping paper.** If shipping paper not available or no answer, refer to appropriate telephone number listed on the inside back cover.
- Keep unauthorized personnel away.
- Stay upwind, uphill and/or upstream.

PROTECTIVE CLOTHING

- Wear positive pressure self-contained breathing apparatus (SCBA).
- Wear chemical protective clothing that is specifically recommended by the manufacturer **when there is NO RISK OF FIRE**.
- Structural firefighters' protective clothing provides thermal protection **but only limited chemical protection**.

EVACUATION

Immediate precautionary measure

- Isolate spill or leak area in all directions for at least 50 meters (150 feet) for liquids and at least 25 meters (75 feet) for solids.

Large Spill

- Consider initial evacuation for at least 250 meters (800 feet) in all directions.

Fire

- If tank, rail car or tank truck is involved in a fire, ISOLATE for 800 meters (1/2 mile) in all directions; also, consider initial evacuation for 800 meters (1/2 mile) in all directions.

EMERGENCY RESPONSE

FIRE

Small Fire

- Water spray or fog is preferred; if water not available use dry chemical, CO_2 or regular foam.

Large Fire

- Flood fire area with water from a distance.
- Use water spray or fog; avoid aiming straight or solid streams directly onto the product.
- Do not move cargo or vehicle if cargo has been exposed to heat.
- If it can be done safely, move undamaged containers away from the area around the fire.

Fire Involving Tanks or Car/Trailer Loads

- Fight fire from maximum distance or use unmanned master stream devices or monitor nozzles.
- Cool containers with flooding quantities of water until well after fire is out.
- ALWAYS stay away from tanks engulfed in fire.
- For massive fire, use unmanned master stream devices or monitor nozzles; if this is impossible, withdraw from area and let fire burn.

SPILL OR LEAK

- ELIMINATE all ignition sources (no smoking, flares, sparks or flames) from immediate area.
- Keep combustibles (wood, paper, oil, etc.) away from spilled material.
- Do not touch damaged containers or spilled material unless wearing appropriate protective clothing.
- Keep substance wet using water spray.
- Stop leak if you can do it without risk.

Small Spill

- Pick up with inert, damp, non-combustible material using clean, non-sparking tools and place into loosely covered plastic containers for later disposal.

Large Spill

- Wet down with water and dike for later disposal.
- Prevent entry into waterways, sewers, basements or confined areas.
- **DO NOT CLEAN-UP OR DISPOSE OF, EXCEPT UNDER SUPERVISION OF A SPECIALIST.**

FIRST AID

- Call 911 or emergency medical service.
- Ensure that medical personnel are aware of the material(s) involved and take precautions to protect themselves.
- Move victim to fresh air if it can be done safely.
- Give artificial respiration if victim is not breathing.
- Administer oxygen if breathing is difficult.
- Remove and isolate contaminated clothing and shoes.
- Contaminated clothing may be a fire risk when dry.
- Remove material from skin immediately.
- In case of contact with substance, immediately flush skin or eyes with running water for at least 20 minutes.
- Keep victim calm and warm.

GUIDE 146 ORGANIC PEROXIDES (HEAT, CONTAMINATION AND FRICTION SENSITIVE)

POTENTIAL HAZARDS

FIRE OR EXPLOSION

- May explode from heat, shock, friction or contamination.
- May ignite combustibles (wood, paper, oil, clothing, etc.).
- May be ignited by heat, sparks or flames.
- May burn rapidly with flare-burning effect.
- Containers may explode when heated.
- Runoff may create fire or explosion hazard.

HEALTH

- Fire may produce irritating, corrosive and/or toxic gases.
- Ingestion or contact (skin, eyes) with substance may cause severe injury or burns.
- Runoff from fire control or dilution water may cause environmental contamination.

PUBLIC SAFETY

- **CALL 911. Then call emergency response telephone number on shipping paper.** If shipping paper not available or no answer, refer to appropriate telephone number listed on the inside back cover.
- Keep unauthorized personnel away.
- Stay upwind, uphill and/or upstream.

PROTECTIVE CLOTHING

- Wear positive pressure self-contained breathing apparatus (SCBA).
- Wear chemical protective clothing that is specifically recommended by the manufacturer **when there is NO RISK OF FIRE**.
- Structural firefighters' protective clothing provides thermal protection **but only limited chemical protection**.

EVACUATION

Immediate precautionary measure

- Isolate spill or leak area in all directions for at least 50 meters (150 feet) for liquids and at least 25 meters (75 feet) for solids.

Large Spill

- Consider initial evacuation for at least 250 meters (800 feet) in all directions.

Fire

- If tank, rail car or tank truck is involved in a fire, ISOLATE for 800 meters (1/2 mile) in all directions; also, consider initial evacuation for 800 meters (1/2 mile) in all directions.

In Canada, an Emergency Response Assistance Plan (ERAP) may be required for this product. Please consult the shipping paper and/or the ERAP Program Section (page 390).

EMERGENCY RESPONSE

FIRE

Small Fire

- Water spray or fog is preferred; if water not available use dry chemical, CO_2 or regular foam.

Large Fire

- Flood fire area with water from a distance.
- Use water spray or fog; avoid aiming straight or solid streams directly onto the product.
- Do not move cargo or vehicle if cargo has been exposed to heat.
- If it can be done safely, move undamaged containers away from the area around the fire.

Fire Involving Tanks or Car/Trailer Loads

- Fight fire from maximum distance or use unmanned master stream devices or monitor nozzles.
- Cool containers with flooding quantities of water until well after fire is out.
- ALWAYS stay away from tanks engulfed in fire.
- For massive fire, use unmanned master stream devices or monitor nozzles; if this is impossible, withdraw from area and let fire burn.

SPILL OR LEAK

- ELIMINATE all ignition sources (no smoking, flares, sparks or flames) from immediate area.
- Keep combustibles (wood, paper, oil, etc.) away from spilled material.
- Do not touch damaged containers or spilled material unless wearing appropriate protective clothing.
- Keep substance wet using water spray.
- Stop leak if you can do it without risk.

Small Spill

- Pick up with inert, damp, non-combustible material using clean, non-sparking tools and place into loosely covered plastic containers for later disposal.

Large Spill

- Wet down with water and dike for later disposal.
- Prevent entry into waterways, sewers, basements or confined areas.
- **DO NOT CLEAN-UP OR DISPOSE OF, EXCEPT UNDER SUPERVISION OF A SPECIALIST.**

FIRST AID

- Call 911 or emergency medical service.
- Ensure that medical personnel are aware of the material(s) involved and take precautions to protect themselves.
- Move victim to fresh air if it can be done safely.
- Give artificial respiration if victim is not breathing.
- Administer oxygen if breathing is difficult.
- Remove and isolate contaminated clothing and shoes.
- Contaminated clothing may be a fire risk when dry.
- Remove material from skin immediately.
- In case of contact with substance, immediately flush skin or eyes with running water for at least 20 minutes.
- Keep victim calm and warm.

GUIDE 147 Lithium Ion Batteries

POTENTIAL HAZARDS

FIRE OR EXPLOSION

- Lithium ion batteries contain flammable liquid electrolyte that may vent, ignite and produce sparks when subjected to high temperatures (> 150°C (302°F)), when damaged or abused (e.g., mechanical damage or electrical overcharging).
- May burn rapidly with flare-burning effect.
- May ignite other batteries in close proximity.

HEALTH

- Contact with battery electrolyte may be irritating to skin, eyes and mucous membranes.
- Fire will produce irritating, corrosive and/or toxic gases.
- Burning batteries may produce toxic hydrogen fluoride gas (see GUIDE 125).
- Fumes may cause dizziness or asphyxiation.

PUBLIC SAFETY

- **CALL 911. Then call emergency response telephone number on shipping paper.** If shipping paper not available or no answer, refer to appropriate telephone number listed on the inside back cover.
- Keep unauthorized personnel away.
- Stay upwind, uphill and/or upstream.
- Ventilate closed spaces before entering, but only if properly trained and equipped.

PROTECTIVE CLOTHING

- Wear positive pressure self-contained breathing apparatus (SCBA).
- Structural firefighters' protective clothing provides thermal protection **but only limited chemical protection**.

EVACUATION

Immediate precautionary measure

- Isolate spill or leak area for at least 25 meters (75 feet) in all directions.

Large Spill

- Consider initial downwind evacuation for at least 100 meters (330 feet).

Fire

- If rail car or trailer is involved in a fire, ISOLATE for 500 meters (1/3 mile) in all directions; also initiate evacuation including emergency responders for 500 meters (1/3 mile) in all directions.

EMERGENCY RESPONSE

FIRE

Small Fire

- Dry chemical, CO_2, water spray or regular foam.

Large Fire

- Water spray, fog or regular foam.
- If it can be done safely, move undamaged containers away from the area around the fire.

SPILL OR LEAK

- ELIMINATE all ignition sources (no smoking, flares, sparks or flames) from immediate area.
- Do not touch or walk through spilled material.
- Absorb with earth, sand or other non-combustible material.
- Leaking batteries and contaminated absorbent material should be placed in metal containers.

FIRST AID

- Call 911 or emergency medical service.
- Ensure that medical personnel are aware of the material(s) involved and take precautions to protect themselves.
- Move victim to fresh air if it can be done safely.
- Give artificial respiration if victim is not breathing.
- Administer oxygen if breathing is difficult.
- Remove and isolate contaminated clothing and shoes.
- In case of contact with substance, immediately flush skin or eyes with running water for at least 20 minutes.

GUIDE 148 ORGANIC PEROXIDES (HEAT AND CONTAMINATION SENSITIVE/TEMPERATURE CONTROLLED)

POTENTIAL HAZARDS

FIRE OR EXPLOSION

- May explode from heat, contamination or loss of temperature control.
- These materials are particularly sensitive to temperature rises. Above a given "Control Temperature" they decompose violently and catch fire.
- May ignite combustibles (wood, paper, oil, clothing, etc.).
- May ignite spontaneously if exposed to air.
- May be ignited by heat, sparks or flames.
- May burn rapidly with flare-burning effect.
- Containers may explode when heated.
- Runoff may create fire or explosion hazard.

HEALTH

- Fire may produce irritating, corrosive and/or toxic gases.
- Ingestion or contact (skin, eyes) with substance may cause severe injury or burns.
- Runoff from fire control or dilution water may cause environmental contamination.

PUBLIC SAFETY

- **CALL 911. Then call emergency response telephone number on shipping paper.** If shipping paper not available or no answer, refer to appropriate telephone number listed on the inside back cover.
- Keep unauthorized personnel away.
- Stay upwind, uphill and/or upstream.

PROTECTIVE CLOTHING

- Wear positive pressure self-contained breathing apparatus (SCBA).
- Wear chemical protective clothing that is specifically recommended by the manufacturer **when there is NO RISK OF FIRE**.
- Structural firefighters' protective clothing provides thermal protection **but only limited chemical protection**.

EVACUATION

Immediate precautionary measure

- Isolate spill or leak area in all directions for at least 50 meters (150 feet) for liquids and at least 25 meters (75 feet) for solids.

Large Spill

- Consider initial evacuation for at least 250 meters (800 feet) in all directions.

Fire

- If tank, rail car or tank truck is involved in a fire, ISOLATE for 800 meters (1/2 mile) in all directions; also, consider initial evacuation for 800 meters (1/2 mile) in all directions.

In Canada, an Emergency Response Assistance Plan (ERAP) may be required for this product. Please consult the shipping paper and/or the ERAP Program Section (page 390).

EMERGENCY RESPONSE

FIRE

- **The temperature of the substance must be maintained at or below the "Control Temperature" at all times.**

Small Fire

- Water spray or fog is preferred; if water not available use dry chemical, CO_2 or regular foam.

Large Fire

- Flood fire area with water from a distance.
- Use water spray or fog; avoid aiming straight or solid streams directly onto the product.
- Do not move cargo or vehicle if cargo has been exposed to heat.
- If it can be done safely, move undamaged containers away from the area around the fire.

Fire Involving Tanks or Car/Trailer Loads

- Fight fire from maximum distance or use unmanned master stream devices or monitor nozzles.
- Cool containers with flooding quantities of water until well after fire is out.
- **BEWARE OF POSSIBLE CONTAINER EXPLOSION.**
- ALWAYS stay away from tanks engulfed in fire.
- For massive fire, use unmanned master stream devices or monitor nozzles; if this is impossible, withdraw from area and let fire burn.

SPILL OR LEAK

- **DO NOT allow the substance to warm up. Use a coolant agent such as dry ice or ice (wear thermal protective gloves). If this is not possible or none can be obtained, evacuate the area immediately.**
- ELIMINATE all ignition sources (no smoking, flares, sparks or flames) from immediate area.
- Keep combustibles (wood, paper, oil, etc.) away from spilled material.
- Do not touch or walk through spilled material.
- Stop leak if you can do it without risk.

Small Spill

- Pick up with inert, damp, non-combustible material using clean, non-sparking tools and place into loosely covered plastic containers for later disposal.

Large Spill

- Dike far ahead of liquid spill for later disposal.
- Prevent entry into waterways, sewers, basements or confined areas.
- **DO NOT CLEAN-UP OR DISPOSE OF, EXCEPT UNDER SUPERVISION OF A SPECIALIST.**

FIRST AID

- Call 911 or emergency medical service.
- Ensure that medical personnel are aware of the material(s) involved and take precautions to protect themselves.
- Move victim to fresh air if it can be done safely.
- Give artificial respiration if victim is not breathing.
- Administer oxygen if breathing is difficult.
- Remove and isolate contaminated clothing and shoes.
- Contaminated clothing may be a fire risk when dry.
- Remove material from skin immediately.
- In case of contact with substance, immediately flush skin or eyes with running water for at least 20 minutes.
- Keep victim calm and warm.

GUIDE 149 SUBSTANCES (SELF-REACTIVE)

POTENTIAL HAZARDS

FIRE OR EXPLOSION

- **Self-decomposition, self-polymerization, or self-ignition may be triggered by heat, chemical reaction, friction or impact.**
- May be ignited by heat, sparks or flames.
- Some may decompose explosively when heated or involved in a fire.
- Those substances designated with a **(P)** may polymerize explosively when heated or involved in a fire.
- May burn violently. Decomposition or polymerization may be self-accelerating and produce large amounts of gases.
- Vapors or dust may form explosive mixtures with air.

HEALTH

- Inhalation or contact with vapors, substance or decomposition products may cause severe injury or death.
- May produce irritating, toxic and/or corrosive gases.
- Runoff from fire control or dilution water may cause environmental contamination.

PUBLIC SAFETY

- **CALL 911. Then call emergency response telephone number on shipping paper.** If shipping paper not available or no answer, refer to appropriate telephone number listed on the inside back cover.
- Keep unauthorized personnel away.
- Stay upwind, uphill and/or upstream.

PROTECTIVE CLOTHING

- Wear positive pressure self-contained breathing apparatus (SCBA).
- Wear chemical protective clothing that is specifically recommended by the manufacturer **when there is NO RISK OF FIRE**.
- Structural firefighters' protective clothing provides thermal protection **but only limited chemical protection**.

EVACUATION

Immediate precautionary measure

- Isolate spill or leak area in all directions for at least 50 meters (150 feet) for liquids and at least 25 meters (75 feet) for solids.

Large Spill

- Consider initial evacuation for at least 250 meters (800 feet) in all directions.

Fire

- If tank, rail car or tank truck is involved in a fire, ISOLATE for 800 meters (1/2 mile) in all directions; also, consider initial evacuation for 800 meters (1/2 mile) in all directions.

In Canada, an Emergency Response Assistance Plan (ERAP) may be required for this product. Please consult the shipping paper and/or the ERAP Program Section (page 390).

EMERGENCY RESPONSE

FIRE

Small Fire

- Dry chemical, CO_2, water spray or regular foam.

Large Fire

- Flood fire area with water from a distance.
- If it can be done safely, move undamaged containers away from the area around the fire.

Fire Involving Tanks or Car/Trailer Loads

- **BEWARE OF POSSIBLE CONTAINER EXPLOSION.**
- Fight fire from maximum distance or use unmanned master stream devices or monitor nozzles.
- Cool containers with flooding quantities of water until well after fire is out.
- Withdraw immediately in case of rising sound from venting safety devices or discoloration of tank.
- ALWAYS stay away from tanks engulfed in fire.

SPILL OR LEAK

- ELIMINATE all ignition sources (no smoking, flares, sparks or flames) from immediate area.
- Do not touch or walk through spilled material.
- Stop leak if you can do it without risk.

Small Spill

- Pick up with inert, damp, non-combustible material using clean, non-sparking tools and place into loosely covered plastic containers for later disposal.
- Prevent entry into waterways, sewers, basements or confined areas.

FIRST AID

- Call 911 or emergency medical service.
- Ensure that medical personnel are aware of the material(s) involved and take precautions to protect themselves.
- Move victim to fresh air if it can be done safely.
- Give artificial respiration if victim is not breathing.
- Administer oxygen if breathing is difficult.
- Remove and isolate contaminated clothing and shoes.
- In case of contact with substance, immediately flush skin or eyes with running water for at least 20 minutes.
- Keep victim calm and warm.

GUIDE 150 SUBSTANCES (SELF-REACTIVE/ TEMPERATURE CONTROLLED)

POTENTIAL HAZARDS

FIRE OR EXPLOSION

- **Self-decomposition, self-polymerization, or self-ignition may be triggered by heat, chemical reaction, friction or impact.**
- Self-accelerating decomposition may occur if the specific control temperature is not maintained.
- These materials are particularly sensitive to temperature rises. Above a given "Control Temperature" they decompose or polymerize violently and may catch fire.
- May be ignited by heat, sparks or flames.
- Those substances designated with a **(P)** may polymerize explosively when heated or involved in a fire.
- Some may decompose explosively when heated or involved in a fire.
- May burn violently. Decomposition or polymerization may be self-accelerating and produce large amounts of gases.
- Vapors or dust may form explosive mixtures with air.

HEALTH

- Inhalation or contact with vapors, substance or decomposition products may cause severe injury or death.
- May produce irritating, toxic and/or corrosive gases.
- Runoff from fire control or dilution water may cause environmental contamination.

PUBLIC SAFETY

- **CALL 911. Then call emergency response telephone number on shipping paper.** If shipping paper not available or no answer, refer to appropriate telephone number listed on the inside back cover.
- Keep unauthorized personnel away.
- Stay upwind, uphill and/or upstream.

PROTECTIVE CLOTHING

- Wear positive pressure self-contained breathing apparatus (SCBA).
- Wear chemical protective clothing that is specifically recommended by the manufacturer **when there is NO RISK OF FIRE**.
- Structural firefighters' protective clothing provides thermal protection **but only limited chemical protection**.

EVACUATION

Immediate precautionary measure

- Isolate spill or leak area in all directions for at least 50 meters (150 feet) for liquids and at least 25 meters (75 feet) for solids.

Large Spill

- Consider initial evacuation for at least 250 meters (800 feet) in all directions.

Fire

- If tank, rail car or tank truck is involved in a fire, ISOLATE for 800 meters (1/2 mile) in all directions; also, consider initial evacuation for 800 meters (1/2 mile) in all directions.

In Canada, an Emergency Response Assistance Plan (ERAP) may be required for this product. Please consult the shipping paper and/or the ERAP Program Section (page 390).

EMERGENCY RESPONSE

FIRE

- **The temperature of the substance must be maintained at or below the "Control Temperature" at all times.**

Small Fire

- Dry chemical, CO_2, water spray or regular foam.

Large Fire

- Flood fire area with water from a distance.
- If it can be done safely, move undamaged containers away from the area around the fire.

Fire Involving Tanks or Car/Trailer Loads

- **BEWARE OF POSSIBLE CONTAINER EXPLOSION.**
- Fight fire from maximum distance or use unmanned master stream devices or monitor nozzles.
- Cool containers with flooding quantities of water until well after fire is out.
- Withdraw immediately in case of rising sound from venting safety devices or discoloration of tank.
- ALWAYS stay away from tanks engulfed in fire.

SPILL OR LEAK

- **DO NOT allow the substance to warm up. Use a coolant agent such as dry ice or ice (wear thermal protective gloves). If this is not possible or none can be obtained, evacuate the area immediately.**
- ELIMINATE all ignition sources (no smoking, flares, sparks or flames) from immediate area.
- Do not touch or walk through spilled material.
- Stop leak if you can do it without risk.

Small Spill

- Pick up with inert, damp, non-combustible material using clean, non-sparking tools and place into loosely covered plastic containers for later disposal.
- Prevent entry into waterways, sewers, basements or confined areas.
- **DO NOT CLEAN-UP OR DISPOSE OF, EXCEPT UNDER SUPERVISION OF A SPECIALIST.**

FIRST AID

- Call 911 or emergency medical service.
- Ensure that medical personnel are aware of the material(s) involved and take precautions to protect themselves.
- Move victim to fresh air if it can be done safely.
- Give artificial respiration if victim is not breathing.
- Administer oxygen if breathing is difficult.
- Remove and isolate contaminated clothing and shoes.
- In case of contact with substance, immediately flush skin or eyes with running water for at least 20 minutes.
- Keep victim calm and warm.

GUIDE 151 SUBSTANCES - TOXIC (NON-COMBUSTIBLE)

POTENTIAL HAZARDS

HEALTH

- **Highly toxic**, may be fatal if inhaled, ingested or absorbed through skin.
- Avoid any skin contact.
- Effects of contact or inhalation may be delayed.
- Fire may produce irritating, corrosive and/or toxic gases.
- Runoff from fire control or dilution water may be corrosive and/or toxic and cause environmental contamination.

FIRE OR EXPLOSION

- Non-combustible, substance itself does not burn but may decompose upon heating to produce corrosive and/or toxic fumes.
- Containers may explode when heated.
- Runoff may pollute waterways.

PUBLIC SAFETY

- **CALL 911. Then call emergency response telephone number on shipping paper.** If shipping paper not available or no answer, refer to appropriate telephone number listed on the inside back cover.
- Keep unauthorized personnel away.
- Stay upwind, uphill and/or upstream.

PROTECTIVE CLOTHING

- Wear positive pressure self-contained breathing apparatus (SCBA).
- Wear chemical protective clothing that is specifically recommended by the manufacturer **when there is NO RISK OF FIRE**.
- Structural firefighters' protective clothing provides thermal protection **but only limited chemical protection**.

EVACUATION

Immediate precautionary measure

- Isolate spill or leak area in all directions for at least 50 meters (150 feet) for liquids and at least 25 meters (75 feet) for solids.

Spill

- For highlighted materials: see Table 1 - Initial Isolation and Protective Action Distances.
- For non-highlighted materials: increase the immediate precautionary measure distance, in the downwind direction, as necessary.

Fire

- If tank, rail car or tank truck is involved in a fire, ISOLATE for 800 meters (1/2 mile) in all directions; also, consider initial evacuation for 800 meters (1/2 mile) in all directions.

In Canada, an Emergency Response Assistance Plan (ERAP) may be required for this product. Please consult the shipping paper and/or the ERAP Program Section (page 390).

EMERGENCY RESPONSE

FIRE

Small Fire
- Dry chemical, CO_2 or water spray.

Large Fire
- Water spray, fog or regular foam.
- If it can be done safely, move undamaged containers away from the area around the fire.
- Dike runoff from fire control for later disposal.
- Avoid aiming straight or solid streams directly onto the product.

Fire Involving Tanks or Car/Trailer Loads
- Fight fire from maximum distance or use unmanned master stream devices or monitor nozzles.
- Do not get water inside containers.
- Cool containers with flooding quantities of water until well after fire is out.
- Withdraw immediately in case of rising sound from venting safety devices or discoloration of tank.
- ALWAYS stay away from tanks engulfed in fire.
- For massive fire, use unmanned master stream devices or monitor nozzles; if this is impossible, withdraw from area and let fire burn.

SPILL OR LEAK

- Do not touch damaged containers or spilled material unless wearing appropriate protective clothing.
- Stop leak if you can do it without risk.
- Prevent entry into waterways, sewers, basements or confined areas.
- Cover with plastic sheet to prevent spreading.
- Absorb or cover with dry earth, sand or other non-combustible material and transfer to containers.
- DO NOT GET WATER INSIDE CONTAINERS.

FIRST AID

- Call 911 or emergency medical service.
- Ensure that medical personnel are aware of the material(s) involved and take precautions to protect themselves.
- Move victim to fresh air if it can be done safely.
- Give artificial respiration if victim is not breathing.
- **Do not perform mouth-to-mouth resuscitation if victim ingested or inhaled the substance; wash face and mouth before giving artificial respiration. Use a pocket mask equipped with a one-way valve or other proper respiratory medical device.**
- Administer oxygen if breathing is difficult.
- Remove and isolate contaminated clothing and shoes.
- In case of contact with substance, immediately flush skin or eyes with running water for at least 20 minutes.
- For minor skin contact, avoid spreading material on unaffected skin.
- Keep victim calm and warm.
- Effects of exposure (inhalation, ingestion or skin contact) to substance may be delayed.

GUIDE 152 SUBSTANCES - TOXIC (COMBUSTIBLE)

POTENTIAL HAZARDS

HEALTH

- **Highly toxic,** may be fatal if inhaled, ingested or absorbed through skin.
- Contact with molten substance may cause severe burns to skin and eyes.
- Avoid any skin contact.
- Effects of contact or inhalation may be delayed.
- Fire may produce irritating, corrosive and/or toxic gases.
- Runoff from fire control or dilution water may be corrosive and/or toxic and cause environmental contamination.

FIRE OR EXPLOSION

- Combustible material: may burn but does not ignite readily.
- Containers may explode when heated.
- Runoff may pollute waterways.
- Substance may be transported in a molten form.

PUBLIC SAFETY

- **CALL 911. Then call emergency response telephone number on shipping paper.** If shipping paper not available or no answer, refer to appropriate telephone number listed on the inside back cover.
- Keep unauthorized personnel away.
- Stay upwind, uphill and/or upstream.

PROTECTIVE CLOTHING

- Wear positive pressure self-contained breathing apparatus (SCBA).
- Wear chemical protective clothing that is specifically recommended by the manufacturer **when there is NO RISK OF FIRE**.
- Structural firefighters' protective clothing provides thermal protection **but only limited chemical protection**.

EVACUATION

Immediate precautionary measure

- Isolate spill or leak area in all directions for at least 50 meters (150 feet) for liquids and at least 25 meters (75 feet) for solids.

Spill

- For highlighted materials: see Table 1 - Initial Isolation and Protective Action Distances.
- For non-highlighted materials: increase the immediate precautionary measure distance, in the downwind direction, as necessary.

Fire

- If tank, rail car or tank truck is involved in a fire, ISOLATE for 800 meters (1/2 mile) in all directions; also, consider initial evacuation for 800 meters (1/2 mile) in all directions.

In Canada, an Emergency Response Assistance Plan (ERAP) may be required for this product. Please consult the shipping paper and/or the ERAP Program Section (page 390).

EMERGENCY RESPONSE

FIRE

Small Fire

- Dry chemical, CO_2 or water spray.

Large Fire

- Water spray, fog or regular foam.
- If it can be done safely, move undamaged containers away from the area around the fire.
- Dike runoff from fire control for later disposal.
- Avoid aiming straight or solid streams directly onto the product.

Fire Involving Tanks or Car/Trailer Loads

- Fight fire from maximum distance or use unmanned master stream devices or monitor nozzles.
- Do not get water inside containers.
- Cool containers with flooding quantities of water until well after fire is out.
- Withdraw immediately in case of rising sound from venting safety devices or discoloration of tank.
- ALWAYS stay away from tanks engulfed in fire.
- For massive fire, use unmanned master stream devices or monitor nozzles; if this is impossible, withdraw from area and let fire burn.

SPILL OR LEAK

- ELIMINATE all ignition sources (no smoking, flares, sparks or flames) from immediate area.
- Do not touch damaged containers or spilled material unless wearing appropriate protective clothing.
- Stop leak if you can do it without risk.
- Prevent entry into waterways, sewers, basements or confined areas.
- Cover with plastic sheet to prevent spreading.
- Absorb or cover with dry earth, sand or other non-combustible material and transfer to containers.
- DO NOT GET WATER INSIDE CONTAINERS.

FIRST AID

- Call 911 or emergency medical service.
- Ensure that medical personnel are aware of the material(s) involved and take precautions to protect themselves.
- Move victim to fresh air if it can be done safely.
- Give artificial respiration if victim is not breathing.
- **Do not perform mouth-to-mouth resuscitation if victim ingested or inhaled the substance; wash face and mouth before giving artificial respiration. Use a pocket mask equipped with a one-way valve or other proper respiratory medical device.**
- Administer oxygen if breathing is difficult.
- Remove and isolate contaminated clothing and shoes.
- In case of contact with substance, immediately flush skin or eyes with running water for at least 20 minutes.
- For minor skin contact, avoid spreading material on unaffected skin.
- Keep victim calm and warm.
- Effects of exposure (inhalation, ingestion or skin contact) to substance may be delayed.

GUIDE 153 SUBSTANCES - TOXIC AND/OR CORROSIVE (COMBUSTIBLE)

POTENTIAL HAZARDS

HEALTH

- **TOXIC**; inhalation, ingestion or skin contact with material may cause severe injury or death.
- Contact with molten substance may cause severe burns to skin and eyes.
- Avoid any skin contact.
- Effects of contact or inhalation may be delayed.
- Fire may produce irritating, corrosive and/or toxic gases.
- Runoff from fire control or dilution water may be corrosive and/or toxic and cause environmental contamination.

FIRE OR EXPLOSION

- Combustible material: may burn but does not ignite readily.
- When heated, vapors may form explosive mixtures with air: indoors, outdoors and sewers explosion hazards.
- Those substances designated with a **(P)** may polymerize explosively when heated or involved in a fire.
- Contact with metals may evolve flammable hydrogen gas.
- Containers may explode when heated.
- Runoff may pollute waterways.
- Substance may be transported in a molten form.

PUBLIC SAFETY

- **CALL 911. Then call emergency response telephone number on shipping paper.** If shipping paper not available or no answer, refer to appropriate telephone number listed on the inside back cover.
- Keep unauthorized personnel away.
- Stay upwind, uphill and/or upstream.
- Ventilate closed spaces before entering, but only if properly trained and equipped.

PROTECTIVE CLOTHING

- Wear positive pressure self-contained breathing apparatus (SCBA).
- Wear chemical protective clothing that is specifically recommended by the manufacturer **when there is NO RISK OF FIRE.**
- Structural firefighters' protective clothing provides thermal protection **but only limited chemical protection.**

EVACUATION

Immediate precautionary measure

- Isolate spill or leak area in all directions for at least 50 meters (150 feet) for liquids and at least 25 meters (75 feet) for solids.

Spill

- For highlighted materials: see Table 1 - Initial Isolation and Protective Action Distances.
- For non-highlighted materials: increase the immediate precautionary measure distance, in the downwind direction, as necessary.

Fire

- If tank, rail car or tank truck is involved in a fire, ISOLATE for 800 meters (1/2 mile) in all directions; also, consider initial evacuation for 800 meters (1/2 mile) in all directions.

In Canada, an Emergency Response Assistance Plan (ERAP) may be required for this product. Please consult the shipping paper and/or the ERAP Program Section (page 390).

EMERGENCY RESPONSE

FIRE

Small Fire
- Dry chemical, CO_2 or water spray.

Large Fire
- Dry chemical, CO_2, alcohol-resistant foam or water spray.
- If it can be done safely, move undamaged containers away from the area around the fire.
- Dike runoff from fire control for later disposal.

Fire Involving Tanks or Car/Trailer Loads
- Fight fire from maximum distance or use unmanned master stream devices or monitor nozzles.
- Do not get water inside containers.
- Cool containers with flooding quantities of water until well after fire is out.
- Withdraw immediately in case of rising sound from venting safety devices or discoloration of tank.
- ALWAYS stay away from tanks engulfed in fire.

SPILL OR LEAK

- ELIMINATE all ignition sources (no smoking, flares, sparks or flames) from immediate area.
- Do not touch damaged containers or spilled material unless wearing appropriate protective clothing.
- Stop leak if you can do it without risk.
- Prevent entry into waterways, sewers, basements or confined areas.
- Absorb or cover with dry earth, sand or other non-combustible material and transfer to containers.
- DO NOT GET WATER INSIDE CONTAINERS.

FIRST AID

- Call 911 or emergency medical service.
- Ensure that medical personnel are aware of the material(s) involved and take precautions to protect themselves.
- Move victim to fresh air if it can be done safely.
- Give artificial respiration if victim is not breathing.
- **Do not perform mouth-to-mouth resuscitation if victim ingested or inhaled the substance; wash face and mouth before giving artificial respiration. Use a pocket mask equipped with a one-way valve or other proper respiratory medical device.**
- Administer oxygen if breathing is difficult.
- Remove and isolate contaminated clothing and shoes.
- In case of contact with substance, immediately flush skin or eyes with running water for at least 20 minutes.
- For minor skin contact, avoid spreading material on unaffected skin.
- Keep victim calm and warm.
- Effects of exposure (inhalation, ingestion or skin contact) to substance may be delayed.

GUIDE 154 SUBSTANCES - TOXIC AND/OR CORROSIVE (NON-COMBUSTIBLE)

POTENTIAL HAZARDS

HEALTH

- **TOXIC**; inhalation, ingestion or skin contact with material may cause severe injury or death.
- Contact with molten substance may cause severe burns to skin and eyes.
- Avoid any skin contact.
- Effects of contact or inhalation may be delayed.
- Fire may produce irritating, corrosive and/or toxic gases.
- Runoff from fire control or dilution water may be corrosive and/or toxic and cause environmental contamination.

FIRE OR EXPLOSION

- Non-combustible, substance itself does not burn but may decompose upon heating to produce corrosive and/or toxic fumes.
- Some are oxidizers and may ignite combustibles (wood, paper, oil, clothing, etc.).
- Contact with metals may evolve flammable hydrogen gas.
- Containers may explode when heated.
- For electric vehicles or equipment, GUIDE 147 (lithium ion batteries) or GUIDE 138 (sodium batteries) should also be consulted.

PUBLIC SAFETY

- **CALL 911. Then call emergency response telephone number on shipping paper.** If shipping paper not available or no answer, refer to appropriate telephone number listed on the inside back cover.
- Keep unauthorized personnel away.
- Stay upwind, uphill and/or upstream.
- Ventilate closed spaces before entering, but only if properly trained and equipped.

PROTECTIVE CLOTHING

- Wear positive pressure self-contained breathing apparatus (SCBA).
- Wear chemical protective clothing that is specifically recommended by the manufacturer **when there is NO RISK OF FIRE**.
- Structural firefighters' protective clothing provides thermal protection **but only limited chemical protection**.

EVACUATION

Immediate precautionary measure

- Isolate spill or leak area in all directions for at least 50 meters (150 feet) for liquids and at least 25 meters (75 feet) for solids.

Spill

- For highlighted materials: see Table 1 - Initial Isolation and Protective Action Distances.
- For non-highlighted materials: increase the immediate precautionary measure distance, in the downwind direction, as necessary.

Fire

- If tank, rail car or tank truck is involved in a fire, ISOLATE for 800 meters (1/2 mile) in all directions; also, consider initial evacuation for 800 meters (1/2 mile) in all directions.

In Canada, an Emergency Response Assistance Plan (ERAP) may be required for this product. Please consult the shipping paper and/or the ERAP Program Section (page 390).

EMERGENCY RESPONSE

FIRE

Small Fire

- Dry chemical, CO_2 or water spray.

Large Fire

- Dry chemical, CO_2, alcohol-resistant foam or water spray.
- If it can be done safely, move undamaged containers away from the area around the fire.
- Dike runoff from fire control for later disposal.

Fire Involving Tanks or Car/Trailer Loads

- Fight fire from maximum distance or use unmanned master stream devices or monitor nozzles.
- Do not get water inside containers.
- Cool containers with flooding quantities of water until well after fire is out.
- Withdraw immediately in case of rising sound from venting safety devices or discoloration of tank.
- ALWAYS stay away from tanks engulfed in fire.

SPILL OR LEAK

- ELIMINATE all ignition sources (no smoking, flares, sparks or flames) from immediate area.
- Do not touch damaged containers or spilled material unless wearing appropriate protective clothing.
- Stop leak if you can do it without risk.
- Prevent entry into waterways, sewers, basements or confined areas.
- Absorb or cover with dry earth, sand or other non-combustible material and transfer to containers.
- DO NOT GET WATER INSIDE CONTAINERS.

FIRST AID

- Call 911 or emergency medical service.
- Ensure that medical personnel are aware of the material(s) involved and take precautions to protect themselves.
- Move victim to fresh air if it can be done safely.
- Give artificial respiration if victim is not breathing.
- **Do not perform mouth-to-mouth resuscitation if victim ingested or inhaled the substance; wash face and mouth before giving artificial respiration. Use a pocket mask equipped with a one-way valve or other proper respiratory medical device.**
- Administer oxygen if breathing is difficult.
- Remove and isolate contaminated clothing and shoes.
- In case of contact with substance, immediately flush skin or eyes with running water for at least 20 minutes.
- For minor skin contact, avoid spreading material on unaffected skin.
- Keep victim calm and warm.
- Effects of exposure (inhalation, ingestion or skin contact) to substance may be delayed.

GUIDE 155 SUBSTANCES - TOXIC AND/OR CORROSIVE (FLAMMABLE/WATER-SENSITIVE)

POTENTIAL HAZARDS

FIRE OR EXPLOSION

- **HIGHLY FLAMMABLE: Will be easily ignited by heat, sparks or flames.**
- Vapors form explosive mixtures with air: indoors, outdoors and sewers explosion hazards.
- Most vapors are heavier than air. They will spread along the ground and collect in low or confined areas (sewers, basements, tanks, etc.).
- Vapors may travel to source of ignition and flash back.
- Those substances designated with a **(P)** may polymerize explosively when heated or involved in a fire.
- Substance will react with water (some violently) releasing flammable, toxic or corrosive gases and runoff.
- Contact with metals may evolve flammable hydrogen gas.
- Containers may explode when heated or if contaminated with water.

HEALTH

- **TOXIC**; inhalation, ingestion or contact (skin, eyes) with vapors, dusts or substance may cause severe injury, burns or death.
- **Bromoacetates and chloroacetates are extremely irritating/lachrymators (cause eye irritation and flow of tears).**
- Reaction with water or moist air will release toxic, corrosive or flammable gases.
- Reaction with water may generate much heat that will increase the concentration of fumes in the air.
- Fire will produce irritating, corrosive and/or toxic gases.
- Runoff from fire control or dilution water may be corrosive and/or toxic and cause environmental contamination.

PUBLIC SAFETY

- **CALL 911. Then call emergency response telephone number on shipping paper.** If shipping paper not available or no answer, refer to appropriate telephone number listed on the inside back cover.
- Keep unauthorized personnel away.
- Stay upwind, uphill and/or upstream.
- Ventilate closed spaces before entering, but only if properly trained and equipped.

PROTECTIVE CLOTHING

- Wear positive pressure self-contained breathing apparatus (SCBA).
- Wear chemical protective clothing that is specifically recommended by the manufacturer **when there is NO RISK OF FIRE**.
- Structural firefighters' protective clothing provides thermal protection **but only limited chemical protection**.

EVACUATION

Immediate precautionary measure

- Isolate spill or leak area in all directions for at least 50 meters (150 feet) for liquids and at least 25 meters (75 feet) for solids.

Spill

- For highlighted materials: see Table 1 - Initial Isolation and Protective Action Distances.
- For non-highlighted materials: increase the immediate precautionary measure distance, in the downwind direction, as necessary.

Fire

- If tank, rail car or tank truck is involved in a fire, ISOLATE for 800 meters (1/2 mile) in all directions; also, consider initial evacuation for 800 meters (1/2 mile) in all directions.

In Canada, an Emergency Response Assistance Plan (ERAP) may be required for this product. Please consult the shipping paper and/or the ERAP Program Section (page 390).

EMERGENCY RESPONSE

FIRE

- Note: Most foams will react with the material and release corrosive/toxic gases.

CAUTION: For Acetyl chloride (UN1717), use CO_2 or dry chemical only.

Small Fire

- CO_2, dry chemical, dry sand, alcohol-resistant foam.

Large Fire

- Water spray, fog or alcohol-resistant foam.
- **FOR CHLOROSILANES, DO NOT USE WATER**; use AFFF alcohol-resistant medium-expansion foam.
- If it can be done safely, move undamaged containers away from the area around the fire.
- Avoid aiming straight or solid streams directly onto the product.

Fire Involving Tanks or Car/Trailer Loads

- Fight fire from maximum distance or use unmanned master stream devices or monitor nozzles.
- Do not get water inside containers.
- Cool containers with flooding quantities of water until well after fire is out.
- Withdraw immediately in case of rising sound from venting safety devices or discoloration of tank.
- ALWAYS stay away from tanks engulfed in fire.

SPILL OR LEAK

- ELIMINATE all ignition sources (no smoking, flares, sparks or flames) from immediate area.
- All equipment used when handling the product must be grounded.
- Do not touch damaged containers or spilled material unless wearing appropriate protective clothing.
- Stop leak if you can do it without risk.
- A vapor-suppressing foam may be used to reduce vapors.
- **FOR CHLOROSILANES**, use AFFF alcohol-resistant medium-expansion foam to reduce vapors.
- **DO NOT GET WATER on spilled substance or inside containers.**
- Use water spray to reduce vapors or divert vapor cloud drift. Avoid allowing water runoff to contact spilled material.
- Prevent entry into waterways, sewers, basements or confined areas.

Small Spill

- Cover with DRY earth, DRY sand or other non-combustible material followed with plastic sheet to minimize spreading or contact with rain.
- Use clean, non-sparking tools to collect material and place it into loosely covered plastic containers for later disposal.

FIRST AID

- Call 911 or emergency medical service.
- Ensure that medical personnel are aware of the material(s) involved and take precautions to protect themselves.
- Move victim to fresh air if it can be done safely.
- Give artificial respiration if victim is not breathing.
- **Do not perform mouth-to-mouth resuscitation if victim ingested or inhaled the substance; wash face and mouth before giving artificial respiration. Use a pocket mask equipped with a one-way valve or other proper respiratory medical device.**
- Administer oxygen if breathing is difficult.
- Remove and isolate contaminated clothing and shoes.
- In case of contact with substance, immediately flush skin or eyes with running water for at least 20 minutes.
- For minor skin contact, avoid spreading material on unaffected skin.
- Keep victim calm and warm.
- Effects of exposure (inhalation, ingestion or skin contact) to substance may be delayed.

GUIDE 156 SUBSTANCES - TOXIC AND/OR CORROSIVE (COMBUSTIBLE/WATER-SENSITIVE)

POTENTIAL HAZARDS

FIRE OR EXPLOSION

- Combustible material: may burn but does not ignite readily.
- Substance will react with water (some violently) releasing flammable, toxic or corrosive gases and runoff.
- When heated, vapors may form explosive mixtures with air: indoors, outdoors and sewers explosion hazards.
- Most vapors are heavier than air. They will spread along the ground and collect in low or confined areas (sewers, basements, tanks, etc.).
- Vapors may travel to source of ignition and flash back.
- Contact with metals may evolve flammable hydrogen gas.
- Containers may explode when heated or if contaminated with water.

HEALTH

- **TOXIC;** inhalation, ingestion or contact (skin, eyes) with vapors, dusts or substance may cause severe injury, burns or death.
- Contact with molten substance may cause severe burns to skin and eyes.
- Reaction with water or moist air will release toxic, corrosive or flammable gases.
- Reaction with water may generate much heat that will increase the concentration of fumes in the air.
- Fire will produce irritating, corrosive and/or toxic gases.
- Runoff from fire control or dilution water may be corrosive and/or toxic and cause environmental contamination.

PUBLIC SAFETY

- **CALL 911. Then call emergency response telephone number on shipping paper.** If shipping paper not available or no answer, refer to appropriate telephone number listed on the inside back cover.
- Keep unauthorized personnel away.
- Stay upwind, uphill and/or upstream.
- Ventilate closed spaces before entering, but only if properly trained and equipped.

PROTECTIVE CLOTHING

- Wear positive pressure self-contained breathing apparatus (SCBA).
- Wear chemical protective clothing that is specifically recommended by the manufacturer **when there is NO RISK OF FIRE**.
- Structural firefighters' protective clothing provides thermal protection **but only limited chemical protection**.

EVACUATION

Immediate precautionary measure

- Isolate spill or leak area in all directions for at least 50 meters (150 feet) for liquids and at least 25 meters (75 feet) for solids.

Spill

- For highlighted materials: see Table 1 - Initial Isolation and Protective Action Distances.
- For non-highlighted materials: increase the immediate precautionary measure distance, in the downwind direction, as necessary.

Fire

- If tank, rail car or tank truck is involved in a fire, ISOLATE for 800 meters (1/2 mile) in all directions; also, consider initial evacuation for 800 meters (1/2 mile) in all directions.

In Canada, an Emergency Response Assistance Plan (ERAP) may be required for this product. Please consult the shipping paper and/or the ERAP Program Section (page 390).

EMERGENCY RESPONSE

FIRE

- Note: Most foams will react with the material and release corrosive/toxic gases.

Small Fire

- CO_2, dry chemical, dry sand, alcohol-resistant foam.

Large Fire

- Water spray, fog or alcohol-resistant foam.
- **FOR CHLOROSILANES, DO NOT USE WATER**; use AFFF alcohol-resistant medium-expansion foam.
- If it can be done safely, move undamaged containers away from the area around the fire.
- Avoid aiming straight or solid streams directly onto the product.

Fire Involving Tanks or Car/Trailer Loads

- Fight fire from maximum distance or use unmanned master stream devices or monitor nozzles.
- Do not get water inside containers.
- Cool containers with flooding quantities of water until well after fire is out.
- Withdraw immediately in case of rising sound from venting safety devices or discoloration of tank.
- ALWAYS stay away from tanks engulfed in fire.

SPILL OR LEAK

- ELIMINATE all ignition sources (no smoking, flares, sparks or flames) from immediate area.
- All equipment used when handling the product must be grounded.
- Do not touch damaged containers or spilled material unless wearing appropriate protective clothing.
- Stop leak if you can do it without risk.
- A vapor-suppressing foam may be used to reduce vapors.
- **FOR CHLOROSILANES**, use AFFF alcohol-resistant medium-expansion foam to reduce vapors.
- **DO NOT GET WATER on spilled substance or inside containers.**
- Use water spray to reduce vapors or divert vapor cloud drift. Avoid allowing water runoff to contact spilled material.
- Prevent entry into waterways, sewers, basements or confined areas.

Small Spill

- Cover with DRY earth, DRY sand or other non-combustible material followed with plastic sheet to minimize spreading or contact with rain.
- Use clean, non-sparking tools to collect material and place it into loosely covered plastic containers for later disposal.

FIRST AID

- Call 911 or emergency medical service.
- Ensure that medical personnel are aware of the material(s) involved and take precautions to protect themselves.
- Move victim to fresh air if it can be done safely.
- Give artificial respiration if victim is not breathing.
- **Do not perform mouth-to-mouth resuscitation if victim ingested or inhaled the substance; wash face and mouth before giving artificial respiration. Use a pocket mask equipped with a one-way valve or other proper respiratory medical device.**
- Administer oxygen if breathing is difficult.
- Remove and isolate contaminated clothing and shoes.
- In case of contact with substance, immediately flush skin or eyes with running water for at least 20 minutes.
- For minor skin contact, avoid spreading material on unaffected skin.
- Keep victim calm and warm.
- Effects of exposure (inhalation, ingestion or skin contact) to substance may be delayed.

GUIDE 157 SUBSTANCES - TOXIC AND/OR CORROSIVE (NON-COMBUSTIBLE/WATER-SENSITIVE)

POTENTIAL HAZARDS

HEALTH

- **TOXIC**; inhalation, ingestion or contact (skin, eyes) with vapors, dusts or substance may cause severe injury, burns or death.
- Reaction with water or moist air may release toxic, corrosive or flammable gases.
- Reaction with water may generate much heat that will increase the concentration of fumes in the air.
- Fire will produce irritating, corrosive and/or toxic gases.
- Runoff from fire control or dilution water may be corrosive and/or toxic and cause environmental contamination.

FIRE OR EXPLOSION

- Non-combustible, substance itself does not burn but may decompose upon heating to produce corrosive and/or toxic fumes.
- UN1796, UN1802, UN1826, UN2032, UN3084, UN3085, and, at concentrations above 65%, UN2031 may act as oxidizers. Also consult GUIDE 140.
- Vapors may accumulate in confined areas (basement, tanks, hopper/tank cars, etc.).
- Substance may react with water (some violently), releasing corrosive and/or toxic gases and runoff.
- Contact with metals may evolve flammable hydrogen gas.
- Containers may explode when heated or if contaminated with water.

PUBLIC SAFETY

- **CALL 911. Then call emergency response telephone number on shipping paper.** If shipping paper not available or no answer, refer to appropriate telephone number listed on the inside back cover.
- Keep unauthorized personnel away.
- Stay upwind, uphill and/or upstream.
- Ventilate closed spaces before entering, but only if properly trained and equipped.

PROTECTIVE CLOTHING

- Wear positive pressure self-contained breathing apparatus (SCBA).
- Wear chemical protective clothing that is specifically recommended by the manufacturer **when there is NO RISK OF FIRE**.
- Structural firefighters' protective clothing provides thermal protection **but only limited chemical protection**.

EVACUATION

Immediate precautionary measure

- Isolate spill or leak area in all directions for at least 50 meters (150 feet) for liquids and at least 25 meters (75 feet) for solids.

Spill

- For highlighted materials: see Table 1 - Initial Isolation and Protective Action Distances.
- For non-highlighted materials: increase the immediate precautionary measure distance, in the downwind direction, as necessary.

Fire

- If tank, rail car or tank truck is involved in a fire, ISOLATE for 800 meters (1/2 mile) in all directions; also, consider initial evacuation for 800 meters (1/2 mile) in all directions.

In Canada, an Emergency Response Assistance Plan (ERAP) may be required for this product. Please consult the shipping paper and/or the ERAP Program Section (page 390).

EMERGENCY RESPONSE

FIRE

- Note: Some foams will react with the material and release corrosive/toxic gases.

Small Fire

- CO_2 (except for Cyanides), dry chemical, dry sand, alcohol-resistant foam.

Large Fire

- Water spray, fog or alcohol-resistant foam.
- If it can be done safely, move undamaged containers away from the area around the fire.
- Avoid aiming straight or solid streams directly onto the product.
- Dike runoff from fire control for later disposal.

Fire Involving Tanks or Car/Trailer Loads

- Fight fire from maximum distance or use unmanned master stream devices or monitor nozzles.
- Do not get water inside containers.
- Cool containers with flooding quantities of water until well after fire is out.
- Withdraw immediately in case of rising sound from venting safety devices or discoloration of tank.
- ALWAYS stay away from tanks engulfed in fire.

SPILL OR LEAK

- ELIMINATE all ignition sources (no smoking, flares, sparks or flames) from immediate area.
- All equipment used when handling the product must be grounded.
- Do not touch damaged containers or spilled material unless wearing appropriate protective clothing.
- Stop leak if you can do it without risk.
- A vapor-suppressing foam may be used to reduce vapors.
- DO NOT GET WATER INSIDE CONTAINERS.
- Use water spray to reduce vapors or divert vapor cloud drift. Avoid allowing water runoff to contact spilled material.
- Prevent entry into waterways, sewers, basements or confined areas.

Small Spill

- Cover with DRY earth, DRY sand or other non-combustible material followed with plastic sheet to minimize spreading or contact with rain.
- Use clean, non-sparking tools to collect material and place it into loosely covered plastic containers for later disposal.

FIRST AID

- Call 911 or emergency medical service.
- Ensure that medical personnel are aware of the material(s) involved and take precautions to protect themselves.
- Move victim to fresh air if it can be done safely.
- Give artificial respiration if victim is not breathing.
- **Do not perform mouth-to-mouth resuscitation if victim ingested or inhaled the substance; wash face and mouth before giving artificial respiration. Use a pocket mask equipped with a one-way valve or other proper respiratory medical device.**
- Administer oxygen if breathing is difficult.
- Remove and isolate contaminated clothing and shoes.
- In case of contact with substance, immediately flush skin or eyes with running water for at least 20 minutes.
- **In case of skin contact with Hydrofluoric acid (UN1790)**, if calcium gluconate gel is available, rinse 5 minutes, then apply gel. Otherwise, continue rinsing until medical treatment is available.
- For minor skin contact, avoid spreading material on unaffected skin.
- Keep victim calm and warm.
- Effects of exposure (inhalation, ingestion or skin contact) to substance may be delayed.

GUIDE 158 Infectious Substances

POTENTIAL HAZARDS

HEALTH

- Inhalation or contact with substance may cause infection, disease or death.
- Category A Infectious Substances (UN2814, UN2900 or UN3549) are more hazardous, or are in a more hazardous form, than infectious substances shipped as Category B Biological Substances (UN3373) or clinical waste/medical waste (UN3291).
- Runoff from fire control or dilution water may cause environmental contamination.
- Damaged packages containing solid CO_2 as a refrigerant may produce water or frost from condensation of air. Do not touch this liquid as it could be contaminated by the contents of the parcel.
- Contact with solid CO_2 may cause burns, severe injury and/or frostbite.

FIRE OR EXPLOSION

- Some of these materials may burn, but none ignite readily.
- Some may be transported in flammable liquids.

PUBLIC SAFETY

- **CALL 911. Then call emergency response telephone number on shipping paper.** If shipping paper not available or no answer, refer to appropriate telephone number listed on the inside back cover.
- Keep unauthorized personnel away.
- Stay upwind, uphill and/or upstream.
- Consult the shipping paper to identify the substance involved.

PROTECTIVE CLOTHING

- Use judgement based on the amount of material present and the possible routes of exposure to select protective clothing.
- Wear appropriate respiratory protection, such as fit-tested N95 respirator (at minimum), powered air purifying respirator (PAPR), or positive pressure self-contained breathing apparatus (SCBA).
- Wear full coverage body protection (e.g., Tyvek suit), faceshield, and disposable fluid-resistant gloves (e.g., latex or nitrile).
- Wear appropriate footwear; disposable shoe covers can be worn to protect against contamination.
- Puncture- and cut-resistant gloves should be worn over fluid-resistant gloves if sharp objects (e.g., broken glass, needles) are present.
- Wear insulated gloves (e.g. cryo gloves) over fluid-resistant gloves when handling dry ice (UN1845).
- Decontaminate protective clothing and personal protective equipment after use and before cleaning or disposal with a compatible chemical disinfectant (e.g., 10% solution of bleach, equivalent to 0.5% sodium hypochlorite) or through a validated decontamination technology (e.g., autoclave) or process.
- Structural firefighters' protective clothing provides thermal protection **but only limited chemical protection**.
- For more information on decontamination, consult p. 362

EVACUATION

Immediate precautionary measure

- Isolate spill or leak area for at least 25 meters (75 feet) in all directions.

In Canada, an Emergency Response Assistance Plan (ERAP) may be required for this product. Please consult the shipping paper and/or the ERAP Program Section (page 390).

EMERGENCY RESPONSE

FIRE

Small Fire

- Dry chemical, soda ash, lime or sand.

Large Fire

- Use extinguishing agent suitable for type of surrounding fire.
- Do not scatter spilled material with high-pressure water streams.
- If it can be done safely, move undamaged containers away from the area around the fire.

SPILL OR LEAK

- Do not touch or walk through spilled material.
- Do not touch damaged containers or spilled material unless wearing appropriate protective clothing.
- Absorb with earth, sand or other non-combustible material.
- Cover damaged package or spilled material with absorbent material such as paper towel, towel or rag to absorb any liquids, and, beginning from outside edge, pour liquid bleach or other chemical disinfectant to saturate. Keep wet with liquid bleach or other disinfectant.
- **DO NOT CLEAN-UP OR DISPOSE OF, EXCEPT UNDER SUPERVISION OF A SPECIALIST.**

FIRST AID

- Call 911 or emergency medical service.
- Ensure that medical personnel are aware of the material(s) involved and take precautions to protect themselves.
- Move victim to a safe isolated area if it can be done safely.

CAUTION: Victim may be a source of contamination.

- Remove and isolate contaminated clothing and shoes.
- In case of contact with substance, immediately flush eyes with running water and wash skin with soap and water for at least 20 minutes. Take caution not to break the skin.
- Effects of exposure (inhalation, ingestion, injection/inoculation or skin contact) to substance may be delayed. Victim should consult medical professional for information regarding symptoms and treatment.
- **For further assistance, contact your local Poison Control Center.**

GUIDE 159 SUBSTANCES (IRRITATING)

POTENTIAL HAZARDS

HEALTH

- Inhalation of vapors or dust is extremely irritating.
- May cause burning of eyes and lachrymation (flow of tears).
- May cause coughing, difficult breathing and nausea.
- Brief exposure effects last only a few minutes.
- Exposure in an enclosed area may be very harmful.
- Fire will produce irritating, corrosive and/or toxic gases.
- Runoff from fire control or dilution water may cause environmental contamination.

FIRE OR EXPLOSION

- Some of these materials may burn, but none ignite readily.
- Containers may explode when heated.

PUBLIC SAFETY

- **CALL 911. Then call emergency response telephone number on shipping paper.** If shipping paper not available or no answer, refer to appropriate telephone number listed on the inside back cover.
- Keep unauthorized personnel away.
- Stay upwind, uphill and/or upstream.
- Ventilate closed spaces before entering, but only if properly trained and equipped.

PROTECTIVE CLOTHING

- Wear positive pressure self-contained breathing apparatus (SCBA).
- Wear chemical protective clothing that is specifically recommended by the manufacturer **when there is NO RISK OF FIRE**.
- Structural firefighters' protective clothing provides thermal protection **but only limited chemical protection**.

EVACUATION

Immediate precautionary measure

- Isolate spill or leak area in all directions for at least 50 meters (150 feet) for liquids and at least 25 meters (75 feet) for solids.

Spill

- For highlighted materials: see Table 1 - Initial Isolation and Protective Action Distances.
- For non-highlighted materials: increase the immediate precautionary measure distance, in the downwind direction, as necessary.

Fire

- If tank, rail car or tank truck is involved in a fire, ISOLATE for 800 meters (1/2 mile) in all directions; also, consider initial evacuation for 800 meters (1/2 mile) in all directions.

In Canada, an Emergency Response Assistance Plan (ERAP) may be required for this product. Please consult the shipping paper and/or the ERAP Program Section (page 390).

EMERGENCY RESPONSE

FIRE

Small Fire

- Dry chemical, CO_2, water spray or regular foam.

Large Fire

- Water spray, fog or regular foam.
- If it can be done safely, move undamaged containers away from the area around the fire.
- Dike runoff from fire control for later disposal.

Fire Involving Tanks or Car/Trailer Loads

- Fight fire from maximum distance or use unmanned master stream devices or monitor nozzles.
- Do not get water inside containers.
- Cool containers with flooding quantities of water until well after fire is out.
- Withdraw immediately in case of rising sound from venting safety devices or discoloration of tank.
- ALWAYS stay away from tanks engulfed in fire.
- For massive fire, use unmanned master stream devices or monitor nozzles; if this is impossible, withdraw from area and let fire burn.

SPILL OR LEAK

- Do not touch or walk through spilled material.
- Stop leak if you can do it without risk.

Small Spill

- Pick up with sand or other non-combustible absorbent material and place into containers for later disposal.

Large Spill

- Dike far ahead of liquid spill for later disposal.
- Prevent entry into waterways, sewers, basements or confined areas.

FIRST AID

- Call 911 or emergency medical service.
- Ensure that medical personnel are aware of the material(s) involved and take precautions to protect themselves.
- Move victim to fresh air if it can be done safely.
- Give artificial respiration if victim is not breathing.
- **Do not perform mouth-to-mouth resuscitation if victim ingested or inhaled the substance; wash face and mouth before giving artificial respiration. Use a pocket mask equipped with a one-way valve or other proper respiratory medical device.**
- Administer oxygen if breathing is difficult.
- Remove and isolate contaminated clothing and shoes.
- In case of contact with substance, immediately flush skin or eyes with running water for at least 20 minutes.
- For minor skin contact, avoid spreading material on unaffected skin.
- Keep victim calm and warm.
- Effects should disappear after individual has been exposed to fresh air for approximately 10 minutes.

GUIDE 160 HALOGENATED SOLVENTS

POTENTIAL HAZARDS

HEALTH

- Toxic by ingestion.
- Vapors may cause dizziness or asphyxiation.
- Exposure in an enclosed area may be very harmful.
- Contact may irritate or burn skin and eyes.
- Fire may produce irritating and/or toxic gases.
- Runoff from fire control or dilution water may cause environmental contamination.

FIRE OR EXPLOSION

- Some of these materials may burn, but none ignite readily.
- Most vapors are heavier than air.
- Air/vapor mixtures may explode when ignited.
- Container may explode in heat of fire.

PUBLIC SAFETY

- **CALL 911. Then call emergency response telephone number on shipping paper.** If shipping paper not available or no answer, refer to appropriate telephone number listed on the inside back cover.
- Keep unauthorized personnel away.
- Stay upwind, uphill and/or upstream.
- Many gases are heavier than air and will spread along the ground and collect in low or confined areas (sewers, basements, tanks, etc.).
- Ventilate closed spaces before entering, but only if properly trained and equipped.

PROTECTIVE CLOTHING

- Wear positive pressure self-contained breathing apparatus (SCBA).
- Wear chemical protective clothing that is specifically recommended by the manufacturer **when there is NO RISK OF FIRE**.
- Structural firefighters' protective clothing provides thermal protection **but only limited chemical protection**.

EVACUATION

Immediate precautionary measure

- Isolate spill or leak area for at least 50 meters (150 feet) in all directions.

Large Spill

- Consider initial downwind evacuation for at least 100 meters (330 feet).

Fire

- If tank, rail car or tank truck is involved in a fire, ISOLATE for 800 meters (1/2 mile) in all directions; also, consider initial evacuation for 800 meters (1/2 mile) in all directions.

EMERGENCY RESPONSE

FIRE

Small Fire

- Dry chemical, CO_2 or water spray.

Large Fire

- Dry chemical, CO_2, alcohol-resistant foam or water spray.
- If it can be done safely, move undamaged containers away from the area around the fire.
- Dike runoff from fire control for later disposal.

Fire Involving Tanks or Car/Trailer Loads

- Fight fire from maximum distance or use unmanned master stream devices or monitor nozzles.
- Cool containers with flooding quantities of water until well after fire is out.
- Withdraw immediately in case of rising sound from venting safety devices or discoloration of tank.
- ALWAYS stay away from tanks engulfed in fire.

SPILL OR LEAK

- ELIMINATE all ignition sources (no smoking, flares, sparks or flames) from immediate area.
- Stop leak if you can do it without risk.

Small Liquid Spill

- Pick up with sand, earth or other non-combustible absorbent material.

Large Spill

- Dike far ahead of liquid spill for later disposal.
- Prevent entry into waterways, sewers, basements or confined areas.

FIRST AID

- Call 911 or emergency medical service.
- Ensure that medical personnel are aware of the material(s) involved and take precautions to protect themselves.
- Move victim to fresh air if it can be done safely.
- Give artificial respiration if victim is not breathing.
- Administer oxygen if breathing is difficult.
- Remove and isolate contaminated clothing and shoes.
- In case of contact with substance, immediately flush skin or eyes with running water for at least 20 minutes.
- For minor skin contact, avoid spreading material on unaffected skin.
- Wash skin with soap and water.
- Keep victim calm and warm.

GUIDE 161 RADIOACTIVE MATERIALS (LOW LEVEL RADIATION)

POTENTIAL HAZARDS

HEALTH

- Radiation presents minimal risk to transport workers, emergency response personnel and the public during transportation accidents. Packaging durability increases as potential hazard of radioactive content increases.
- Very low levels of contained radioactive materials and low radiation levels outside packages result in low risks to people. Damaged packages may release measurable amounts of radioactive material, but the resulting risks are expected to be low.
- Some radioactive materials cannot be detected by commonly available instruments.
- Packages do not have RADIOACTIVE I, II, or III labels. Some may have EMPTY labels or may have the word "Radioactive" in the package marking.

FIRE OR EXPLOSION

- Some of these materials may burn, but most do not ignite readily.
- Many have cardboard outer packaging; content (physically large or small) can be of many different physical forms.
- Radioactivity does not change flammability or other properties of materials.

PUBLIC SAFETY

- **CALL 911. Then call emergency response telephone number on shipping paper.** If shipping paper not available or no answer, refer to appropriate telephone number listed on the inside back cover.
- **Priorities for rescue, life-saving, first aid, fire control and other hazards are higher than the priority for measuring radiation levels.**
- Radiation Authority must be notified of accident conditions. Radiation Authority is usually responsible for decisions about radiological consequences and closure of emergencies.
- Stay upwind, uphill and/or upstream.
- Keep unauthorized personnel away.
- Detain or isolate uninjured persons or equipment suspected to be contaminated; delay decontamination and cleanup until instructions are received from Radiation Authority.

PROTECTIVE CLOTHING

- Positive pressure self-contained breathing apparatus (SCBA) and structural firefighters' protective clothing will provide adequate protection.

EVACUATION

Immediate precautionary measure

- Isolate spill or leak area for at least 25 meters (75 feet) in all directions.

Large Spill

- Consider initial downwind evacuation for at least 100 meters (330 feet).

Fire

- When a large quantity of this material is involved in a major fire, consider an initial evacuation distance of 300 meters (1000 feet) in all directions.

EMERGENCY RESPONSE

FIRE

- Presence of radioactive material will not influence the fire control processes and should not influence selection of techniques.
- If it can be done safely, move undamaged containers away from the area around the fire.
- Do not move damaged packages; move undamaged packages out of fire zone.

Small Fire

- Dry chemical, CO_2, water spray or regular foam.

Large Fire

- Water spray, fog (flooding amounts).

SPILL OR LEAK

- Do not touch damaged packages or spilled material.
- Cover liquid spill with sand, earth or other non-combustible absorbent material.
- Cover powder spill with plastic sheet or tarp to minimize spreading.

FIRST AID

- Call 911 or emergency medical service.
- Ensure that medical personnel are aware of the material(s) involved and take precautions to protect themselves.
- Medical problems take priority over radiological concerns.
- Use first aid treatment according to the nature of the injury.
- Do not delay care and transport of a seriously injured person.
- Give artificial respiration if victim is not breathing.
- Administer oxygen if breathing is difficult.
- In case of contact with substance, immediately flush skin or eyes with running water for at least 20 minutes.
- Injured persons contaminated by contact with released material are not a serious hazard to health care personnel, equipment or facilities.

GUIDE 162 RADIOACTIVE MATERIALS (LOW TO MODERATE LEVEL RADIATION)

POTENTIAL HAZARDS

HEALTH

- Radiation presents minimal risk to transport workers, emergency response personnel and the public during transportation accidents. Packaging durability increases as potential hazard of radioactive content increases.
- Undamaged packages are safe. Contents of damaged packages may cause higher external radiation exposure, or both external and internal radiation exposure if contents are released.
- Low radiation hazard when material is inside container. If material is released from package or bulk container, hazard will vary from low to moderate. Level of hazard will depend on the type and amount of radioactivity, the kind of material it is in, and/or the surfaces it is on.
- Some material may be released from packages during accidents of moderate severity but risks to people are not great.
- Released radioactive materials or contaminated objects usually will be visible if packaging fails.
- Some exclusive use shipments of bulk and packaged materials will not have “RADIOACTIVE” labels. Placards, markings and shipping papers provide identification.
- Some packages may have a “RADIOACTIVE” label and a second hazard label. The second hazard is usually greater than the radiation hazard; so follow this GUIDE as well as the response GUIDE for the second hazard class label.
- Some radioactive materials cannot be detected by commonly available instruments.
- Runoff from control of cargo fire may cause low-level pollution.

FIRE OR EXPLOSION

- Some of these materials may burn, but most do not ignite readily.
- Uranium and Thorium metal cuttings may ignite spontaneously if exposed to air (see GUIDE 136).
- Nitrates are oxidizers and may ignite other combustibles (see GUIDE 141).

PUBLIC SAFETY

- **CALL 911. Then call emergency response telephone number on shipping paper.** If shipping paper not available or no answer, refer to appropriate telephone number listed on the inside back cover.
- **Priorities for rescue, life-saving, first aid, fire control and other hazards are higher than the priority for measuring radiation levels.**
- Radiation Authority must be notified of accident conditions. Radiation Authority is usually responsible for decisions about radiological consequences and closure of emergencies.
- Stay upwind, uphill and/or upstream.
- Keep unauthorized personnel away.
- Detain or isolate uninjured persons or equipment suspected to be contaminated; delay decontamination and cleanup until instructions are received from Radiation Authority.

PROTECTIVE CLOTHING

- Positive pressure self-contained breathing apparatus (SCBA) and structural firefighters' protective clothing will provide adequate protection.

EVACUATION

Immediate precautionary measure

- Isolate spill or leak area for at least 25 meters (75 feet) in all directions.

Large Spill

- Consider initial downwind evacuation for at least 100 meters (330 feet).

Fire

- When a large quantity of this material is involved in a major fire, consider an initial evacuation distance of 300 meters (1000 feet) in all directions.

In Canada, an Emergency Response Assistance Plan (ERAP) may be required for this product. Please consult the shipping paper and/or the ERAP Program Section (page 390).

EMERGENCY RESPONSE

FIRE

- Presence of radioactive material will not influence the fire control processes and should not influence selection of techniques.
- If it can be done safely, move undamaged containers away from the area around the fire.
- Do not move damaged packages; move undamaged packages out of fire zone.

Small Fire

- Dry chemical, CO_2, water spray or regular foam.

Large Fire

- Water spray, fog (flooding amounts).
- Dike runoff from fire control for later disposal.

SPILL OR LEAK

- Do not touch damaged packages or spilled material.
- Cover liquid spill with sand, earth or other non-combustible absorbent material.
- Dike to collect large liquid spills.
- Cover powder spill with plastic sheet or tarp to minimize spreading.

FIRST AID

- Call 911 or emergency medical service.
- Ensure that medical personnel are aware of the material(s) involved and take precautions to protect themselves.
- Medical problems take priority over radiological concerns.
- Use first aid treatment according to the nature of the injury.
- Do not delay care and transport of a seriously injured person.
- Give artificial respiration if victim is not breathing.
- Administer oxygen if breathing is difficult.
- In case of contact with substance, wipe from skin immediately; flush skin or eyes with running water for at least 20 minutes.
- Injured persons contaminated by contact with released material are not a serious hazard to health care personnel, equipment or facilities.

GUIDE 163 RADIOACTIVE MATERIALS (LOW TO HIGH LEVEL RADIATION)

POTENTIAL HAZARDS

HEALTH

- Radiation presents minimal risk to transport workers, emergency response personnel and the public during transportation accidents. Packaging durability increases as potential hazard of radioactive content increases.
- Undamaged packages are safe. Contents of damaged packages may cause higher external radiation exposure, or both external and internal radiation exposure if contents are released.
- Type A packages (cartons, boxes, drums, articles, etc.) identified as "Type A" by marking on packages or by shipping papers contain non-life-endangering amounts. Partial releases might be expected if "Type A" packages are damaged in moderately severe accidents.
- Type B packages, and the rarely occurring Type C packages (large and small, usually metal), contain the most hazardous amounts. They can be identified by package markings or by shipping papers. Life-threatening conditions may exist only if contents are released or package shielding fails. Because of design, evaluation and testing of packages, these conditions would be expected only for accidents of utmost severity.
- The rarely occurring "Special Arrangement" shipments may be of Type A, Type B or Type C packages. Package type will be marked on packages, and shipment details will be on shipping papers.
- Radioactive White-I labels indicate radiation levels outside single, isolated, undamaged packages are very low (less than 0.005 mSv/h (0.5 mrem/h)).
- Radioactive Yellow-II and Yellow-III labeled packages have higher radiation levels. The transport index (TI) on the label identifies the maximum radiation level in mrem/h one meter from a single, isolated, undamaged package.
- Some radioactive materials cannot be detected by commonly available instruments.
- Water from cargo fire control may cause pollution.

FIRE OR EXPLOSION

- Some of these materials may burn, but most do not ignite readily.
- Radioactivity does not change flammability or other properties of materials.
- Type B packages are designed and evaluated to withstand total engulfment in flames at temperatures of 800°C (1475°F) for a period of 30 minutes.

PUBLIC SAFETY

- **CALL 911. Then call emergency response telephone number on shipping paper.** If shipping paper not available or no answer, refer to appropriate telephone number listed on the inside back cover.
- **Priorities for rescue, life-saving, first aid, fire control and other hazards are higher than the priority for measuring radiation levels.**
- Radiation Authority must be notified of accident conditions. Radiation Authority is usually responsible for decisions about radiological consequences and closure of emergencies.
- Stay upwind, uphill and/or upstream.
- Keep unauthorized personnel away.
- Detain or isolate uninjured persons or equipment suspected to be contaminated; delay decontamination and cleanup until instructions are received from Radiation Authority.

PROTECTIVE CLOTHING

- Positive pressure self-contained breathing apparatus (SCBA) and structural firefighters' protective clothing will provide adequate protection against internal radiation exposure, but not external radiation exposure.

EVACUATION

Immediate precautionary measure

- Isolate spill or leak area for at least 25 meters (75 feet) in all directions.

Large Spill

- Consider initial downwind evacuation for at least 100 meters (330 feet).

Fire

- When a large quantity of this material is involved in a major fire, consider an initial evacuation distance of 300 meters (1000 feet) in all directions.

EMERGENCY RESPONSE

FIRE

- Presence of radioactive material will not influence the fire control processes and should not influence selection of techniques.
- If it can be done safely, move undamaged containers away from the area around the fire.
- Do not move damaged packages; move undamaged packages out of fire zone.

Small Fire

- Dry chemical, CO_2, water spray or regular foam.

Large Fire

- Water spray, fog (flooding amounts).
- Dike runoff from fire control for later disposal.

SPILL OR LEAK

- Do not touch damaged packages or spilled material.
- Damp surfaces on undamaged or slightly damaged packages are seldom an indication of packaging failure. Most packaging for liquid content have inner containers and/or inner absorbent materials.
- Cover liquid spill with sand, earth or other non-combustible absorbent material.

FIRST AID

- Call 911 or emergency medical service.
- Ensure that medical personnel are aware of the material(s) involved and take precautions to protect themselves.
- Medical problems take priority over radiological concerns.
- Use first aid treatment according to the nature of the injury.
- Do not delay care and transport of a seriously injured person.
- Give artificial respiration if victim is not breathing.
- Administer oxygen if breathing is difficult.
- In case of contact with substance, immediately flush skin or eyes with running water for at least 20 minutes.
- Injured persons contaminated by contact with released material are not a serious hazard to health care personnel, equipment or facilities.

GUIDE 164 RADIOACTIVE MATERIALS (SPECIAL FORM/ LOW TO HIGH LEVEL EXTERNAL RADIATION)

POTENTIAL HAZARDS

HEALTH

- Radiation presents minimal risk to transport workers, emergency response personnel and the public during transportation accidents. Packaging durability increases as potential hazard of radioactive content increases.
- Undamaged packages are safe; contents of damaged packages may cause external radiation exposure, and much higher external exposure if contents (source capsules) are released.
- Contamination and internal radiation hazards are not expected, but not impossible.
- Type A packages (cartons, boxes, drums, articles, etc.) identified as "Type A" by marking on packages or by shipping papers contain non-life-endangering amounts. Radioactive sources may be released if "Type A" packages are damaged in moderately severe accidents.
- Type B packages, and the rarely occurring Type C packages, (large and small, usually metal) contain the most hazardous amounts. They can be identified by package markings or by shipping papers. Life-threatening conditions may exist only if contents are released or package shielding fails. Because of design, evaluation and testing of packages, these conditions would be expected only for accidents of utmost severity.
- Radioactive White-I labels indicate radiation levels outside single, isolated, undamaged packages are very low (less than 0.005 mSv/h (0.5 mrem/h)).
- Radioactive Yellow-II and Yellow-III labeled packages have higher radiation levels. The transport index (TI) on the label identifies the maximum radiation level in mrem/h one meter from a single, isolated, undamaged package.
- Radiation from the package contents, usually in durable metal capsules, can be detected by most radiation instruments.
- Water from cargo fire control is not expected to cause pollution.

FIRE OR EXPLOSION

- Packagings can burn completely without risk of content loss from sealed source capsule.
- Radioactivity does not change flammability or other properties of materials.
- Radioactive source capsules and Type B packages are designed and evaluated to withstand total engulfment in flames at temperatures of 800°C (1475°F) for a period of 30 minutes.

PUBLIC SAFETY

- **CALL 911. Then call emergency response telephone number on shipping paper.** If shipping paper not available or no answer, refer to appropriate telephone number listed on the inside back cover.
- **Priorities for rescue, life-saving, first aid, fire control and other hazards are higher than the priority for measuring radiation levels.**
- Radiation Authority must be notified of accident conditions. Radiation Authority is usually responsible for decisions about radiological consequences and closure of emergencies.
- Stay upwind, uphill and/or upstream.
- Keep unauthorized personnel away.
- Delay final cleanup until instructions or advice is received from Radiation Authority.

PROTECTIVE CLOTHING

- Positive pressure self-contained breathing apparatus (SCBA) and structural firefighters' protective clothing will provide adequate protection against internal radiation exposure, but not external radiation exposure.

EVACUATION

Immediate precautionary measure

- Isolate spill or leak area for at least 25 meters (75 feet) in all directions.

Large Spill

- Consider initial downwind evacuation for at least 100 meters (330 feet).

Fire

- When a large quantity of this material is involved in a major fire, consider an initial evacuation distance of 300 meters (1000 feet) in all directions.

EMERGENCY RESPONSE

FIRE

- Presence of radioactive material will not influence the fire control processes and should not influence selection of techniques.
- If it can be done safely, move undamaged containers away from the area around the fire.
- Do not move damaged packages; move undamaged packages out of fire zone.

Small Fire

- Dry chemical, CO_2, water spray or regular foam.

Large Fire

- Water spray, fog (flooding amounts).

SPILL OR LEAK

- Do not touch damaged packages or spilled material.
- Damp surfaces on undamaged or slightly damaged packages are seldom an indication of packaging failure. Contents are seldom liquid. Content is usually a metal capsule, easily seen if released from package.
- If source capsule is identified as being out of package, **DO NOT TOUCH**. Stay away and await advice from Radiation Authority.

FIRST AID

- Call 911 or emergency medical service.
- Ensure that medical personnel are aware of the material(s) involved and take precautions to protect themselves.
- Medical problems take priority over radiological concerns.
- Use first aid treatment according to the nature of the injury.
- Do not delay care and transport of a seriously injured person.
- Persons exposed to special form sources are not likely to be contaminated with radioactive material.
- Give artificial respiration if victim is not breathing.
- Administer oxygen if breathing is difficult.
- Injured persons contaminated by contact with released material are not a serious hazard to health care personnel, equipment or facilities.

GUIDE 165 Radioactive Materials (Fissile/Low to High Level Radiation)

POTENTIAL HAZARDS

HEALTH

- Radiation presents minimal risk to transport workers, emergency response personnel and the public during transportation accidents. Packaging durability increases as potential radiation and criticality hazards of the content increase.
- Undamaged packages are safe. Contents of damaged packages may cause higher external radiation exposure, or both external and internal radiation exposure if contents are released.
- Type AF or IF packages, identified by package markings, do not contain life-threatening amounts of material. External radiation levels are low and packages are designed, evaluated and tested to control releases and to prevent a fission chain reaction under severe transport conditions.
- Type B(U)F, B(M)F and CF packages (identified by markings on packages or shipping papers) contain potentially life-endangering amounts. Because of design, evaluation and testing of packages, fission chain reactions are prevented and releases are not expected to be life-endangering for all accidents except those of utmost severity.
- The rarely occurring "Special Arrangement" shipments may be of Type AF, BF or CF packages. Package type will be marked on packages, and shipment details will be on shipping papers.
- The transport index (TI) shown on labels or a shipping paper might not indicate the radiation level at one meter from a single, isolated, undamaged package; instead, it might relate to controls needed during transport because of the fissile properties of the materials. Alternatively, the fissile nature of the contents may be indicated by a criticality safety index (CSI) on a special FISSILE label or on the shipping paper.
- Some radioactive materials cannot be detected by commonly available instruments.
- Water from cargo fire control is not expected to cause pollution.

FIRE OR EXPLOSION

- These materials are seldom flammable. Packages are designed to withstand fires without damage to contents.
- Radioactivity does not change flammability or other properties of materials.
- Type AF, IF, B(U)F, B(M)F and CF packages are designed and evaluated to withstand total engulfment in flames at temperatures of 800°C (1475°F) for a period of 30 minutes.

PUBLIC SAFETY

- **CALL 911. Then call emergency response telephone number on shipping paper.** If shipping paper not available or no answer, refer to appropriate telephone number listed on the inside back cover.
- **Priorities for rescue, life-saving, first aid, fire control and other hazards are higher than the priority for measuring radiation levels.** • Radiation Authority must be notified of accident conditions. Radiation Authority is usually responsible for decisions about radiological consequences and closure of emergencies.
- Stay upwind, uphill and/or upstream. • Keep unauthorized personnel away.
- Detain or isolate uninjured persons or equipment suspected to be contaminated; delay decontamination and cleanup until instructions are received from Radiation Authority.

PROTECTIVE CLOTHING

- Positive pressure self-contained breathing apparatus (SCBA) and structural firefighters' protective clothing will provide adequate protection against internal radiation exposure, but not external radiation exposure.

EVACUATION

Immediate precautionary measure

- Isolate spill or leak area for at least 25 meters (75 feet) in all directions.

Large Spill

- Consider initial downwind evacuation for at least 100 meters (330 feet).

Fire

- When a large quantity of this material is involved in a major fire, consider an initial evacuation distance of 300 meters (1000 feet) in all directions.

In Canada, an Emergency Response Assistance Plan (ERAP) may be required for this product. Please consult the shipping paper and/or the ERAP Program Section (page 390).

EMERGENCY RESPONSE

FIRE

- Presence of radioactive material will not influence the fire control processes and should not influence selection of techniques.
- If it can be done safely, move undamaged containers away from the area around the fire.
- Do not move damaged packages; move undamaged packages out of fire zone.

Small Fire

- Dry chemical, CO_2, water spray or regular foam.

Large Fire

- Water spray, fog (flooding amounts).

SPILL OR LEAK

- Do not touch damaged packages or spilled material.
- Damp surfaces on undamaged or slightly damaged packages are seldom an indication of packaging failure. Most packaging for liquid content have inner containers and/or inner absorbent materials.

Liquid Spill

- Package contents are seldom liquid. If any radioactive contamination resulting from a liquid release is present, it probably will be low-level.

FIRST AID

- Call 911 or emergency medical service.
- Ensure that medical personnel are aware of the material(s) involved and take precautions to protect themselves.
- Medical problems take priority over radiological concerns.
- Use first aid treatment according to the nature of the injury.
- Do not delay care and transport of a seriously injured person.
- Give artificial respiration if victim is not breathing.
- Administer oxygen if breathing is difficult.
- In case of contact with substance, immediately flush skin or eyes with running water for at least 20 minutes.
- Injured persons contaminated by contact with released material are not a serious hazard to health care personnel, equipment or facilities.

GUIDE 166 RADIOACTIVE MATERIALS - CORROSIVE (URANIUM HEXAFLUORIDE/WATER-SENSITIVE)

POTENTIAL HAZARDS

HEALTH

- Radiation presents minimal risk to transport workers, emergency response personnel and the public during transportation accidents. Packaging durability increases as potential radiation and criticality hazards of the content increase.
- **Chemical hazard greatly exceeds radiation hazard.**
- Substance reacts with water and water vapor in air to form **toxic and corrosive hydrogen fluoride gas, hydrofluoric acid**, and an extremely irritating and corrosive, white-colored, water-soluble residue.
- If inhaled, may be fatal.
- Direct contact causes burns to skin, eyes, and respiratory tract.
- Low-level radioactive material; very low radiation hazard to people.
- Runoff from control of cargo fire may cause low-level pollution.

FIRE OR EXPLOSION

- Substance does not burn.
- The material may react violently with fuels.
- Product will decompose to produce toxic and/or corrosive fumes.
- Containers in protective overpacks (horizontal cylindrical shape with short legs for tie-downs), are identified with "AF", "B(U)F" or "H(U)" on shipping papers or by markings on the overpacks. They are designed and evaluated to withstand severe conditions including total engulfment in flames at temperatures of 800°C (1475°F) for a period of 30 minutes.
- Bare filled cylinders, identified with UN2978 as part of the marking (may also be marked H(U) or H(M)), may rupture in heat of engulfing fire; bare empty (except for residue) cylinders will not rupture in fires.
- Radioactivity does not change flammability or other properties of materials.

PUBLIC SAFETY

- **CALL 911. Then call emergency response telephone number on shipping paper.** If shipping paper not available or no answer, refer to appropriate telephone number listed on the inside back cover.
- **Priorities for rescue, life-saving, first aid, fire control and other hazards are higher than the priority for measuring radiation levels.**
- Radiation Authority must be notified of accident conditions. Radiation Authority is usually responsible for decisions about radiological consequences and closure of emergencies.
- Stay upwind, uphill and/or upstream.
- Keep unauthorized personnel away.
- Detain or isolate uninjured persons or equipment suspected to be contaminated; delay decontamination and cleanup until instructions are received from Radiation Authority.

PROTECTIVE CLOTHING

- Wear positive pressure self-contained breathing apparatus (SCBA).
- Wear chemical protective clothing that is specifically recommended by the manufacturer **when there is NO RISK OF FIRE**.
- Structural firefighters' protective clothing provides thermal protection **but only limited chemical protection**.

EVACUATION

Immediate precautionary measure

- Isolate spill or leak area for at least 25 meters (75 feet) in all directions.

Spill

- See Table 1 - Initial Isolation and Protective Action Distances.

Fire

- When a large quantity of this material is involved in a major fire, consider an initial evacuation distance of 300 meters (1000 feet) in all directions.

In Canada, an Emergency Response Assistance Plan (ERAP) may be required for this product. Please consult the shipping paper and/or the ERAP Program Section (page 390).

EMERGENCY RESPONSE

FIRE

- DO NOT USE WATER OR FOAM ON MATERIAL ITSELF.
- If it can be done safely, move undamaged containers away from the area around the fire.

Small Fire

- Dry chemical or CO_2.

Large Fire

- Water spray, fog or regular foam.
- Cool containers with flooding quantities of water until well after fire is out.
- If this is impossible, withdraw from area and let fire burn.
- ALWAYS stay away from tanks engulfed in fire.

SPILL OR LEAK

- Do not touch damaged packages or spilled material.
- DO NOT GET WATER INSIDE CONTAINERS.
- Without fire or smoke, leak will be evident by visible and irritating vapors and residue forming at the point of release.
- Use fine water spray to reduce vapors; do not put water directly on point of material release from container.
- Residue buildup may self-seal small leaks.
- Dike far ahead of spill to collect runoff water.

FIRST AID

- Call 911 or emergency medical service.
- Ensure that medical personnel are aware of the material(s) involved and take precautions to protect themselves.
- Medical problems take priority over radiological concerns.
- Use first aid treatment according to the nature of the injury.
- **In case of skin contact with hydrogen fluoride gas and/or Hydrofluoric acid**, if calcium gluconate gel is available, rinse 5 minutes, then apply gel. Otherwise, continue rinsing until medical treatment is available.
- Do not delay care and transport of a seriously injured person.
- Give artificial respiration if victim is not breathing.
- Administer oxygen if breathing is difficult.
- In case of contact with substance, immediately flush skin or eyes with running water for at least 20 minutes.
- Effects of exposure (inhalation, ingestion or skin contact) to substance may be delayed.
- Keep victim calm and warm.

Page intentionally left blank

There are no materials that refer to this guide.

Page intentionally left blank

There are no materials that refer to this guide.

GUIDE 168 CARBON MONOXIDE (REFRIGERATED LIQUID)

POTENTIAL HAZARDS

HEALTH

- **TOXIC; Extremely Hazardous.**
- Inhalation extremely dangerous; may be fatal.
- Contact with gas or liquefied gas may cause burns, severe injury and/or frostbite.
- Odorless, will not be detected by sense of smell.

FIRE OR EXPLOSION

- **EXTREMELY FLAMMABLE.**

CAUTION: Flame can be invisible. Use an alternate method of detection (thermal camera, broom handle, etc.)

- May be ignited by heat, sparks or flames.
- Containers may explode when heated.
- Vapor explosion and poison hazard indoors, outdoors or in sewers.
- Vapors from liquefied gas are initially heavier than air and spread along ground.
- Vapors may travel to source of ignition and flash back.
- Runoff may create fire or explosion hazard.

PUBLIC SAFETY

- **CALL 911. Then call emergency response telephone number on shipping paper.** If shipping paper not available or no answer, refer to appropriate telephone number listed on the inside back cover.
- Keep unauthorized personnel away.
- Stay upwind, uphill and/or upstream.
- Many gases are heavier than air and will spread along the ground and collect in low or confined areas (sewers, basements, tanks, etc.).
- Ventilate closed spaces before entering, but only if properly trained and equipped.

PROTECTIVE CLOTHING

- Wear positive pressure self-contained breathing apparatus (SCBA).
- Wear chemical protective clothing that is specifically recommended by the manufacturer **when there is NO RISK OF FIRE**.
- Structural firefighters' protective clothing provides thermal protection **but only limited chemical protection**.
- Always wear thermal protective clothing when handling refrigerated/cryogenic liquids.

EVACUATION

Immediate precautionary measure

- Isolate spill or leak area for at least 100 meters (330 feet) in all directions.

Spill

- See Table 1 - Initial Isolation and Protective Action Distances.

Fire

- If tank, rail car or tank truck is involved in a fire, ISOLATE for 800 meters (1/2 mile) in all directions; also, consider initial evacuation for 800 meters (1/2 mile) in all directions.

EMERGENCY RESPONSE

FIRE

CAUTION: Flame can be invisible. Use an alternate method of detection (thermal camera, broom handle, etc.)

- **DO NOT EXTINGUISH A LEAKING GAS FIRE UNLESS LEAK CAN BE STOPPED.**

Small Fire

- Dry chemical, CO_2 or water spray.

Large Fire

- Water spray, fog or regular foam.
- If it can be done safely, move undamaged containers away from the area around the fire.

Fire Involving Tanks

- Fight fire from maximum distance or use unmanned master stream devices or monitor nozzles.
- Cool containers with flooding quantities of water until well after fire is out.
- Do not direct water at source of leak or safety devices; icing may occur.
- Withdraw immediately in case of rising sound from venting safety devices or discoloration of tank.
- ALWAYS stay away from tanks engulfed in fire.

SPILL OR LEAK

- ELIMINATE all ignition sources (no smoking, flares, sparks or flames) from immediate area.
- All equipment used when handling the product must be grounded.
- Do not touch or walk through spilled material.
- Stop leak if you can do it without risk.
- Use water spray to reduce vapors or divert vapor cloud drift. Avoid allowing water runoff to contact spilled material.
- Do not direct water at spill or source of leak.
- If possible, turn leaking containers so that gas escapes rather than liquid.
- Prevent entry into waterways, sewers, basements or confined areas.
- Isolate area until gas has dispersed.

FIRST AID

- Call 911 or emergency medical service.
- Ensure that medical personnel are aware of the material(s) involved and take precautions to protect themselves.
- Move victim to fresh air if it can be done safely.
- Give artificial respiration if victim is not breathing.
- Administer oxygen if breathing is difficult.
- Remove and isolate contaminated clothing and shoes.
- In case of contact with substance, immediately flush skin or eyes with running water for at least 20 minutes.
- In case of contact with liquefied gas, thaw frosted parts with lukewarm water.
- Keep victim calm and warm.
- Keep victim under observation.
- Effects of contact or inhalation may be delayed.

GUIDE 169 Aluminum (Molten)

POTENTIAL HAZARDS

FIRE OR EXPLOSION

- Substance is transported in molten form at a temperature above 705°C (1300°F).
- Violent reaction with water; contact may cause an explosion or may produce a flammable gas.
- Will ignite combustible materials (wood, paper, oil, debris, etc.).
- Contact with nitrates or other oxidizers may cause an explosion.
- Contact with containers or other materials, including cold, wet or dirty tools, may cause an explosion.
- Contact with concrete will cause spalling and small pops.

HEALTH

- Contact causes severe burns to skin and eyes.
- Fire may produce irritating and/or toxic gases.

PUBLIC SAFETY

- **CALL 911. Then call emergency response telephone number on shipping paper.** If shipping paper not available or no answer, refer to appropriate telephone number listed on the inside back cover.
- Stay upwind, uphill and/or upstream.
- Keep unauthorized personnel away.
- Ventilate closed spaces before entering, but only if properly trained and equipped.

PROTECTIVE CLOTHING

- Wear positive pressure self-contained breathing apparatus (SCBA).
- Wear flame-retardant structural firefighters' protective clothing, including faceshield, helmet and gloves, as this will provide limited thermal protection.

EVACUATION

Immediate precautionary measure

- Isolate spill or leak area for at least 50 meters (150 feet) in all directions.

EMERGENCY RESPONSE

FIRE

- **Do not use water, except in life-threatening situations and then only in a fine spray.**
- **Do not use halogenated extinguishing agents or foam.**
- Move combustibles out of path of advancing pool if you can do so without risk.
- Extinguish fires started by molten material by using appropriate method for the burning material; keep water, halogenated extinguishing agents and foam away from the molten material.

SPILL OR LEAK

- Do not touch or walk through spilled material.
- Do not attempt to stop leak, due to danger of explosion.
- Keep combustibles (wood, paper, oil, etc.) away from spilled material.
- Substance is very fluid, spreads quickly, and may splash. Do not try to stop it with shovels or other objects.
- Dike far ahead of spill; use dry sand to contain the flow of material.
- Where possible allow molten material to solidify naturally.
- Avoid contact even after material solidifies. Molten, heated and cold aluminum look alike; do not touch unless you know it is cold.
- Clean up under the supervision of an expert after material has solidified.

FIRST AID

- Call 911 or emergency medical service.
- Ensure that medical personnel are aware of the material(s) involved and take precautions to protect themselves.
- Move victim to fresh air if it can be done safely.
- Give artificial respiration if victim is not breathing.
- Administer oxygen if breathing is difficult.
- For severe burns, immediate medical attention is required.
- Removal of solidified molten material from skin requires medical assistance.
- Remove and isolate contaminated clothing and shoes.
- In case of contact with substance, immediately flush skin or eyes with running water for at least 20 minutes.
- Keep victim calm and warm.

GUIDE 170 METALS (POWDERS, DUSTS, SHAVINGS, BORINGS, TURNINGS, OR CUTTINGS, ETC.)

POTENTIAL HAZARDS

FIRE OR EXPLOSION

- May react violently or explosively on contact with water.
- Some are transported in flammable liquids.
- May be ignited by friction, heat, sparks or flames.
- Some of these materials will burn with intense heat.
- Dusts or fumes may form explosive mixtures in air.
- Containers may explode when heated.
- May re-ignite after fire is extinguished.

HEALTH

- Oxides from metallic fires are a severe health hazard.
- Inhalation or contact with substance or decomposition products may cause severe injury or death.
- Fire may produce irritating, corrosive and/or toxic gases.
- Runoff from fire control or dilution water may cause environmental contamination.

PUBLIC SAFETY

- **CALL 911. Then call emergency response telephone number on shipping paper.** If shipping paper not available or no answer, refer to appropriate telephone number listed on the inside back cover.
- Stay upwind, uphill and/or upstream.
- Keep unauthorized personnel away.

PROTECTIVE CLOTHING

- Wear positive pressure self-contained breathing apparatus (SCBA).
- Structural firefighters' protective clothing provides thermal protection **but only limited chemical protection**.

EVACUATION

Immediate precautionary measure

- Isolate spill or leak area in all directions for at least 50 meters (150 feet) for liquids and at least 25 meters (75 feet) for solids.

Large Spill

- Consider initial downwind evacuation for at least 50 meters (160 feet).

Fire

- If tank, rail car or tank truck is involved in a fire, ISOLATE for 800 meters (1/2 mile) in all directions; also, consider initial evacuation for 800 meters (1/2 mile) in all directions.

In Canada, an Emergency Response Assistance Plan (ERAP) may be required for this product. Please consult the shipping paper and/or the ERAP Program Section (page 390).

EMERGENCY RESPONSE

FIRE

- **DO NOT USE WATER, FOAM OR CO_2.**
- Dousing metallic fires with water will generate hydrogen gas, an extremely dangerous explosion hazard, particularly if fire is in a confined environment (i.e., building, cargo hold, etc.).
- Use DRY sand, graphite powder, dry sodium chloride-based extinguishers, or class D extinguishers.
- Confining and smothering metal fires is preferable rather than applying water.
- If it can be done safely, move undamaged containers away from the area around the fire.

Fire Involving Tanks or Car/Trailer Loads

- If impossible to extinguish, protect surroundings and allow fire to burn itself out.

SPILL OR LEAK

- ELIMINATE all ignition sources (no smoking, flares, sparks or flames) from immediate area.
- Do not touch or walk through spilled material.
- Stop leak if you can do it without risk.
- Prevent entry into waterways, sewers, basements or confined areas.

FIRST AID

- Call 911 or emergency medical service.
- Ensure that medical personnel are aware of the material(s) involved and take precautions to protect themselves.
- Move victim to fresh air if it can be done safely.
- Give artificial respiration if victim is not breathing.
- Administer oxygen if breathing is difficult.
- Remove and isolate contaminated clothing and shoes.
- In case of contact with substance, immediately flush skin or eyes with running water for at least 20 minutes.
- Keep victim calm and warm.

GUIDE 171 SUBSTANCES (LOW TO MODERATE HAZARD)

POTENTIAL HAZARDS

FIRE OR EXPLOSION

- Some may burn but none ignite readily.
- Containers may explode when heated.
- Some may be transported hot.
- For UN3508, Capacitor, asymmetric, be aware of possible short circuiting as this product is transported in a charged state.
- Polymeric beads, expandable (UN2211) may evolve flammable vapours.

HEALTH

- Inhalation of material may be harmful.
- Contact may cause burns to skin and eyes.
- Inhalation of Asbestos dust may have a damaging effect on the lungs.
- Fire may produce irritating, corrosive and/or toxic gases.
- Some liquids produce vapors that may cause dizziness or asphyxiation.
- Runoff from fire control or dilution water may cause environmental contamination.

PUBLIC SAFETY

- **CALL 911. Then call emergency response telephone number on shipping paper.** If shipping paper not available or no answer, refer to appropriate telephone number listed on the inside back cover.
- Keep unauthorized personnel away.
- Stay upwind, uphill and/or upstream.

PROTECTIVE CLOTHING

- Wear positive pressure self-contained breathing apparatus (SCBA).
- Structural firefighters' protective clothing provides thermal protection **but only limited chemical protection**.

EVACUATION

Immediate precautionary measure

- Isolate spill or leak area in all directions for at least 50 meters (150 feet) for liquids and at least 25 meters (75 feet) for solids.

Spill

- For highlighted materials: see Table 1 - Initial Isolation and Protective Action Distances.
- For non-highlighted materials: increase the immediate precautionary measure distance, in the downwind direction, as necessary.

Fire

- If tank, rail car or tank truck is involved in a fire, ISOLATE for 800 meters (1/2 mile) in all directions; also, consider initial evacuation for 800 meters (1/2 mile) in all directions.

EMERGENCY RESPONSE

FIRE

Small Fire

- Dry chemical, CO_2, water spray or regular foam.

Large Fire

- Water spray, fog or regular foam.
- Do not scatter spilled material with high-pressure water streams.
- If it can be done safely, move undamaged containers away from the area around the fire.
- Dike runoff from fire control for later disposal.

Fire Involving Tanks

- Cool containers with flooding quantities of water until well after fire is out.
- Withdraw immediately in case of rising sound from venting safety devices or discoloration of tank.
- ALWAYS stay away from tanks engulfed in fire.

SPILL OR LEAK

- Do not touch or walk through spilled material.
- Stop leak if you can do it without risk.
- Prevent dust cloud.
- For Asbestos, avoid inhalation of dust. Cover spill with plastic sheet or tarp to minimize spreading. Do not clean up or dispose of, except under supervision of a specialist.

Small Dry Spill

- With clean shovel, place material into clean, dry container and cover loosely; move containers from spill area.

Small Spill

- Pick up with sand or other non-combustible absorbent material and place into containers for later disposal.

Large Spill

- Dike far ahead of liquid spill for later disposal.
- Cover powder spill with plastic sheet or tarp to minimize spreading.
- Prevent entry into waterways, sewers, basements or confined areas.

FIRST AID

- Call 911 or emergency medical service.
- Ensure that medical personnel are aware of the material(s) involved and take precautions to protect themselves.
- Move victim to fresh air if it can be done safely.
- Give artificial respiration if victim is not breathing.
- Administer oxygen if breathing is difficult.
- Remove and isolate contaminated clothing and shoes.
- In case of contact with substance, immediately flush skin or eyes with running water for at least 20 minutes.

GUIDE 172 GALLIUM AND MERCURY

POTENTIAL HAZARDS

HEALTH

- Inhalation of vapors or contact with substance will result in contamination and potential harmful effects.
- Fire will produce irritating, corrosive and/or toxic gases.

FIRE OR EXPLOSION

- Non-combustible, substance itself does not burn but may react upon heating to produce corrosive and/or toxic fumes.
- Runoff may pollute waterways.

PUBLIC SAFETY

- **CALL 911. Then call emergency response telephone number on shipping paper.** If shipping paper not available or no answer, refer to appropriate telephone number listed on the inside back cover.
- Stay upwind, uphill and/or upstream.
- Keep unauthorized personnel away.

PROTECTIVE CLOTHING

- Wear positive pressure self-contained breathing apparatus (SCBA).
- Structural firefighters' protective clothing provides thermal protection **but only limited chemical protection**.

EVACUATION

Immediate precautionary measure

- Isolate spill or leak area for at least 50 meters (150 feet) in all directions.

Large Spill

- Consider initial downwind evacuation for at least 100 meters (330 feet).

Fire

- When any large container is involved in a fire, consider initial evacuation for 500 meters (1/3 mile) in all directions.

EMERGENCY RESPONSE

FIRE

- Use extinguishing agent suitable for type of surrounding fire.
- **Do not direct water at the heated metal.**

SPILL OR LEAK

- Do not touch or walk through spilled material.
- Do not touch damaged containers or spilled material unless wearing appropriate protective clothing.
- Stop leak if you can do it without risk.
- Prevent entry into waterways, sewers, basements or confined areas.
- Do not use steel or aluminum tools or equipment.
- Cover with earth, sand or other non-combustible material followed with plastic sheet to minimize spreading or contact with rain.
- For mercury, use a mercury spill kit.
- Mercury spill areas may be subsequently treated with calcium sulphide/calcium sulfide or with sodium thiosulphate/sodium thiosulfate wash to neutralize any residual mercury.

FIRST AID

- Call 911 or emergency medical service.
- Ensure that medical personnel are aware of the material(s) involved and take precautions to protect themselves.
- Move victim to fresh air if it can be done safely.
- Give artificial respiration if victim is not breathing.
- Administer oxygen if breathing is difficult.
- Remove and isolate contaminated clothing and shoes.
- In case of contact with substance, immediately flush skin or eyes with running water for at least 20 minutes.
- Keep victim calm and warm.

GUIDE 173 ADSORBED GASES - TOXIC*

POTENTIAL HAZARDS

HEALTH

- **TOXIC; may be fatal if inhaled or absorbed through skin.**
- Vapors may be irritating.
- Contact with gas may cause burns and injury.
- Fire will produce irritating, corrosive and/or toxic gases.
- Runoff from fire control or dilution water may cause environmental contamination.

FIRE OR EXPLOSION

- Some gases may burn or be ignited by heat, sparks or flames.
- May form explosive mixtures with air.
- Oxidizers may ignite combustibles (wood, paper, oil, clothing, etc.) but NOT readily due to low transportation pressures.
- Vapors may travel to source of ignition and flash back.
- Some of these materials may react violently with water.
- Cylinders exposed to fire may vent and release toxic and flammable gas through pressure relief devices.
- Runoff may create fire hazard.

PUBLIC SAFETY

- **CALL 911. Then call emergency response telephone number on shipping paper.** If shipping paper not available or no answer, refer to appropriate telephone number listed on the inside back cover.
- Keep unauthorized personnel away.
- Stay upwind, uphill and/or upstream.
- Many gases are heavier than air and will spread along the ground and collect in low or confined areas (sewers, basements, tanks, etc.).
- Ventilate closed spaces before entering, but only if properly trained and equipped.

PROTECTIVE CLOTHING

- Wear positive pressure self-contained breathing apparatus (SCBA).
- Wear chemical protective clothing that is specifically recommended by the manufacturer **when there is NO RISK OF FIRE**.
- Structural firefighters' protective clothing provides thermal protection **but only limited chemical protection**.

EVACUATION

Immediate precautionary measure

- Isolate spill or leak area for at least 100 meters (330 feet) in all directions.

Spill

- See Table 1 - Initial Isolation and Protective Action Distances.

Fire

- If several small packages (inside a railcar or trailer) are involved in a fire, ISOLATE for 1600 meters (1 mile) in all directions; also, consider initial evacuation for 1600 meters (1 mile) in all directions.

In Canada, an Emergency Response Assistance Plan (ERAP) may be required for this product. Please consult the shipping paper and/or the ERAP Program Section (page 390).

* SOME SUBSTANCES MAY ALSO BE FLAMMABLE, CORROSIVE AND/OR OXIDIZING

EMERGENCY RESPONSE

FIRE

- **DO NOT EXTINGUISH A LEAKING GAS FIRE UNLESS LEAK CAN BE STOPPED.**

Small Fire

- Dry chemical, CO_2, water spray or alcohol-resistant foam.
- **For UN3515, UN3518, UN3520**, use water only; no dry chemical, CO_2 or Halon®.

Large Fire

- Water spray, fog or alcohol-resistant foam.
- Do not get water inside containers.
- If it can be done safely, move undamaged containers away from the area around the fire.
- Damaged cylinders should be handled only by specialists.

Fire Involving Several Small Packages (inside a railcar or trailer)

- Fight fire from maximum distance or use unmanned master stream devices or monitor nozzles.
- Cool containers with flooding quantities of water until well after fire is out.
- Do not direct water at source of leak or safety devices.
- Withdraw immediately in case of rising sound from venting safety devices or discoloration of tank.
- ALWAYS stay away from tanks engulfed in fire.

SPILL OR LEAK

- Some gases may be flammable. ELIMINATE all ignition sources (no smoking, flares, sparks or flames) from immediate area.
- For flammable gases, all equipment used when handling the product must be grounded.
- For oxidizing substances, keep combustibles (wood, paper, oil, etc.) away from spilled material.
- Do not touch or walk through spilled material.
- Stop leak if you can do it without risk.
- Do not direct water at spill or source of leak.
- Use water spray to reduce vapors or divert vapor cloud drift. Avoid allowing water runoff to contact spilled material.
- Prevent entry into waterways, sewers, basements or confined areas.
- Isolate area until gas has dispersed.

FIRST AID

- Call 911 or emergency medical service.
- Ensure that medical personnel are aware of the material(s) involved and take precautions to protect themselves.
- Move victim to fresh air if it can be done safely.
- Give artificial respiration if victim is not breathing.
- **Do not perform mouth-to-mouth resuscitation if victim ingested or inhaled the substance; wash face and mouth before giving artificial respiration. Use a pocket mask equipped with a one-way valve or other proper respiratory medical device.**
- Administer oxygen if breathing is difficult.
- Remove and isolate contaminated clothing and shoes.
- In case of contact with substance, immediately flush skin or eyes with running water for at least 20 minutes.
- In case of burns, immediately cool affected skin for as long as possible with cold water. Do not remove clothing if adhering to skin.
- Keep victim calm and warm.
- Keep victim under observation.
- Effects of contact or inhalation may be delayed.

GUIDE 174 ADSORBED GASES - FLAMMABLE OR OXIDIZING

POTENTIAL HAZARDS

FIRE OR EXPLOSION

- Some gases will be ignited by heat, sparks or flames.
- Substance does not burn but will support combustion.
- Vapors may travel to source of ignition and flash back.
- Cylinders exposed to fire may vent and release flammable gas through pressure relief devices.
- Containers may explode when exposed to prolonged direct flame impingement.

HEALTH

- Vapors may cause dizziness or asphyxiation without warning.
- Some may be irritating if inhaled at high concentrations.
- Contact with gas may cause burns and injury.
- Fire may produce irritating and/or toxic gases.

PUBLIC SAFETY

- **CALL 911. Then call emergency response telephone number on shipping paper.** If shipping paper not available or no answer, refer to appropriate telephone number listed on the inside back cover.
- Keep unauthorized personnel away.
- Stay upwind, uphill and/or upstream.
- Many gases are heavier than air and will spread along the ground and collect in low or confined areas (sewers, basements, tanks, etc.).
- Ventilate closed spaces before entering, but only if properly trained and equipped.

PROTECTIVE CLOTHING

- Wear positive pressure self-contained breathing apparatus (SCBA).
- Structural firefighters' protective clothing provides thermal protection **but only limited chemical protection**.

EVACUATION

Immediate precautionary measure

- Isolate spill or leak area for at least 100 meters (330 feet) in all directions.

Large Spill

- Consider initial downwind evacuation for at least 800 meters (1/2 mile).

Fire

- If several small packages (inside a railcar or trailer) are involved in a fire, ISOLATE for 1600 meters (1 mile) in all directions; also, consider initial evacuation for 1600 meters (1 mile) in all directions.

In Canada, an Emergency Response Assistance Plan (ERAP) may be required for this product. Please consult the shipping paper and/or the ERAP Program Section (page 390).

EMERGENCY RESPONSE

FIRE

- **DO NOT EXTINGUISH A LEAKING GAS FIRE UNLESS LEAK CAN BE STOPPED.**
- Use extinguishing agent suitable for type of surrounding fire.

Small Fire

- Dry chemical or CO_2.

Large Fire

- Water spray or fog.
- If it can be done safely, move undamaged containers away from the area around the fire.
- Damaged cylinders should be handled only by specialists.

Fire Involving Several Small Packages (inside a railcar or trailer)

- Fight fire from maximum distance or use unmanned master stream devices or monitor nozzles.
- Cool containers with flooding quantities of water until well after fire is out.
- Do not direct water at source of leak or safety devices.
- Withdraw immediately in case of rising sound from venting safety devices or discoloration of tank.
- ALWAYS stay away from tanks engulfed in fire.
- For massive fire, use unmanned master stream devices or monitor nozzles; if this is impossible, withdraw from area and let fire burn.

SPILL OR LEAK

- For flammable gases, ELIMINATE all ignition sources (no smoking, flares, sparks or flames) from immediate area.
- For oxidizing substances, keep combustibles (wood, paper, oil, etc.) away from spilled material.
- All equipment used when handling the product must be grounded.
- Do not touch or walk through spilled material.
- Stop leak if you can do it without risk.
- Use water spray to reduce vapors or divert vapor cloud drift. Avoid allowing water runoff to contact spilled material.
- Do not direct water at spill or source of leak.
- Prevent spreading of vapors through sewers, ventilation systems and confined areas.
- Ventilate the area.
- Isolate area until gas has dispersed.

FIRST AID

- Call 911 or emergency medical service.
- Ensure that medical personnel are aware of the material(s) involved and take precautions to protect themselves.
- Move victim to fresh air if it can be done safely.
- Give artificial respiration if victim is not breathing.
- Administer oxygen if breathing is difficult.
- Remove and isolate contaminated clothing and shoes.
- In case of burns, immediately cool affected skin for as long as possible with cold water. Do not remove clothing if adhering to skin.
- Keep victim calm and warm.

INTRODUCTION TO GREEN TABLES

TABLE 1 - INITIAL ISOLATION AND PROTECTIVE ACTION DISTANCES

This table suggests distances useful to protect people from vapors/gases resulting from spills involving:

- materials that are considered toxic by inhalation (TIH) (PIH in the US)
- materials that produce toxic gases upon contact with water
- chemical warfare agents

This table provides first responders with initial guidance until technically qualified emergency response personnel are available. For each material, first responders will find distances for the following zones:

- The **Initial Isolation Zone** defines an area **surrounding** the incident in which people may be exposed to dangerous (upwind) and life-threatening (downwind) concentrations of material.
- The **Protective Action Zone** defines an area **downwind** from the incident in which people may become incapacitated and unable to take protective action and/or incur serious or irreversible health effects. Table 1 provides specific guidance for small and large spills occurring day or night.

Adjusting distances for a specific incident involves many interdependent variables. These adjustments should only be made by technically qualified personnel. For this reason, no precise guidance can be provided in this document to aid in adjusting the table distances; however, general guidance follows.

Factors that May Change the Protective Action Distances

Fire

In the **orange-bordered pages**, under **EVACUATION – Fire**, the evacuation distance required to protect against fragmentation hazard of a large container is clearly indicated. If involved in a fire, the toxic hazard may be less dangerous than the fire or explosion hazard.

In these cases, the **fire hazard distance should be used** as an isolation distance and Table 1 should be used to protect downwind for residual material release.

Worst-case scenario: terrorism, sabotage or catastrophic accident

Initial isolation and protective action distances are derived from historical data on transportation incidents and the use of statistical models. For worst-case scenarios involving the instantaneous release of the entire contents of a package (e.g., as a result of terrorism, sabotage or catastrophic accident), the distances may increase substantially.

For such events, **doubling** the initial isolation and protective action distances is appropriate in absence of other information.

When more than one large package is leaking

If more than one rail car, tank truck, tank or large cylinder, containing TIH materials is leaking, **large spill** distances may need to be increased.

Other factors that can increase the protective action distance:

- If a material has a **protective action distance of 11.0+ km (7.0+ miles)**, the actual distance can be larger in certain atmospheric conditions.
- If the material's vapor plume is **channeled in a valley** or **between many tall buildings**, protective action distances may be larger than shown due to less mixing of the plume with the atmosphere.
- If there is a **daytime spill** in a region with known **strong temperature inversions** or **snow cover**, or it occurs **near sunset**, this may require an increase of the protective action distance because airborne contaminants mix and disperse more slowly and may travel much farther downwind.
  - In such cases, the nighttime protective action distances may be more appropriate.
- If the temperature of the **liquid spill** or the **outdoor temperature exceeds 30°C (86°F)**, the protective action distance may be larger.

Water-reactive materials

Materials that react with water to produce large amounts of toxic gases are included in Table 1. Some of these materials have 2 entries in Table 1. They are identified by **(when spilled on land)** since they are TIH products and **(when spilled in water)** because they produce additional toxic gases when spilled in water.

Choose the **larger protective action distance** if:

- it is not clear whether the spill is on land or in water
- the spill occurs both on land and in water

TABLE 2 - WATER-REACTIVE MATERIALS WHICH PRODUCE TOXIC GASES

This table lists materials that produce large amounts of Toxic Inhalation Hazard gases (TIH) when spilled in water as well as the TIH gases that are produced.

NOTE: The produced TIH gases indicated in Table 2 are for information purposes only. In Table 1, the initial isolation and protective action distances have already taken into consideration the produced TIH gas.

When a water-reactive TIH-producing material is spilled into a river or stream, the source of the toxic gas may flow downstream for a great distance.

TABLE 3 - INITIAL ISOLATION AND PROTECTIVE ACTION DISTANCES FOR LARGE SPILLS FOR DIFFERENT QUANTITIES OF SIX COMMON TIH (PIH IN THE US) GASES

This table lists materials that may be more commonly encountered. These materials are:

- UN1005 - Ammonia, anhydrous
- UN1017 - Chlorine
- UN1040 - Ethylene oxide and UN1040 - Ethylene oxide with nitrogen

- UN1050 - Hydrogen chloride, anhydrous and UN2186 - Hydrogen chloride, refrigerated liquid
- UN1052 - Hydrogen fluoride, anhydrous
- UN1079 - Sulfur dioxide/Sulphur dioxide

This table provides initial isolation and protective action distances for large spills (more than 208 liters or 55 US gallons):

- involving different container types (therefore different volume capacities)
- for daytime and nighttime situations
- for different wind speeds (low, moderate and high)

PROTECTIVE ACTIONS

Protective actions are the steps taken to preserve the health and safety of emergency responders and the public during an incident involving releases of hazardous materials/ dangerous goods.

Table 1 - Initial Isolation and Protective Action Distances (green-bordered pages) predicts the size of the area that could be affected by a cloud of toxic gas. People in this area should be evacuated and/or sheltered-in-place inside buildings.

Isolate hazard area and deny entry means to keep everybody away from the area if they are not directly involved in emergency response operations. Unprotected emergency responders should not be allowed to enter the isolation zone.

This "isolation" task is done to establish control over the area of operations. This is the first step for any protective actions that may follow.

Evacuate means to move all people from a threatened area to a safer place. To perform an evacuation, there must be enough time for people to be warned, get ready, and leave an area. If there is enough time, evacuation is the best protective action.

Begin evacuating people nearby and those who are outdoors in direct view of the scene. When additional help arrives, expand the area to be evacuated downwind and crosswind to at least the extent recommended in this guidebook.

Even after people move to the distances recommended, they may not be completely safe from harm. They should not be permitted to gather at such distances. Send evacuees to a definite place, by a specific route, far enough away so they will not have to be moved again if the wind shifts.

Shelter-in-place means people should seek shelter inside a building and remain inside until the danger passes. **It is vital for first responders to maintain communications with sheltered-in-place people** so that they are advised about changing conditions.

Sheltering-in-place is used either when:

- evacuating the public would cause greater risk than staying where they are
- an evacuation cannot be performed

Direct the people inside to:

- close all doors and windows
- shut off all ventilating, heating and cooling systems
- stay far from windows to avoid shattered glass and projectile metal fragments in the event of a fire and/or explosion
- tune in to local radio or TV stations, and stay inside until told it is safe to leave by first responders

Shelter-in-place may not be the best option if:

- the vapors are flammable

- it will take a long time for the gas to clear the area
- buildings cannot be closed tightly

Vehicles can offer some protection for a short period if the windows are closed and the ventilation systems are shut off. Vehicles are not as effective as buildings for in-place protection.

NOTE: Every hazardous materials/dangerous goods incident is different. Each will have special problems and concerns. Actions to protect the public must be carefully selected. These pages can help with **initial** decisions on how to protect the public. Officials must continue to gather information and monitor the situation until the threat is removed.

PROTECTIVE ACTION DECISION FACTORS TO CONSIDER

The choice of protective actions for a given situation depends on a number of factors. For some cases, evacuation may be the best option; in others, sheltering-in-place may be the best course. Sometimes, these two actions may be used in combination. In any emergency, officials need to quickly give the public instructions. The public will need continuing information and instructions while being evacuated or sheltered-in-place.

Proper evaluation of the factors listed below will determine the effectiveness of evacuation or in-place protection (shelter-in-place). The importance of these factors can vary with emergency conditions. In specific emergencies, other factors may need to be identified and considered as well. This list indicates what kind of information may be needed to make the initial decision.

The hazardous materials/dangerous goods:

- degree of health hazard
- chemical and physical properties
- amount involved
- containment/control of release
- rate of vapor movement

The population threatened:

- location
- number of people
- time available to evacuate or shelter-in-place
- ability to control evacuation or shelter-in-place
- building types and availability
- special institutions or populations, e.g., nursing homes, hospitals, prisons

The weather conditions:

- effect on vapor and cloud movement
- potential for change
- effect on evacuation or shelter-in-place

BACKGROUND ON TABLE 1 – INITIAL ISOLATION AND PROTECTIVE ACTION DISTANCES

Initial isolation and protective action distances in this guidebook were determined for small and large spills occurring during day or night. The overall analysis, statistical in nature, was conducted using:

- state-of-the-art emission rate and dispersion models
- statistical release data from the U.S. Department of Transportation (DOT) Hazardous Materials Information System (HMIS) database
- meteorological observations from more than 120 locations in the United States, Canada, and Mexico
- the most current toxicological exposure guidelines

For each chemical, thousands of hypothetical releases were modeled to account for the statistical variance in both release amount and atmospheric conditions. Based on this statistical sample, they selected the 90th percentile protective action distance for each chemical and category to appear in the table. A brief description of the analysis is provided below.

A detailed report outlining the methodology and data used to generate the initial isolation and protective action distances may be obtained from the U.S. DOT, Pipeline and Hazardous Materials Safety Administration (PHMSA).

DESCRIPTION OF THE ANALYSIS

Release amounts and emission rates into the atmosphere were statistically modeled based on:

- data from the U.S. DOT HMIS database
- container types and sizes authorized for transport as specified in 49 CFR §172.101 and Part 173
- physical properties of the individual materials
- atmospheric data from a historical database

For liquefied gases, which can flash to form both a vapor/aerosol mixture and an evaporating pool, the emission model calculated one or both of:

- the release of vapor due to evaporation of pools on the ground
- direct release of vapors from the container

The emission model also calculated the emission of toxic vapor by-products generated from spilling water-reactive materials in water.

Small spills involve 208 liters (55 US gallons) or less.

Large spills involve greater quantities.

The exceptions are the entries at the beginning of Table 1 marked **(when used as a weapon)**. The volumes used for these calculations varies, but in most cases:

- Small spills include releases up to 2 kg (4.4 lbs.).
- Large spills include releases up to 25 kg (55 lbs.).

Downwind dispersion of the vapor was estimated for each case modeled. Using a database containing hourly meteorological data from 120 American, Canadian, and Mexican cities, the atmospheric parameters affecting the dispersion and the emission rate were selected.

The dispersion calculation accounted for both the:

- time-dependent emission rate from the source
- density of the vapor plume (i.e., heavy gas effects)

Since atmospheric mixing is less effective at dispersing vapor plumes during nighttime, day and night were separated in the analysis.

In the table:

- **day** refers to time periods after sunrise and before sunset
- **night** includes all hours between sunset and sunrise

Toxicological short-term exposure guidelines for the materials were applied to determine the downwind distance to which people may:

- become incapacitated and unable to take protective action
- incur serious health effects after a single, or rare, exposure

When available, toxicological exposure guidelines were chosen from AEGL-2 or ERPG-2 emergency response guidelines. AEGL-2 values were the first choice.

For materials without AEGL-2 or ERPG-2 values, emergency response guidelines were estimated based on lethal concentration limits derived from animal-based-studies. This approach was recommended by an independent panel of toxicological experts from industry and academia.

HOW TO USE TABLE 1 – INITIAL ISOLATION AND PROTECTIVE ACTION DISTANCES

(1) The responder should already have:

- identified the material by its ID number and name (if you cannot find an ID number, use the Name of Material index in the blue-bordered pages to find that number);
- confirmed that the material is highlighted in green in the yellow or blue-bordered pages. If not, Table 1 doesn't apply;
- found the three-digit guide for the material, in order to consult emergency actions it recommends along with this table; and
- **noted the wind direction**

(2) Look in Table 1 (green-bordered pages) for the ID number and name of the material involved. Some ID numbers have more than one shipping name listed. Look for the specific name of the material. If you do not know the shipping name and Table 1 lists more than one name for the same ID number, use the entry with the largest distances.

(3) Determine if the incident involves a SMALL or LARGE spill and if it is DAY or NIGHT. A SMALL SPILL consists of a release of 208 liters (55 US gallons) or less. This generally corresponds to a spill from a single small package (for example, a drum), a small cylinder, or a small leak from a large package. A LARGE SPILL consists of a release of more than 208 liters (55 US gallons). This usually involves a spill from a large package, or multiple spills from many small packages. DAY is any time after sunrise and before sunset. NIGHT is any time between sunset and sunrise.

(4) Look up the INITIAL ISOLATION DISTANCE. This distance defines the radius of a zone (initial isolation zone) surrounding the spill in ALL DIRECTIONS. In this zone, protective clothing and respiratory protection is required. Evacuate the general public in a direction perpendicular to wind direction (crosswind) and away from the spill.

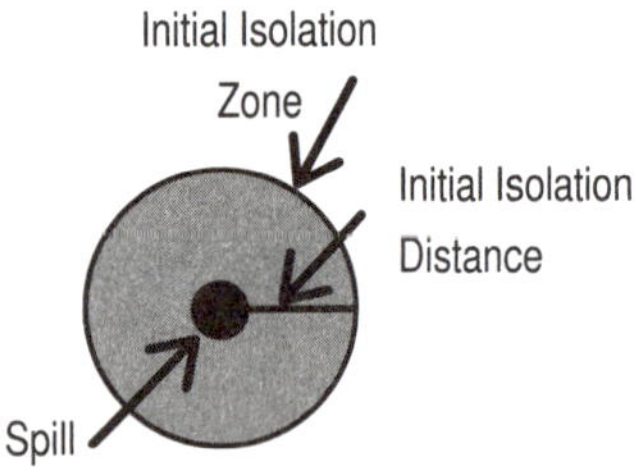

(5) Look up the PROTECTIVE ACTION DISTANCE.
For a given material, spill size, and whether day or night, Table 1 gives the downwind distance—in kilometers and miles—from the spill or leak source, for which you should consider protective actions. For practical purposes, the protective action zone (i.e., the area in which people are at risk of harmful exposure) is a square. Its length and width are the same as the downwind distance shown in Table 1. Protective actions are the

steps you take to preserve the health and safety of emergency responders and the public. People in this area should be evacuated and/or sheltered-in-place. Consult pages 289-291.

(6) Initiate protective actions beginning with those closest to the spill site and working away in a downwind direction. When a water-reactive TIH (PIH in the US) producing material is spilled into a river or stream, the source of the toxic gas may move with the current or stretch from the spill point downstream for a large distance.

In the figure below, the spill is located at the center of the small black circle. The larger circle represents the initial isolation zone around the spill. The square (the protective action zone) is the area in which you should take protective actions.

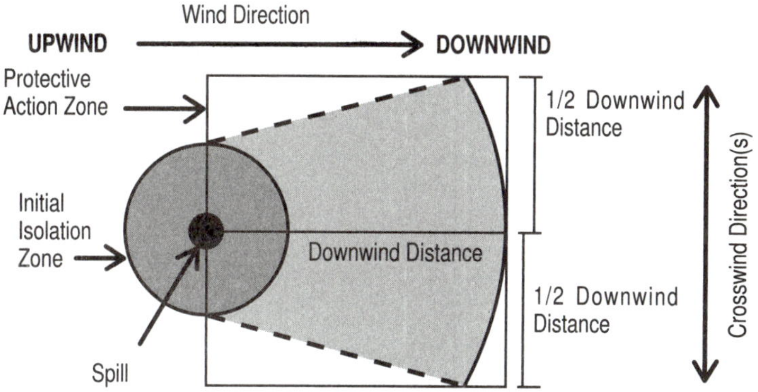

Note 1: For factors that may change the protective action distances, see "Introduction to Green Tables" (page 286).

Note 2: When a product in Table 1 has the mention (when spilled in water), you can refer to Table 2 for the list of gases produced when these materials are spilled in water. The TIH gases indicated in Table 2 are for information purposes only.

For more information on the material, safety precautions and mitigation procedures, call the emergency response telephone number listed on the shipping paper or the appropriate response agency as soon as possible.

TABLE 1 - INITIAL ISOLATION AND PROTECTIVE ACTION DISTANCES

			SMALL SPILLS (From a small package or small leak from a large package)			LARGE SPILLS (From a large package or from many small packages)		
			First ISOLATE in all Directions	Then PROTECT persons Downwind during		First ISOLATE in all Directions	Then PROTECT persons Downwind during	
ID No.	Guide	NAME OF MATERIAL	Meters (Feet)	DAY Kilometers (Miles)	NIGHT Kilometers (Miles)	Meters (Feet)	DAY Kilometers (Miles)	NIGHT Kilometers (Miles)
—	117	AC (when used as a weapon)	60 m (200 ft)	0.3 km (0.2 mi)	1.0 km (0.6 mi)	1000 m (3000 ft)	3.7 km (2.3 mi)	8.4 km (5.3 mi)
—	154	Adamsite (when used as a weapon)	30 m (100 ft)	0.1 km (0.1 mi)	0.3 km (0.2 mi)	60 m (200 ft)	0.3 km (0.2 mi)	1.4 km (0.9 mi)
—	153	Buzz (when used as a weapon)	60 m (200 ft)	0.4 km (0.2 mi)	1.7 km (1.1 mi)	400 m (1250 ft)	2.2 km (1.4 mi)	8.1 km (5.0 mi)
—	153	BZ (when used as a weapon)	60 m (200 ft)	0.4 km (0.2 mi)	1.7 km (1.1 mi)	400 m (1250 ft)	2.2 km (1.4 mi)	8.1 km (5.0 mi)
—	159	CA (when used as a weapon)	30 m (100 ft)	0.1 km (0.1 mi)	0.4 km (0.3 mi)	100 m (300 ft)	0.5 km (0.4 mi)	2.6 km (1.6 mi)
—	125	CG (when used as a weapon)	150 m (500 ft)	0.8 km (0.5 mi)	3.2 km (2.0 mi)	1000 m (3000 ft)	7.5 km (4.7 mi)	11.0+ km (7.0+ mi)
—	125	CK (when used as a weapon)	30 m (100 ft)	0.2 km (0.2 mi)	1.4 km (0.9 mi)	300 m (1000 ft)	1.4 km (0.9 mi)	6.1 km (3.8 mi)
—	153	CN (when used as a weapon)	30 m (100 ft)	0.1 km (0.1 mi)	0.2 km (0.1 mi)	60 m (200 ft)	0.3 km (0.2 mi)	1.2 km (0.8 mi)
—	153	CS (when used as a weapon)	30 m (100 ft)	0.1 km (0.1 mi)	0.6 km (0.4 mi)	100 m (300 ft)	0.4 km (0.3 mi)	1.9 km (1.2 mi)
—	154	CX (when used as a weapon)	60 m (200 ft)	0.2 km (0.2 mi)	1.1 km (0.7 mi)	200 m (600 ft)	1.2 km (0.7 mi)	5.1 km (3.2 mi)
—	151	DA (when used as a weapon)	30 m (100 ft)	0.2 km (0.1 mi)	0.8 km (0.5 mi)	300 m (1000 ft)	1.9 km (1.2 mi)	7.5 km (4.7 mi)
—	153	DC (when used as a weapon)	30 m (100 ft)	0.1 km (0.1 mi)	0.6 km (0.4 mi)	60 m (200 ft)	0.4 km (0.3 mi)	1.8 km (1.1 mi)
—	154	DM (when used as a weapon)	30 m (100 ft)	0.1 km (0.1 mi)	0.3 km (0.2 mi)	60 m (200 ft)	0.3 km (0.2 mi)	1.4 km (0.9 mi)
—	125	DP (when used as a weapon)	30 m (100 ft)	0.2 km (0.1 mi)	0.7 km (0.4 mi)	200 m (600 ft)	1.0 km (0.7 mi)	2.4 km (1.5 mi)
—	151	ED (when used as a weapon)	150 m (500 ft)	0.9 km (0.6 mi)	2.1 km (1.3 mi)	1000 m (3000 ft)	5.9 km (3.7 mi)	8.3 km (5.2 mi)
—	153	GA (when used as a weapon)	30 m (100 ft)	0.2 km (0.1 mi)	0.2 km (0.1 mi)	100 m (300 ft)	0.5 km (0.4 mi)	0.6 km (0.4 mi)

—	153	GB **(when used as a weapon)**	60 m	(200 ft)	0.4 km	(0.3 mi)	1.1 km	(0.7 mi)	400 m	(1250 ft)	2.1 km	(1.3 mi)	4.9 km	(3.0 mi)
—	153	GD **(when used as a weapon)**	60 m	(200 ft)	0.4 km	(0.3 mi)	0.7 km	(0.5 mi)	300 m	(1000 ft)	1.8 km	(1.1 mi)	2.7 km	(1.7 mi)
—	153	GF **(when used as a weapon)**	30 m	(100 ft)	0.2 km	(0.2 mi)	0.3 km	(0.2 mi)	150 m	(500 ft)	0.8 km	(0.5 mi)	1.0 km	(0.6 mi)
—	153	H **(when used as a weapon)**	30 m	(100 ft)	0.1 km	(0.1 mi)	0.1 km	(0.1 mi)	60 m	(200 ft)	0.3 km	(0.2 mi)	0.4 km	(0.3 mi)
—	153	HD **(when used as a weapon)**	30 m	(100 ft)	0.1 km	(0.1 mi)	0.1 km	(0.1 mi)	60 m	(200 ft)	0.3 km	(0.2 mi)	0.4 km	(0.3 mi)
—	153	HL **(when used as a weapon)**	30 m	(100 ft)	0.1 km	(0.1 mi)	0.3 km	(0.2 mi)	100 m	(300 ft)	0.5 km	(0.3 mi)	1.0 km	(0.6 mi)
—	153	HN-1 **(when used as a weapon)**	60 m	(200 ft)	0.3 km	(0.2 mi)	0.5 km	(0.3 mi)	200 m	(600 ft)	1.1 km	(0.7 mi)	1.8 km	(1.1 mi)
—	153	HN-2 **(when used as a weapon)**	60 m	(200 ft)	0.3 km	(0.2 mi)	0.6 km	(0.4 mi)	300 m	(1000 ft)	1.3 km	(0.8 mi)	2.1 km	(1.3 mi)
—	153	HN-3 **(when used as a weapon)**	30 m	(100 ft)	0.1 km	(0.1 mi)	0.1 km	(0.1 mi)	60 m	(200 ft)	0.3 km	(0.2 mi)	0.3 km	(0.2 mi)
—	153	L (Lewisite) **(when used as a weapon)**	30 m	(100 ft)	0.1 km	(0.1 mi)	0.3 km	(0.2 mi)	100 m	(300 ft)	0.5 km	(0.3 mi)	1.0 km	(0.6 mi)
—	153	Lewisite **(when used as a weapon)**	30 m	(100 ft)	0.1 km	(0.1 mi)	0.3 km	(0.2 mi)	100 m	(300 ft)	0.5 km	(0.3 mi)	1.0 km	(0.6 mi)
—	152	MD **(when used as a weapon)**	300 m	(1000 ft)	1.6 km	(1.0 mi)	4.3 km	(2.7 mi)	1000 m	(3000 ft)	11.0+ km	(7.0+ mi)	11.0+ km	(7.0+ mi)
—	153	Mustard **(when used as a weapon)**	30 m	(100 ft)	0.1 km	(0.1 mi)	0.1 km	(0.1 mi)	60 m	(200 ft)	0.3 km	(0.2 mi)	0.4 km	(0.3 mi)
—	153	Mustard Lewisite **(when used as a weapon)**	30 m	(100 ft)	0.1 km	(0.1 mi)	0.3 km	(0.2 mi)	100 m	(300 ft)	0.5 km	(0.3 mi)	1.0 km	(0.6 mi)
—	152	PD **(when used as a weapon)**	60 m	(200 ft)	0.4 km	(0.3 mi)	0.4 km	(0.3 mi)	300 m	(1000 ft)	1.6 km	(1.0 mi)	1.6 km	(1.0 mi)
—	119	SA **(when used as a weapon)**	300 m	(1000 ft)	1.9 km	(1.2 mi)	5.7 km	(3.6 mi)	1000 m	(3000 ft)	8.9 km	(5.6 mi)	11.0+ km	(7.0+ mi)
—	153	Sarin **(when used as a weapon)**	60 m	(200 ft)	0.4 km	(0.3 mi)	1.1 km	(0.7 mi)	400 m	(1250 ft)	2.1 km	(1.3 mi)	4.9 km	(3.0 mi)

"+" means distance can be larger in certain atmospheric conditions

TABLE 1

TABLE 1 - INITIAL ISOLATION AND PROTECTIVE ACTION DISTANCES

			SMALL SPILLS (From a small package or small leak from a large package)			LARGE SPILLS (From a large package or from many small packages)		
			First **ISOLATE** in all Directions	Then **PROTECT** persons Downwind during		First **ISOLATE** in all Directions	Then **PROTECT** persons Downwind during	
ID No.	Guide	NAME OF MATERIAL	Meters (Feet)	**DAY** Kilometers (Miles)	**NIGHT** Kilometers (Miles)	Meters (Feet)	**DAY** Kilometers (Miles)	**NIGHT** Kilometers (Miles)
—	**153**	Soman **(when used as a weapon)**	60 m (200 ft)	0.4 km (0.3 mi)	0.7 km (0.5 mi)	300 m (1000 ft)	1.8 km (1.1 mi)	2.7 km (1.7 mi)
—	**153**	Tabun **(when used as a weapon)**	30 m (100 ft)	0.2 km (0.1 mi)	0.2 km (0.1 mi)	100 m (300 ft)	0.5 km (0.4 mi)	0.6 km (0.4 mi)
—	**153**	Thickened GD **(when used as a weapon)**	60 m (200 ft)	0.4 km (0.3 mi)	0.7 km (0.5 mi)	300 m (1000 ft)	1.8 km (1.1 mi)	2.7 km (1.7 mi)
—	**153**	VX **(when used as a weapon)**	30 m (100 ft)	0.1 km (0.1 mi)	0.1 km (0.1 mi)	60 m (200 ft)	0.4 km (0.2 mi)	0.3 km (0.2 mi)
1005 1005	**125** **125**	Ammonia, anhydrous Anhydrous ammonia	30 m (100 ft)	0.1 km (0.1 mi)	0.2 km (0.1 mi)	**Refer to table 3**		
1008 1008	**125** **125**	Boron trifluoride Boron trifluoride, compressed	30 m (100 ft)	0.2 km (0.1 mi)	0.7 km (0.5 mi)	400 m (1250 ft)	2.3 km (1.4 mi)	5.1 km (3.2 mi)
1016 1016	**119** **119**	Carbon monoxide Carbon monoxide, compressed	30 m (100 ft)	0.1 km (0.1 mi)	0.2 km (0.1 mi)	200 m (600 ft)	1.2 km (0.7 mi)	4.3 km (2.7 mi)
1017	**124**	Chlorine	60 m (200 ft)	0.3 km (0.2 mi)	1.4 km (0.9 mi)	**Refer to table 3**		
1026	**119**	Cyanogen	30 m (100 ft)	0.1 km (0.1 mi)	0.4 km (0.3 mi)	60 m (200 ft)	0.3 km (0.2 mi)	1.1 km (0.7 mi)
1040 1040	**119P** **119P**	Ethylene oxide Ethylene oxide with Nitrogen	30 m (100 ft)	0.1 km (0.1 mi)	0.2 km (0.2 mi)	**Refer to table 3**		
1045 1045	**124** **124**	Fluorine Fluorine, compressed	30 m (100 ft)	0.1 km (0.1 mi)	0.2 km (0.1 mi)	100 m (300 ft)	0.5 km (0.3 mi)	2.3 km (1.4 mi)
1048	**125**	Hydrogen bromide, anhydrous	30 m (100 ft)	0.1 km (0.1 mi)	0.2 km (0.2 mi)	150 m (500 ft)	1.0 km (0.6 mi)	3.4 km (2.1 mi)
1050	**125**	Hydrogen chloride, anhydrous	30 m (100 ft)	0.1 km (0.1 mi)	0.3 km (0.2 mi)	**Refer to table 3**		

1051 1051	**117P** **117P**	Hydrogen cyanide, anhydrous, stabilized Hydrogen cyanide, stabilized	60 m (200 ft)	0.2 km (0.1 mi)	0.6 km (0.4 mi)	200 m (600 ft)	0.7 km (0.5 mi)	1.7 km (1.1 mi)
1052	**125**	Hydrogen fluoride, anhydrous	30 m (100 ft)	0.1 km (0.1 mi)	0.5 km (0.3 mi)	**Refer to table 3**		
1053 1053	**117** **117**	Hydrogen sulfide Hydrogen sulphide	30 m (100 ft)	0.1 km (0.1 mi)	0.5 km (0.3 mi)	400 m (1250 ft)	2.2 km (1.4 mi)	6.3 km (3.9 mi)
1061	**118**	Methylamine, anhydrous	30 m (100 ft)	0.1 km (0.1 mi)	0.2 km (0.1 mi)	200 m (600 ft)	0.7 km (0.4 mi)	2.1 km (1.3 mi)
1062	**123**	Methyl bromide	30 m (100 ft)	0.1 km (0.1 mi)	0.1 km (0.1 mi)	150 m (500 ft)	0.3 km (0.2 mi)	0.8 km (0.5 mi)
1064	**117**	Methyl mercaptan	30 m (100 ft)	0.1 km (0.1 mi)	0.3 km (0.2 mi)	200 m (600 ft)	1.3 km (0.8 mi)	4.1 km (2.6 mi)
1067 1067	**124** **124**	Dinitrogen tetroxide Nitrogen dioxide	30 m (100 ft)	0.1 km (0.1 mi)	0.4 km (0.3 mi)	400 m (1250 ft)	1.4 km (0.9 mi)	3.3 km (2.1 mi)
1069	**125**	Nitrosyl chloride	30 m (100 ft)	0.2 km (0.2 mi)	1.0 km (0.6 mi)	800 m (2500 ft)	4.3 km (2.7 mi)	10.8 km (6.7 mi)
1076	**125**	Phosgene	100 m (300 ft)	0.6 km (0.4 mi)	2.4 km (1.5 mi)	500 m (1500 ft)	2.9 km (1.8 mi)	9.2 km (5.7 mi)
1079 1079	**125** **125**	Sulfur dioxide Sulphur dioxide	100 m (300 ft)	0.6 km (0.4 mi)	2.5 km (1.6 mi)	**Refer to table 3**		
1082 1082	**119P** **119P**	Refrigerant gas R-1113 Trifluorochloroethylene, stabilized	30 m (100 ft)	0.1 km (0.1 mi)	0.1 km (0.1 mi)	60 m (200 ft)	0.4 km (0.2 mi)	0.8 km (0.5 mi)
1092	**131P**	Acrolein, stabilized	100 m (300 ft)	1.2 km (0.8 mi)	3.3 km (2.1 mi)	500 m (1500 ft)	6.1 km (3.8 mi)	10.8 km (6.7 mi)
1093	**131P**	Acrylonitrile, stabilized	30 m (100 ft)	0.2 km (0.2 mi)	0.6 km (0.4 mi)	100 m (300 ft)	1.2 km (0.8 mi)	2.3 km (1.4 mi)
1098	**131**	Allyl alcohol	30 m (100 ft)	0.2 km (0.1 mi)	0.3 km (0.2 mi)	60 m (200 ft)	0.7 km (0.5 mi)	1.2 km (0.8 mi)
1135	**131**	Ethylene chlorohydrin	30 m (100 ft)	0.1 km (0.1 mi)	0.1 km (0.1 mi)	30 m (100 ft)	0.1 km (0.1 mi)	0.1 km (0.1 mi)
1143 1143	**131P** **131P**	Crotonaldehyde Crotonaldehyde, stabilized	30 m (100 ft)	0.1 km (0.1 mi)	0.2 km (0.1 mi)	60 m (200 ft)	0.5 km (0.3 mi)	0.7 km (0.5 mi)

"+" means distance can be larger in certain atmospheric conditions

TABLE 1

TABLE 1 - INITIAL ISOLATION AND PROTECTIVE ACTION DISTANCES

ID No.	Guide	NAME OF MATERIAL	SMALL SPILLS (From a small package or small leak from a large package) First ISOLATE in all Directions Meters (Feet)	SMALL SPILLS Then PROTECT persons Downwind during DAY Kilometers (Miles)	SMALL SPILLS Then PROTECT persons Downwind during NIGHT Kilometers (Miles)	LARGE SPILLS (From a large package or from many small packages) First ISOLATE in all Directions Meters (Feet)	LARGE SPILLS Then PROTECT persons Downwind during DAY Kilometers (Miles)	LARGE SPILLS Then PROTECT persons Downwind during NIGHT Kilometers (Miles)
1162	**155**	Dimethyldichlorosilane **(when spilled in water)**	30 m (100 ft)	0.1 km (0.1 mi)	0.2 km (0.2 mi)	60 m (200 ft)	0.6 km (0.4 mi)	1.8 km (1.1 mi)
1163	**131**	Dimethylhydrazine, unsymmetrical	30 m (100 ft)	0.2 km (0.1 mi)	0.5 km (0.3 mi)	100 m (300 ft)	1.0 km (0.6 mi)	1.8 km (1.1 mi)
1182	**155**	Ethyl chloroformate	30 m (100 ft)	0.2 km (0.1 mi)	0.3 km (0.2 mi)	60 m (200 ft)	0.6 km (0.4 mi)	0.9 km (0.6 mi)
1183	**139**	Ethyldichlorosilane **(when spilled in water)**	30 m (100 ft)	0.1 km (0.1 mi)	0.1 km (0.1 mi)	60 m (200 ft)	0.6 km (0.4 mi)	2.0 km (1.3 mi)
1185	**131P**	Ethyleneimine, stabilized	30 m (100 ft)	0.2 km (0.1 mi)	0.5 km (0.3 mi)	200 m (600 ft)	0.9 km (0.6 mi)	1.8 km (1.1 mi)
1196	**155**	Ethyltrichlorosilane **(when spilled in water)**	30 m (100 ft)	0.1 km (0.1 mi)	0.5 km (0.3 mi)	200 m (600 ft)	2.1 km (1.3 mi)	5.8 km (3.6 mi)
1238	**155**	Methyl chloroformate	30 m (100 ft)	0.2 km (0.2 mi)	0.5 km (0.4 mi)	150 m (500 ft)	1.1 km (0.7 mi)	2.1 km (1.3 mi)
1239	**131**	Methyl chloromethyl ether	60 m (200 ft)	0.5 km (0.3 mi)	1.5 km (0.9 mi)	300 m (1000 ft)	3.1 km (2.0 mi)	5.8 km (3.6 mi)
1242	**139**	Methyldichlorosilane **(when spilled in water)**	30 m (100 ft)	0.1 km (0.1 mi)	0.1 km (0.1 mi)	60 m (200 ft)	0.8 km (0.5 mi)	2.3 km (1.5 mi)
1244	**131**	Methylhydrazine	30 m (100 ft)	0.3 km (0.2 mi)	0.6 km (0.4 mi)	100 m (300 ft)	1.4 km (0.9 mi)	2.1 km (1.3 mi)
1250	**155**	Methyltrichlorosilane **(when spilled in water)**	30 m (100 ft)	0.1 km (0.1 mi)	0.1 km (0.1 mi)	60 m (200 ft)	0.8 km (0.5 mi)	2.5 km (1.6 mi)
1251	**131P**	Methyl vinyl ketone, stabilized	100 m (300 ft)	0.3 km (0.2 mi)	0.7 km (0.4 mi)	800 m (2500 ft)	1.6 km (1.0 mi)	2.8 km (1.8 mi)
1259	**131**	Nickel carbonyl	100 m (300 ft)	1.3 km (0.8 mi)	5.0 km (3.1 mi)	1000 m (3000 ft)	10.8 km (6.8 mi)	11.0+ km (7.0+ mi)

1295	**139**	Trichlorosilane **(when spilled in water)**	30 m	(100 ft)	0.1 km	(0.1 mi)	0.1 km	(0.1 mi)	60 m	(200 ft)	0.6 km	(0.4 mi)	2.1 km	(1.3 mi)
1298	**155**	Trimethylchlorosilane **(when spilled in water)**	30 m	(100 ft)	0.1 km	(0.1 mi)	0.1 km	(0.1 mi)	60 m	(200 ft)	0.5 km	(0.3 mi)	1.4 km	(0.9 mi)
1305 1305	**155P** **155P**	Vinyltrichlorosilane **(when spilled in water)** Vinyltrichlorosilane, stabilized **(when spilled in water)**	30 m	(100 ft)	0.1 km	(0.1 mi)	0.1 km	(0.1 mi)	60 m	(200 ft)	0.6 km	(0.4 mi)	1.9 km	(1.2 mi)
1340 1340	**139** **139**	Phosphorus pentasulfide, free from yellow and white Phosphorus **(when spilled in water)** Phosphorus pentasulphide, free from yellow and white Phosphorus **(when spilled in water)**	30 m	(100 ft)	0.1 km	(0.1 mi)	0.1 km	(0.1 mi)	60 m	(200 ft)	0.3 km	(0.2 mi)	1.4 km	(0.9 mi)
1360	**139**	Calcium phosphide **(when spilled in water)**	30 m	(100 ft)	0.1 km	(0.1 mi)	0.4 km	(0.3 mi)	300 m	(1000 ft)	1.0 km	(0.6 mi)	3.5 km	(2.2 mi)
1380	**135**	Pentaborane	60 m	(200 ft)	0.6 km	(0.4 mi)	1.9 km	(1.2 mi)	200 m	(600 ft)	2.7 km	(1.7 mi)	6.2 km	(3.9 mi)
1384 1384 1384	**135** **135** **135**	Sodium dithionite **(when spilled in water)** Sodium hydrosulfite **(when spilled in water)** Sodium hydrosulphite **(when spilled in water)**	30 m	(100 ft)	0.1 km	(0.1 mi)	0.4 km	(0.3 mi)	60 m	(200 ft)	0.6 km	(0.4 mi)	2.5 km	(1.6 mi)
1390	**139**	Alkali metal amides **(when spilled in water)**	30 m	(100 ft)	0.1 km	(0.1 mi)	0.3 km	(0.2 mi)	60 m	(200 ft)	0.6 km	(0.4 mi)	2.2 km	(1.4 mi)
1397	**139**	Aluminum phosphide **(when spilled in water)**	30 m	(100 ft)	0.1 km	(0.1 mi)	0.7 km	(0.5 mi)	500 m	(1500 ft)	2.0 km	(1.2 mi)	6.5 km	(4.0 mi)

"+" means distance can be larger in certain atmospheric conditions

TABLE 1

TABLE 1 - INITIAL ISOLATION AND PROTECTIVE ACTION DISTANCES

ID No.	Guide	NAME OF MATERIAL	SMALL SPILLS (From a small package or small leak from a large package) — First ISOLATE in all Directions, Meters (Feet)	Then PROTECT persons Downwind during DAY, Kilometers (Miles)	NIGHT, Kilometers (Miles)	LARGE SPILLS (From a large package or from many small packages) — First ISOLATE in all Directions, Meters (Feet)	Then PROTECT persons Downwind during DAY, Kilometers (Miles)	NIGHT, Kilometers (Miles)
1419	**139**	Magnesium aluminum phosphide **(when spilled in water)**	30 m (100 ft)	0.1 km (0.1 mi)	0.6 km (0.4 mi)	500 m (1500 ft)	1.8 km (1.1 mi)	5.8 km (3.6 mi)
1432	**139**	Sodium phosphide **(when spilled in water)**	30 m (100 ft)	0.1 km (0.1 mi)	0.4 km (0.2 mi)	300 m (1000 ft)	1.3 km (0.8 mi)	3.8 km (2.4 mi)
1510	**143**	Tetranitromethane	30 m (100 ft)	0.2 km (0.1 mi)	0.3 km (0.2 mi)	30 m (100 ft)	0.4 km (0.3 mi)	0.7 km (0.4 mi)
1541	**155**	Acetone cyanohydrin, stabilized **(when spilled in water)**	30 m (100 ft)	0.1 km (0.1 mi)	0.1 km (0.1 mi)	60 m (200 ft)	0.2 km (0.2 mi)	0.8 km (0.5 mi)
1556	**152**	Methyldichloroarsine	100 m (300 ft)	1.4 km (0.9 mi)	2.1 km (1.3 mi)	300 m (1000 ft)	3.8 km (2.4 mi)	5.2 km (3.3 mi)
1560 1560	**157** **157**	Arsenic chloride Arsenic trichloride	30 m (100 ft)	0.2 km (0.1 mi)	0.3 km (0.2 mi)	100 m (300 ft)	1.0 km (0.6 mi)	1.5 km (1.0 mi)
1569	**131**	Bromoacetone	30 m (100 ft)	0.4 km (0.3 mi)	1.2 km (0.7 mi)	150 m (500 ft)	1.6 km (1.0 mi)	3.2 km (2.0 mi)
1580	**154**	Chloropicrin	60 m (200 ft)	0.5 km (0.3 mi)	1.2 km (0.8 mi)	200 m (600 ft)	2.2 km (1.4 mi)	3.6 km (2.3 mi)
1581 1581	**123** **123**	Chloropicrin and Methyl bromide mixture Methyl bromide and Chloropicrin mixture	30 m (100 ft)	0.1 km (0.1 mi)	0.6 km (0.4 mi)	300 m (1000 ft)	2.1 km (1.3 mi)	5.9 km (3.7 mi)
1582 1582	**119** **119**	Chloropicrin and Methyl chloride mixture Methyl chloride and Chloropicrin mixture	30 m (100 ft)	0.1 km (0.1 mi)	0.4 km (0.3 mi)	60 m (200 ft)	0.4 km (0.2 mi)	1.7 km (1.1 mi)
1583	**154**	Chloropicrin mixture, n.o.s.	60 m (200 ft)	0.5 km (0.3 mi)	1.2 km (0.8 mi)	200 m (600 ft)	2.2 km (1.4 mi)	3.6 km (2.3 mi)

1589	**125**	Cyanogen chloride, stabilized	300 m (1000 ft)	1.8 km (1.2 mi)	6.4 km (4.0 mi)	1000 m (3000 ft)	9.7 km (6.0 mi)	11.0+ km (7.0+ mi)
1595 1595	**156** **156**	Dimethyl sulfate Dimethyl sulphate	30 m (100 ft)	0.2 km (0.1 mi)	0.2 km (0.1 mi)	60 m (200 ft)	0.5 km (0.3 mi)	0.6 km (0.4 mi)
1605	**154**	Ethylene dibromide	30 m (100 ft)	0.1 km (0.1 mi)	0.1 km (0.1 mi)	30 m (100 ft)	0.1 km (0.1 mi)	0.2 km (0.1 mi)
1612 1612	**123** **123**	Compressed gas and hexaethyl tetraphosphate mixture Hexaethyl tetraphosphate and compressed gas mixture	100 m (300 ft)	0.8 km (0.5 mi)	2.7 km (1.7 mi)	400 m (1250 ft)	3.5 km (2.2 mi)	8.1 km (5.1 mi)
1613 1613	**154** **154**	Hydrocyanic acid, aqueous solution, with not more than 20% Hydrogen cyanide Hydrogen cyanide, aqueous solution, with not more than 20% Hydrogen cyanide	30 m (100 ft)	0.1 km (0.1 mi)	0.1 km (0.1 mi)	100 m (300 ft)	0.5 km (0.3 mi)	1.1 km (0.7 mi)
1614	**152**	Hydrogen cyanide, stabilized (absorbed)	60 m (200 ft)	0.2 km (0.1 mi)	0.6 km (0.4 mi)	150 m (500 ft)	0.5 km (0.3 mi)	1.5 km (0.9 mi)
1647 1647	**151** **151**	Ethylene dibromide and Methyl bromide mixture, liquid Methyl bromide and Ethylene dibromide mixture, liquid	30 m (100 ft)	0.1 km (0.1 mi)	0.1 km (0.1 mi)	150 m (500 ft)	0.3 km (0.2 mi)	0.8 km (0.5 mi)
1660 1660	**124** **124**	Nitric oxide Nitric oxide, compressed	30 m (100 ft)	0.1 km (0.1 mi)	0.6 km (0.4 mi)	100 m (300 ft)	0.6 km (0.4 mi)	2.2 km (1.4 mi)
1670	**157**	Perchloromethyl mercaptan	30 m (100 ft)	0.2 km (0.2 mi)	0.4 km (0.2 mi)	100 m (300 ft)	0.8 km (0.5 mi)	1.2 km (0.8 mi)
1672	**151**	Phenylcarbylamine chloride	30 m (100 ft)	0.2 km (0.1 mi)	0.2 km (0.1 mi)	60 m (200 ft)	0.5 km (0.3 mi)	0.7 km (0.4 mi)
1680	**157**	Potassium cyanide, solid **(when spilled in water)**	30 m (100 ft)	0.1 km (0.1 mi)	0.1 km (0.1 mi)	60 m (200 ft)	0.2 km (0.2 mi)	1.0 km (0.6 mi)
1689	**157**	Sodium cyanide, solid **(when spilled in water)**	30 m (100 ft)	0.1 km (0.1 mi)	0.1 km (0.1 mi)	100 m (300 ft)	0.3 km (0.2 mi)	1.2 km (0.7 mi)

"+" means distance can be larger in certain atmospheric conditions

TABLE 1

TABLE 1 - INITIAL ISOLATION AND PROTECTIVE ACTION DISTANCES

			SMALL SPILLS (From a small package or small leak from a large package)						LARGE SPILLS (From a large package or from many small packages)					
			First ISOLATE in all Directions		Then PROTECT persons Downwind during				First ISOLATE in all Directions		Then PROTECT persons Downwind during			
					DAY		NIGHT				DAY		NIGHT	
ID No.	Guide	NAME OF MATERIAL	Meters	(Feet)	Kilometers	(Miles)	Kilometers	(Miles)	Meters	(Feet)	Kilometers	(Miles)	Kilometers	(Miles)
1695	**131**	Chloroacetone, stabilized	30 m	(100 ft)	0.1 km	(0.1 mi)	0.2 km	(0.1 mi)	60 m	(200 ft)	0.4 km	(0.3 mi)	0.6 km	(0.4 mi)
1716	**156**	Acetyl bromide **(when spilled in water)**	30 m	(100 ft)	0.1 km	(0.1 mi)	0.1 km	(0.1 mi)	30 m	(100 ft)	0.3 km	(0.2 mi)	0.9 km	(0.6 mi)
1717	**155**	Acetyl chloride **(when spilled in water)**	30 m	(100 ft)	0.1 km	(0.1 mi)	0.1 km	(0.1 mi)	100 m	(300 ft)	0.9 km	(0.6 mi)	2.6 km	(1.6 mi)
1722 1722	**155** **155**	Allyl chlorocarbonate Allyl chloroformate	100 m	(300 ft)	0.3 km	(0.2 mi)	0.8 km	(0.5 mi)	400 m	(1250 ft)	1.4 km	(0.9 mi)	2.4 km	(1.5 mi)
1724	**155**	Allyltrichlorosilane, stabilized **(when spilled in water)**	30 m	(100 ft)	0.1 km	(0.1 mi)	0.1 km	(0.1 mi)	60 m	(200 ft)	0.5 km	(0.3 mi)	1.7 km	(1.1 mi)
1725	**137**	Aluminum bromide, anhydrous **(when spilled in water)**	30 m	(100 ft)	0.1 km	(0.1 mi)	0.1 km	(0.1 mi)	30 m	(100 ft)	0.1 km	(0.1 mi)	0.3 km	(0.2 mi)
1726	**137**	Aluminum chloride, anhydrous **(when spilled in water)**	30 m	(100 ft)	0.1 km	(0.1 mi)	0.2 km	(0.1 mi)	60 m	(200 ft)	0.5 km	(0.3 mi)	2.0 km	(1.2 mi)
1728	**155**	Amyltrichlorosilane **(when spilled in water)**	30 m	(100 ft)	0.1 km	(0.1 mi)	0.1 km	(0.1 mi)	60 m	(200 ft)	0.5 km	(0.3 mi)	1.7 km	(1.0 mi)
1732	**157**	Antimony pentafluoride **(when spilled in water)**	30 m	(100 ft)	0.1 km	(0.1 mi)	0.3 km	(0.2 mi)	100 m	(300 ft)	1.1 km	(0.7 mi)	3.9 km	(2.4 mi)
1741	**125**	Boron trichloride **(when spilled on land)**	30 m	(100 ft)	0.1 km	(0.1 mi)	0.3 km	(0.2 mi)	100 m	(300 ft)	0.6 km	(0.4 mi)	1.4 km	(0.9 mi)
1741	**125**	Boron trichloride **(when spilled in water)**	30 m	(100 ft)	0.1 km	(0.1 mi)	0.3 km	(0.2 mi)	100 m	(300 ft)	1.2 km	(0.8 mi)	3.6 km	(2.2 mi)

1744 1744 1744	**154** **154** **154**	Bromine Bromine, solution Bromine, solution (Inhalation Hazard Zone A)	60 m	(200 ft)	0.8 km	(0.5 mi)	2.3 km	(1.5 mi)	300 m	(1000 ft)	3.8 km	(2.4 mi)	7.5 km	(4.7 mi)
1744	**154**	Bromine, solution (Inhalation Hazard Zone B)	30 m	(100 ft)	0.1 km	(0.1 mi)	0.2 km	(0.2 mi)	30 m	(100 ft)	0.3 km	(0.2 mi)	0.5 km	(0.3 mi)
1745	**144**	Bromine pentafluoride **(when spilled on land)**	100 m	(300 ft)	0.9 km	(0.5 mi)	2.5 km	(1.6 mi)	400 m	(1250 ft)	5.4 km	(3.3 mi)	10.7 km	(6.6 mi)
1745	**144**	Bromine pentafluoride **(when spilled in water)**	30 m	(100 ft)	0.1 km	(0.1 mi)	0.3 km	(0.2 mi)	150 m	(500 ft)	1.2 km	(0.7 mi)	4.0 km	(2.5 mi)
1746	**144**	Bromine trifluoride **(when spilled on land)**	30 m	(100 ft)	0.1 km	(0.1 mi)	0.2 km	(0.1 mi)	30 m	(100 ft)	0.3 km	(0.2 mi)	0.4 km	(0.3 mi)
1746	**144**	Bromine trifluoride **(when spilled in water)**	30 m	(100 ft)	0.1 km	(0.1 mi)	0.3 km	(0.2 mi)	100 m	(300 ft)	1.0 km	(0.7 mi)	3.7 km	(2.3 mi)
1747	**155**	Butyltrichlorosilane **(when spilled in water)**	30 m	(100 ft)	0.1 km	(0.1 mi)	0.1 km	(0.1 mi)	60 m	(200 ft)	0.5 km	(0.3 mi)	1.6 km	(1.0 mi)
1749	**124**	Chlorine trifluoride	60 m	(200 ft)	0.3 km	(0.2 mi)	1.1 km	(0.7 mi)	200 m	(600 ft)	1.4 km	(0.9 mi)	3.6 km	(2.3 mi)
1752	**156**	Chloroacetyl chloride **(when spilled on land)**	30 m	(100 ft)	0.3 km	(0.2 mi)	0.6 km	(0.4 mi)	100 m	(300 ft)	1.1 km	(0.7 mi)	1.9 km	(1.2 mi)
1752	**156**	Chloroacetyl chloride **(when spilled in water)**	30 m	(100 ft)	0.1 km	(0.1 mi)	0.1 km	(0.1 mi)	30 m	(100 ft)	0.2 km	(0.1 mi)	0.6 km	(0.4 mi)
1753	**156**	Chlorophenyltrichlorosilane **(when spilled in water)**	30 m	(100 ft)	0.1 km	(0.1 mi)	0.1 km	(0.1 mi)	30 m	(100 ft)	0.2 km	(0.2 mi)	0.8 km	(0.5 mi)
1754	**137**	Chlorosulfonic acid (with or without sulfur trioxide) **(when spilled on land)**	30 m	(100 ft)	0.1 km	(0.1 mi)	0.1 km	(0.1 mi)	30 m	(100 ft)	0.2 km	(0.2 mi)	0.3 km	(0.2 mi)

"+" means distance can be larger in certain atmospheric conditions

TABLE 1

TABLE 1 - INITIAL ISOLATION AND PROTECTIVE ACTION DISTANCES

ID No.	Guide	NAME OF MATERIAL	SMALL SPILLS (From a small package or small leak from a large package) First ISOLATE in all Directions Meters (Feet)	SMALL SPILLS Then PROTECT persons Downwind during DAY Kilometers (Miles)	SMALL SPILLS Then PROTECT persons Downwind during NIGHT Kilometers (Miles)	LARGE SPILLS (From a large package or from many small packages) First ISOLATE in all Directions Meters (Feet)	LARGE SPILLS Then PROTECT persons Downwind during DAY Kilometers (Miles)	LARGE SPILLS Then PROTECT persons Downwind during NIGHT Kilometers (Miles)
1754	**137**	Chlorosulfonic acid (with or without sulfur trioxide) **(when spilled in water)**	30 m (100 ft)	0.1 km (0.1 mi)	0.1 km (0.1 mi)	60 m (200 ft)	0.7 km (0.4 mi)	2.3 km (1.4 mi)
1754	**137**	Chlorosulphonic acid (with or without sulphur trioxide) **(when spilled on land)**	30 m (100 ft)	0.1 km (0.1 mi)	0.1 km (0.1 mi)	30 m (100 ft)	0.2 km (0.2 mi)	0.3 km (0.2 mi)
1754	**137**	Chlorosulphonic acid (with or without sulphur trioxide) **(when spilled in water)**	30 m (100 ft)	0.1 km (0.1 mi)	0.1 km (0.1 mi)	60 m (200 ft)	0.7 km (0.4 mi)	2.3 km (1.4 mi)
1758	**137**	Chromium oxychloride **(when spilled in water)**	30 m (100 ft)	0.1 km (0.1 mi)	0.1 km (0.1 mi)	30 m (100 ft)	0.1 km (0.1 mi)	0.5 km (0.3 mi)
1762	**156**	Cyclohexenyltrichlorosilane **(when spilled in water)**	30 m (100 ft)	0.1 km (0.1 mi)	0.1 km (0.1 mi)	30 m (100 ft)	0.3 km (0.2 mi)	1.2 km (0.7 mi)
1763	**156**	Cyclohexyltrichlorosilane **(when spilled in water)**	30 m (100 ft)	0.1 km (0.1 mi)	0.1 km (0.1 mi)	30 m (100 ft)	0.3 km (0.2 mi)	1.2 km (0.7 mi)
1765	**156**	Dichloroacetyl chloride **(when spilled in water)**	30 m (100 ft)	0.1 km (0.1 mi)	0.1 km (0.1 mi)	30 m (100 ft)	0.2 km (0.1 mi)	0.7 km (0.5 mi)
1766	**156**	Dichlorophenyltrichlorosilane **(when spilled in water)**	30 m (100 ft)	0.1 km (0.1 mi)	0.1 km (0.1 mi)	60 m (200 ft)	0.5 km (0.4 mi)	2.0 km (1.2 mi)
1767	**155**	Diethyldichlorosilane **(when spilled in water)**	30 m (100 ft)	0.1 km (0.1 mi)	0.1 km (0.1 mi)	30 m (100 ft)	0.3 km (0.2 mi)	0.9 km (0.5 mi)

1769	**156**	Diphenyldichlorosilane **(when spilled in water)**	30 m	(100 ft)	0.1 km	(0.1 mi)	0.1 km	(0.1 mi)	30 m	(100 ft)	0.3 km	(0.2 mi)	1.1 km	(0.7 mi)
1771	**156**	Dodecyltrichlorosilane **(when spilled in water)**	30 m	(100 ft)	0.1 km	(0.1 mi)	0.1 km	(0.1 mi)	30 m	(100 ft)	0.4 km	(0.3 mi)	1.2 km	(0.8 mi)
1777 1777	**137** **137**	Fluorosulfonic acid **(when spilled in water)** Fluorosulphonic acid **(when spilled in water)**	30 m	(100 ft)	0.1 km	(0.1 mi)	0.1 km	(0.1 mi)	30 m	(100 ft)	0.2 km	(0.1 mi)	0.5 km	(0.3 mi)
1781	**156**	Hexadecyltrichlorosilane **(when spilled in water)**	30 m	(100 ft)	0.1 km	(0.1 mi)	0.1 km	(0.1 mi)	30 m	(100 ft)	0.1 km	(0.1 mi)	0.4 km	(0.3 mi)
1784	**156**	Hexyltrichlorosilane **(when spilled in water)**	30 m	(100 ft)	0.1 km	(0.1 mi)	0.1 km	(0.1 mi)	30 m	(100 ft)	0.4 km	(0.2 mi)	1.3 km	(0.8 mi)
1799	**156**	Nonyltrichlorosilane **(when spilled in water)**	30 m	(100 ft)	0.1 km	(0.1 mi)	0.1 km	(0.1 mi)	30 m	(100 ft)	0.4 km	(0.3 mi)	1.4 km	(0.9 mi)
1800	**156**	Octadecyltrichlorosilane **(when spilled in water)**	30 m	(100 ft)	0.1 km	(0.1 mi)	0.1 km	(0.1 mi)	30 m	(100 ft)	0.4 km	(0.3 mi)	1.3 km	(0.8 mi)
1801	**156**	Octyltrichlorosilane **(when spilled in water)**	30 m	(100 ft)	0.1 km	(0.1 mi)	0.1 km	(0.1 mi)	30 m	(100 ft)	0.4 km	(0.3 mi)	1.4 km	(0.9 mi)
1804	**156**	Phenyltrichlorosilane **(when spilled in water)**	30 m	(100 ft)	0.1 km	(0.1 mi)	0.1 km	(0.1 mi)	30 m	(100 ft)	0.4 km	(0.2 mi)	1.3 km	(0.8 mi)
1806	**137**	Phosphorus pentachloride **(when spilled in water)**	30 m	(100 ft)	0.1 km	(0.1 mi)	0.1 km	(0.1 mi)	30 m	(100 ft)	0.3 km	(0.2 mi)	1.3 km	(0.8 mi)
1808	**137**	Phosphorus tribromide **(when spilled in water)**	30 m	(100 ft)	0.1 km	(0.1 mi)	0.1 km	(0.1 mi)	30 m	(100 ft)	0.4 km	(0.3 mi)	1.5 km	(0.9 mi)
1809	**137**	Phosphorus trichloride **(when spilled on land)**	30 m	(100 ft)	0.2 km	(0.2 mi)	0.6 km	(0.4 mi)	100 m	(300 ft)	1.0 km	(0.7 mi)	2.1 km	(1.3 mi)
1809	**137**	Phosphorus trichloride **(when spilled in water)**	30 m	(100 ft)	0.1 km	(0.1 mi)	0.1 km	(0.1 mi)	60 m	(200 ft)	0.7 km	(0.4 mi)	2.4 km	(1.5 mi)

"+" means distance can be larger in certain atmospheric conditions

TABLE 1

TABLE 1 - INITIAL ISOLATION AND PROTECTIVE ACTION DISTANCES

ID No.	Guide	NAME OF MATERIAL	SMALL SPILLS (From a small package or small leak from a large package) First ISOLATE in all Directions Meters (Feet)	SMALL SPILLS Then PROTECT persons Downwind during DAY Kilometers (Miles)	SMALL SPILLS Then PROTECT persons Downwind during NIGHT Kilometers (Miles)	LARGE SPILLS (From a large package or from many small packages) First ISOLATE in all Directions Meters (Feet)	LARGE SPILLS Then PROTECT persons Downwind during DAY Kilometers (Miles)	LARGE SPILLS Then PROTECT persons Downwind during NIGHT Kilometers (Miles)
1810	137	Phosphorus oxychloride **(when spilled on land)**	30 m (100 ft)	0.3 km (0.2 mi)	0.6 km (0.4 mi)	100 m (300 ft)	1.0 km (0.7 mi)	1.9 km (1.2 mi)
1810	137	Phosphorus oxychloride **(when spilled in water)**	30 m (100 ft)	0.1 km (0.1 mi)	0.1 km (0.1 mi)	60 m (200 ft)	0.6 km (0.4 mi)	2.1 km (1.3 mi)
1815	132	Propionyl chloride **(when spilled in water)**	30 m (100 ft)	0.1 km (0.1 mi)	0.1 km (0.1 mi)	30 m (100 ft)	0.2 km (0.1 mi)	0.5 km (0.3 mi)
1816	155	Propyltrichlorosilane **(when spilled in water)**	30 m (100 ft)	0.1 km (0.1 mi)	0.1 km (0.1 mi)	60 m (200 ft)	0.5 km (0.3 mi)	1.9 km (1.2 mi)
1818	157	Silicon tetrachloride **(when spilled in water)**	30 m (100 ft)	0.1 km (0.1 mi)	0.2 km (0.1 mi)	60 m (200 ft)	0.8 km (0.5 mi)	2.7 km (1.7 mi)
1828	137	Sulfur chlorides **(when spilled on land)**	30 m (100 ft)	0.1 km (0.1 mi)	0.1 km (0.1 mi)	60 m (200 ft)	0.3 km (0.2 mi)	0.4 km (0.3 mi)
1828	137	Sulfur chlorides **(when spilled in water)**	30 m (100 ft)	0.1 km (0.1 mi)	0.1 km (0.1 mi)	30 m (100 ft)	0.3 km (0.2 mi)	1.0 km (0.6 mi)
1828	137	Sulphur chlorides **(when spilled on land)**	30 m (100 ft)	0.1 km (0.1 mi)	0.1 km (0.1 mi)	60 m (200 ft)	0.3 km (0.2 mi)	0.4 km (0.3 mi)
1828	137	Sulphur chlorides **(when spilled in water)**	30 m (100 ft)	0.1 km (0.1 mi)	0.1 km (0.1 mi)	30 m (100 ft)	0.3 km (0.2 mi)	1.0 km (0.6 mi)
1829 1829	137 137	Sulfur trioxide, stabilized Sulphur trioxide, stabilized	60 m (200 ft)	0.4 km (0.2 mi)	1.0 km (0.6 mi)	300 m (1000 ft)	2.9 km (1.8 mi)	6.3 km (4.0 mi)
1831 1831	137 137	Sulfuric acid, fuming Sulphuric acid, fuming	60 m (200 ft)	0.4 km (0.2 mi)	1.0 km (0.6 mi)	300 m (1000 ft)	2.9 km (1.8 mi)	6.3 km (4.0 mi)

1834	**137**	Sulfuryl chloride **(when spilled on land)**	30 m	(100 ft)	0.2 km	(0.1 mi)	0.4 km	(0.3 mi)	60 m	(200 ft)	0.8 km	(0.5 mi)	1.5 km	(0.9 mi)
1834	**137**	Sulfuryl chloride **(when spilled in water)**	30 m	(100 ft)	0.1 km	(0.1 mi)	0.1 km	(0.1 mi)	30 m	(100 ft)	0.4 km	(0.3 mi)	1.6 km	(1.0 mi)
1834	**137**	Sulphuryl chloride **(when spilled on land)**	30 m	(100 ft)	0.2 km	(0.1 mi)	0.4 km	(0.3 mi)	60 m	(200 ft)	0.8 km	(0.5 mi)	1.5 km	(0.9 mi)
1834	**137**	Sulphuryl chloride **(when spilled in water)**	30 m	(100 ft)	0.1 km	(0.1 mi)	0.1 km	(0.1 mi)	30 m	(100 ft)	0.4 km	(0.3 mi)	1.6 km	(1.0 mi)
1836	**137**	Thionyl chloride **(when spilled on land)**	30 m	(100 ft)	0.1 km	(0.1 mi)	0.2 km	(0.2 mi)	30 m	(100 ft)	0.3 km	(0.2 mi)	0.5 km	(0.3 mi)
1836	**137**	Thionyl chloride **(when spilled in water)**	100 m	(300 ft)	0.9 km	(0.6 mi)	2.9 km	(1.8 mi)	800 m	(2500 ft)	9.7 km	(6.0 mi)	11.0+ km	(7.0+ mi)
1838	**137**	Titanium tetrachloride **(when spilled on land)**	30 m	(100 ft)	0.1 km	(0.1 mi)	0.2 km	(0.1 mi)	30 m	(100 ft)	0.3 km	(0.2 mi)	0.5 km	(0.3 mi)
1838	**137**	Titanium tetrachloride **(when spilled in water)**	30 m	(100 ft)	0.1 km	(0.1 mi)	0.1 km	(0.1 mi)	60 m	(200 ft)	0.5 km	(0.3 mi)	1.7 km	(1.0 mi)
1859 1859	**125** **125**	Silicon tetrafluoride Silicon tetrafluoride, compressed	30 m	(100 ft)	0.2 km	(0.1 mi)	0.8 km	(0.5 mi)	100 m	(300 ft)	0.5 km	(0.3 mi)	1.8 km	(1.2 mi)
1892	**151**	Ethyldichloroarsine	150 m	(500 ft)	1.5 km	(0.9 mi)	2.1 km	(1.3 mi)	400 m	(1250 ft)	4.6 km	(2.9 mi)	6.4 km	(4.0 mi)
1898	**156**	Acetyl iodide **(when spilled in water)**	30 m	(100 ft)	0.1 km	(0.1 mi)	0.1 km	(0.1 mi)	30 m	(100 ft)	0.4 km	(0.3 mi)	1.1 km	(0.7 mi)
1911 1911 1911	**119** **119** **119**	Diborane Diborane, compressed Diborane mixtures	60 m	(200 ft)	0.3 km	(0.2 mi)	1.2 km	(0.7 mi)	300 m	(1000 ft)	1.5 km	(1.0 mi)	4.6 km	(2.9 mi)

"+" means distance can be larger in certain atmospheric conditions

TABLE 1

TABLE 1 - INITIAL ISOLATION AND PROTECTIVE ACTION DISTANCES

			SMALL SPILLS (From a small package or small leak from a large package)			LARGE SPILLS (From a large package or from many small packages)		
			First ISOLATE in all Directions	Then PROTECT persons Downwind during		First ISOLATE in all Directions	Then PROTECT persons Downwind during	
ID No.	Guide	NAME OF MATERIAL	Meters (Feet)	DAY Kilometers (Miles)	NIGHT Kilometers (Miles)	Meters (Feet)	DAY Kilometers (Miles)	NIGHT Kilometers (Miles)
1923	**135**	Calcium dithionite **(when spilled in water)**	30 m (100 ft)	0.1 km (0.1 mi)	0.4 km (0.3 mi)	60 m (200 ft)	0.7 km (0.4 mi)	2.6 km (1.6 mi)
1923	**135**	Calcium hydrosulfite **(when spilled in water)**						
1923	**135**	Calcium hydrosulphite **(when spilled in water)**						
1929	**135**	Potassium dithionite **(when spilled in water)**	30 m (100 ft)	0.1 km (0.1 mi)	0.4 km (0.2 mi)	60 m (200 ft)	0.6 km (0.4 mi)	2.3 km (1.5 mi)
1929	**135**	Potassium hydrosulfite **(when spilled in water)**						
1929	**135**	Potassium hydrosulphite **(when spilled in water)**						
1931	**171**	Zinc dithionite **(when spilled in water)**	30 m (100 ft)	0.1 km (0.1 mi)	0.4 km (0.3 mi)	60 m (200 ft)	0.6 km (0.4 mi)	2.4 km (1.5 mi)
1931	**171**	Zinc hydrosulfite **(when spilled in water)**						
1931	**171**	Zinc hydrosulphite **(when spilled in water)**						
1953	**119**	Compressed gas, poisonous, flammable, n.o.s.	150 m (500 ft)	1.0 km (0.6 mi)	3.8 km (2.4 mi)	1000 m (3000 ft)	5.7 km (3.6 mi)	10.1 km (6.3 mi)
1953	**119**	Compressed gas, poisonous, flammable, n.o.s. (Inhalation Hazard Zone A)						
1953	**119**	Compressed gas, poisonous, flammable, n.o.s. (Inhalation Hazard Zone B)	30 m (100 ft)	0.1 km (0.1 mi)	0.4 km (0.2 mi)	300 m (1000 ft)	1.3 km (0.8 mi)	3.4 km (2.1 mi)

1953	**119**	Compressed gas, poisonous, flammable, n.o.s. (Inhalation Hazard Zone C)	30 m	(100 ft)	0.1 km	(0.1 mi)	0.3 km	(0.2 mi)	150 m	(500 ft)	1.0 km	(0.6 mi)	2.9 km	(1.8 mi)
1953	**119**	Compressed gas, poisonous, flammable, n.o.s. (Inhalation Hazard Zone D)	30 m	(100 ft)	0.1 km	(0.1 mi)	0.2 km	(0.1 mi)	150 m	(500 ft)	0.8 km	(0.5 mi)	2.0 km	(1.3 mi)
1953 1953	**119** **119**	Compressed gas, toxic, flammable, n.o.s. Compressed gas, toxic, flammable, n.o.s. (Inhalation Hazard Zone A)	150 m	(500 ft)	1.0 km	(0.6 mi)	3.8 km	(2.4 mi)	1000 m	(3000 ft)	5.7 km	(3.6 mi)	10.1 km	(6.3 mi)
1953	**119**	Compressed gas, toxic, flammable, n.o.s. (Inhalation Hazard Zone B)	30 m	(100 ft)	0.1 km	(0.1 mi)	0.4 km	(0.2 mi)	300 m	(1000 ft)	1.3 km	(0.8 mi)	3.4 km	(2.1 mi)
1953	**119**	Compressed gas, toxic, flammable, n.o.s. (Inhalation Hazard Zone C)	30 m	(100 ft)	0.1 km	(0.1 mi)	0.3 km	(0.2 mi)	150 m	(500 ft)	1.0 km	(0.6 mi)	2.9 km	(1.8 mi)
1953	**119**	Compressed gas, toxic, flammable, n.o.s. (Inhalation Hazard Zone D)	30 m	(100 ft)	0.1 km	(0.1 mi)	0.2 km	(0.1 mi)	150 m	(500 ft)	0.8 km	(0.5 mi)	2.0 km	(1.3 mi)
1955 1955	**123** **123**	Compressed gas, poisonous, n.o.s. Compressed gas, poisonous, n.o.s. (Inhalation Hazard Zone A)	100 m	(300 ft)	0.5 km	(0.3 mi)	2.5 km	(1.6 mi)	1000 m	(3000 ft)	5.7 km	(3.6 mi)	10.1 km	(6.3 mi)
1955	**123**	Compressed gas, poisonous, n.o.s. (Inhalation Hazard Zone B)	30 m	(100 ft)	0.2 km	(0.1 mi)	0.9 km	(0.6 mi)	400 m	(1250 ft)	2.3 km	(1.4 mi)	5.1 km	(3.2 mi)
1955	**123**	Compressed gas, poisonous, n.o.s. (Inhalation Hazard Zone C)	30 m	(100 ft)	0.1 km	(0.1 mi)	0.3 km	(0.2 mi)	150 m	(500 ft)	1.0 km	(0.6 mi)	2.9 km	(1.8 mi)

"+" means distance can be larger in certain atmospheric conditions

TABLE 1

TABLE 1 - INITIAL ISOLATION AND PROTECTIVE ACTION DISTANCES

ID No.	Guide	NAME OF MATERIAL	SMALL SPILLS (From a small package or small leak from a large package) First ISOLATE in all Directions Meters (Feet)	SMALL SPILLS Then PROTECT persons Downwind during DAY Kilometers (Miles)	SMALL SPILLS Then PROTECT persons Downwind during NIGHT Kilometers (Miles)	LARGE SPILLS (From a large package or from many small packages) First ISOLATE in all Directions Meters (Feet)	LARGE SPILLS Then PROTECT persons Downwind during DAY Kilometers (Miles)	LARGE SPILLS Then PROTECT persons Downwind during NIGHT Kilometers (Miles)
1955	**123**	Compressed gas, poisonous, n.o.s. (Inhalation Hazard Zone D)	30 m (100 ft)	0.1 km (0.1 mi)	0.2 km (0.1 mi)	150 m (500 ft)	0.8 km (0.5 mi)	2.0 km (1.3 mi)
1955 1955	**123** **123**	Compressed gas, toxic, n.o.s. Compressed gas, toxic, n.o.s. (Inhalation Hazard Zone A)	100 m (300 ft)	0.5 km (0.3 mi)	2.5 km (1.6 mi)	1000 m (3000 ft)	5.7 km (3.6 mi)	10.1 km (6.3 mi)
1955	**123**	Compressed gas, toxic, n.o.s. (Inhalation Hazard Zone B)	30 m (100 ft)	0.2 km (0.1 mi)	0.9 km (0.6 mi)	400 m (1250 ft)	2.3 km (1.4 mi)	5.1 km (3.2 mi)
1955	**123**	Compressed gas, toxic, n.o.s. (Inhalation Hazard Zone C)	30 m (100 ft)	0.1 km (0.1 mi)	0.3 km (0.2 mi)	150 m (500 ft)	1.0 km (0.6 mi)	2.9 km (1.8 mi)
1955	**123**	Compressed gas, toxic, n.o s. (Inhalation Hazard Zone D)	30 m (100 ft)	0.1 km (0.1 mi)	0.2 km (0.1 mi)	150 m (500 ft)	0.8 km (0.5 mi)	2.0 km (1.3 mi)
1955 1955 1955	**123** **123** **123**	Organic phosphate compound mixed with compressed gas Organic phosphate mixed with compressed gas Organic phosphorus compound mixed with compressed gas	100 m (300 ft)	1.0 km (0.7 mi)	3.4 km (2.1 mi)	500 m (1500 ft)	4.4 km (2.7 mi)	9.6 km (6.0 mi)
1967 1967 1967	**123** **123** **123**	Insecticide gas, poisonous, n.o.s. Insecticide gas, toxic, n.o.s. Parathion and compressed gas mixture	100 m (300 ft)	1.0 km (0.7 mi)	3.4 km (2.1 mi)	500 m (1500 ft)	4.4 km (2.7 mi)	9.6 km (6.0 mi)

1975	**124**	Dinitrogen tetroxide and Nitric oxide mixture	30 m	(100 ft)	0.1 km	(0.1 mi)	0.6 km	(0.4 mi)	100 m	(300 ft)	0.6 km	(0.4 mi)	2.2 km	(1.4 mi)
1975	**124**	Nitric oxide and Dinitrogen tetroxide mixture												
1975	**124**	Nitric oxide and Nitrogen dioxide mixture												
1975	**124**	Nitrogen dioxide and Nitric oxide mixture												
1994	**136**	Iron pentacarbonyl	100 m	(300 ft)	0.9 km	(0.6 mi)	2.0 km	(1.2 mi)	400 m	(1250 ft)	4.8 km	(3.0 mi)	7.5 km	(4.7 mi)
2004	**135**	Magnesium diamide **(when spilled in water)**	30 m	(100 ft)	0.1 km	(0.1 mi)	0.3 km	(0.2 mi)	60 m	(200 ft)	0.6 km	(0.4 mi)	2.2 km	(1.4 mi)
2011	**139**	Magnesium phosphide **(when spilled in water)**	30 m	(100 ft)	0.1 km	(0.1 mi)	0.6 km	(0.4 mi)	500 m	(1500 ft)	1.7 km	(1.1 mi)	5.4 km	(3.4 mi)
2012	**139**	Potassium phosphide **(when spilled in water)**	30 m	(100 ft)	0.1 km	(0.1 mi)	0.3 km	(0.2 mi)	300 m	(1000 ft)	1.1 km	(0.7 mi)	3.6 km	(2.2 mi)
2013	**139**	Strontium phosphide **(when spilled in water)**	30 m	(100 ft)	0.1 km	(0.1 mi)	0.3 km	(0.2 mi)	300 m	(1000 ft)	1.1 km	(0.7 mi)	3.4 km	(2.2 mi)
2032	**157**	Nitric acid, red fuming	30 m	(100 ft)	0.1 km	(0.1 mi)	0.1 km	(0.1 mi)	150 m	(500 ft)	0.3 km	(0.2 mi)	0.5 km	(0.3 mi)
2186	**125**	Hydrogen chloride, refrigerated liquid	30 m	(100 ft)	0.1 km	(0.1 mi)	0.3 km	(0.2 mi)	**Refer to table 3**					
2188	**119**	Arsine	150 m	(500 ft)	1.0 km	(0.6 mi)	3.8 km	(2.4 mi)	1000 m	(3000 ft)	5.7 km	(3.6 mi)	10.1 km	(6.3 mi)
2189	**119**	Dichlorosilane	30 m	(100 ft)	0.1 km	(0.1 mi)	0.4 km	(0.2 mi)	300 m	(1000 ft)	1.3 km	(0.8 mi)	3.4 km	(2.1 mi)
2190 2190	**124** **124**	Oxygen difluoride Oxygen difluoride, compressed	300 m	(1000 ft)	1.8 km	(1.1 mi)	7.1 km	(4.4 mi)	1000 m	(3000 ft)	11.0+ km	(7.0+ mi)	11.0+ km	(7.0+ mi)
2191 2191	**123** **123**	Sulfuryl fluoride Sulphuryl fluoride	30 m	(100 ft)	0.1 km	(0.1 mi)	0.5 km	(0.3 mi)	400 m	(1250 ft)	2.2 km	(1.4 mi)	5.3 km	(3.3 mi)
2192	**119**	Germane	150 m	(500 ft)	0.9 km	(0.5 mi)	3.3 km	(2.1 mi)	500 m	(1500 ft)	3.3 km	(2.1 mi)	7.5 km	(4.7 mi)
2194	**125**	Selenium hexafluoride	200 m	(600 ft)	1.1 km	(0.7 mi)	3.5 km	(2.2 mi)	600 m	(2000 ft)	3.5 km	(2.2 mi)	7.9 km	(4.9 mi)

"+" means distance can be larger in certain atmospheric conditions

TABLE 1

TABLE 1 - INITIAL ISOLATION AND PROTECTIVE ACTION DISTANCES

ID No.	Guide	NAME OF MATERIAL	SMALL SPILLS (From a small package or small leak from a large package) First ISOLATE in all Directions Meters (Feet)	SMALL SPILLS Then PROTECT persons Downwind during DAY Kilometers (Miles)	SMALL SPILLS Then PROTECT persons Downwind during NIGHT Kilometers (Miles)	LARGE SPILLS (From a large package or from many small packages) First ISOLATE in all Directions Meters (Feet)	LARGE SPILLS Then PROTECT persons Downwind during DAY Kilometers (Miles)	LARGE SPILLS Then PROTECT persons Downwind during NIGHT Kilometers (Miles)
2195	**125**	Tellurium hexafluoride	1000 m (3000 ft)	5.8 km (3.6 mi)	10.9 km (6.8 mi)	1000 m (3000 ft)	11.0+ km (7.0+ mi)	11.0+ km (7.0+ mi)
2196	**125**	Tungsten hexafluoride	30 m (100 ft)	0.2 km (0.1 mi)	0.8 km (0.5 mi)	150 m (500 ft)	0.8 km (0.5 mi)	2.7 km (1.7 mi)
2197	**125**	Hydrogen iodide, anhydrous	30 m (100 ft)	0.1 km (0.1 mi)	0.3 km (0.2 mi)	150 m (500 ft)	1.0 km (0.6 mi)	2.9 km (1.8 mi)
2198 2198	**125** **125**	Phosphorus pentafluoride Phosphorus pentafluoride, compressed	30 m (100 ft)	0.2 km (0.2 mi)	1.0 km (0.7 mi)	150 m (500 ft)	1.0 km (0.6 mi)	3.5 km (2.2 mi)
2199	**119**	Phosphine	60 m (200 ft)	0.3 km (0.2 mi)	1.1 km (0.7 mi)	300 m (1000 ft)	1.3 km (0.8 mi)	3.7 km (2.3 mi)
2202	**117**	Hydrogen selenide, anhydrous	300 m (1000 ft)	1.7 km (1.1 mi)	6.0 km (3.7 mi)	1000 m (3000 ft)	10.7 km (6.7 mi)	11.0+ km (7.0+ mi)
2204 2204	**119** **119**	Carbonyl sulfide Carbonyl sulphide	30 m (100 ft)	0.1 km (0.1 mi)	0.3 km (0.2 mi)	300 m (1000 ft)	1.6 km (1.0 mi)	3.8 km (2.4 mi)
2232 2232	**153** **153**	Chloroacetaldehyde 2-Chloroethanal	30 m (100 ft)	0.2 km (0.1 mi)	0.3 km (0.2 mi)	60 m (200 ft)	0.6 km (0.4 mi)	1.1 km (0.7 mi)
2285	**156**	Isocyanatobenzotrifluorides	30 m (100 ft)	0.1 km (0.1 mi)	0.2 km (0.1 mi)	30 m (100 ft)	0.4 km (0.3 mi)	0.6 km (0.4 mi)
2308 2308	**157** **157**	Nitrosylsulfuric acid, liquid **(when spilled in water)** Nitrosylsulphuric acid, liquid **(when spilled in water)**	30 m (100 ft)	0.1 km (0.1 mi)	0.3 km (0.2 mi)	300 m (1000 ft)	1.0 km (0.6 mi)	2.9 km (1.8 mi)
2334	**131**	Allylamine	30 m (100 ft)	0.2 km (0.1 mi)	0.5 km (0.4 mi)	150 m (500 ft)	1.4 km (0.9 mi)	2.5 km (1.6 mi)
2337	**131**	Phenyl mercaptan	30 m (100 ft)	0.1 km (0.1 mi)	0.1 km (0.1 mi)	30 m (100 ft)	0.3 km (0.2 mi)	0.4 km (0.2 mi)
2353	**132**	Butyryl chloride **(when spilled in water)**	30 m (100 ft)	0.1 km (0.1 mi)	0.1 km (0.1 mi)	30 m (100 ft)	0.3 km (0.2 mi)	0.7 km (0.5 mi)

2382	**131**	Dimethylhydrazine, symmetrical	30 m	(100 ft)	0.2 km	(0.1 mi)	0.3 km	(0.2 mi)	60 m	(200 ft)	0.7 km	(0.5 mi)	1.3 km	(0.8 mi)
2395	**132**	Isobutyryl chloride **(when spilled in water)**	30 m	(100 ft)	0.1 km	(0.1 mi)	0.1 km	(0.1 mi)	30 m	(100 ft)	0.2 km	(0.1 mi)	0.4 km	(0.3 mi)
2407	**155**	Isopropyl chloroformate	30 m	(100 ft)	0.1 km	(0.1 mi)	0.2 km	(0.2 mi)	60 m	(200 ft)	0.5 km	(0.3 mi)	0.9 km	(0.6 mi)
2417 2417	**125** **125**	Carbonyl fluoride Carbonyl fluoride, compressed	150 m	(500 ft)	0.7 km	(0.5 mi)	2.5 km	(1.6 mi)	600 m	(2000 ft)	3.6 km	(2.3 mi)	7.8 km	(4.9 mi)
2418 2418	**125** **125**	Sulfur tetrafluoride Sulphur tetrafluoride	100 m	(300 ft)	0.5 km	(0.3 mi)	2.3 km	(1.5 mi)	400 m	(1250 ft)	2.1 km	(1.3 mi)	6.0 km	(3.7 mi)
2420	**125**	Hexafluoroacetone	100 m	(300 ft)	0.7 km	(0.4 mi)	2.7 km	(1.7 mi)	1000 m	(3000 ft)	11.0+ km	(7.0+ mi)	11.0+ km	(7.0+ mi)
2421	**124**	Nitrogen trioxide	60 m	(200 ft)	0.3 km	(0.2 mi)	1.2 km	(0.7 mi)	200 m	(600 ft)	1.2 km	(0.8 mi)	4.2 km	(2.6 mi)
2434	**156**	Dibenzyldichlorosilane **(when spilled in water)**	30 m	(100 ft)	0.1 km	(0.1 mi)	0.1 km	(0.1 mi)	30 m	(100 ft)	0.1 km	(0.1 mi)	0.4 km	(0.3 mi)
2435	**156**	Ethylphenyldichlorosilane **(when spilled in water)**	30 m	(100 ft)	0.1 km	(0.1 mi)	0.1 km	(0.1 mi)	30 m	(100 ft)	0.3 km	(0.2 mi)	0.9 km	(0.6 mi)
2437	**156**	Methylphenyldichlorosilane **(when spilled in water)**	30 m	(100 ft)	0.1 km	(0.1 mi)	0.1 km	(0.1 mi)	30 m	(100 ft)	0.4 km	(0.2 mi)	1.2 km	(0.8 mi)
2438	**131**	Trimethylacetyl chloride	60 m	(200 ft)	0.5 km	(0.3 mi)	1.0 km	(0.6 mi)	200 m	(600 ft)	2.1 km	(1.3 mi)	3.3 km	(2.1 mi)
2442	**156**	Trichloroacetyl chloride	30 m	(100 ft)	0.2 km	(0.1 mi)	0.3 km	(0.2 mi)	60 m	(200 ft)	0.7 km	(0.4 mi)	1.1 km	(0.7 mi)
2474	**157**	Thiophosgene	60 m	(200 ft)	0.6 km	(0.4 mi)	1.7 km	(1.1 mi)	200 m	(600 ft)	2.1 km	(1.3 mi)	4.0 km	(2.5 mi)
2477	**131**	Methyl isothiocyanate	30 m	(100 ft)	0.1 km	(0.1 mi)	0.1 km	(0.1 mi)	30 m	(100 ft)	0.3 km	(0.2 mi)	0.4 km	(0.3 mi)

"+" means distance can be larger in certain atmospheric conditions

TABLE 1

TABLE 1 - INITIAL ISOLATION AND PROTECTIVE ACTION DISTANCES

ID No.	Guide	NAME OF MATERIAL	SMALL SPILLS (From a small package or small leak from a large package) — First ISOLATE in all Directions: Meters (Feet)	SMALL SPILLS — Then PROTECT persons Downwind during DAY: Kilometers (Miles)	SMALL SPILLS — Then PROTECT persons Downwind during NIGHT: Kilometers (Miles)	LARGE SPILLS (From a large package or from many small packages) — First ISOLATE in all Directions: Meters (Feet)	LARGE SPILLS — Then PROTECT persons Downwind during DAY: Kilometers (Miles)	LARGE SPILLS — Then PROTECT persons Downwind during NIGHT: Kilometers (Miles)
2478	**155**	Isocyanate solution, flammable, poisonous, n.o.s.	60 m (200 ft)	0.8 km (0.5 mi)	1.8 km (1.1 mi)	400 m (1250 ft)	4.4 km (2.7 mi)	7.0 km (4.3 mi)
2478	**155**	Isocyanate solution, flammable, toxic, n.o.s.						
2478	**155**	Isocyanates, flammable, poisonous, n.o.s.						
2478	**155**	Isocyanates, flammable, toxic, n.o.s.						
2480	**155P**	Methyl isocyanate	150 m (500 ft)	1.7 km (1.1 mi)	5.0 km (3.1 mi)	1000 m (3000 ft)	11.0+ km (7.0+ mi)	11.0+ km (7.0+ mi)
2481	**155**	Ethyl isocyanate	150 m (500 ft)	2.0 km (1.2 mi)	5.1 km (3.2 mi)	1000 m (3000 ft)	11.0+ km (7.0+ mi)	11.0+ km (7.0+ mi)
2482	**155P**	n-Propyl isocyanate	100 m (300 ft)	1.3 km (0.8 mi)	2.7 km (1.7 mi)	600 m (2000 ft)	7.4 km (4.6 mi)	10.8 km (6.7 mi)
2483	**155P**	Isopropyl isocyanate	150 m (500 ft)	1.5 km (0.9 mi)	3.2 km (2.0 mi)	1000 m (3000 ft)	11.0 km (6.9 mi)	11.0+ km (7.0+ mi)
2484	**155**	tert-Butyl isocyanate	60 m (200 ft)	0.8 km (0.5 mi)	1.8 km (1.1 mi)	400 m (1250 ft)	4.4 km (2.7 mi)	7.0 km (4.3 mi)
2485	**155P**	n-Butyl isocyanate	60 m (200 ft)	0.6 km (0.4 mi)	1.1 km (0.7 mi)	200 m (600 ft)	2.6 km (1.7 mi)	4.0 km (2.5 mi)
2486	**155P**	Isobutyl isocyanate	60 m (200 ft)	0.6 km (0.4 mi)	1.2 km (0.8 mi)	300 m (1000 ft)	3.1 km (1.9 mi)	4.7 km (3.0 mi)
2487	**155**	Phenyl isocyanate	100 m (300 ft)	0.9 km (0.6 mi)	1.4 km (0.9 mi)	300 m (1000 ft)	3.7 km (2.3 mi)	5.4 km (3.4 mi)
2488	**155**	Cyclohexyl isocyanate	30 m (100 ft)	0.3 km (0.2 mi)	0.4 km (0.3 mi)	100 m (300 ft)	1.0 km (0.6 mi)	1.4 km (0.9 mi)
2495	**144**	Iodine pentafluoride **(when spilled in water)**	30 m (100 ft)	0.1 km (0.1 mi)	0.3 km (0.2 mi)	100 m (300 ft)	1.1 km (0.7 mi)	4.1 km (2.6 mi)
2521	**131P**	Diketene, stabilized	30 m (100 ft)	0.2 km (0.1 mi)	0.3 km (0.2 mi)	60 m (200 ft)	0.6 km (0.4 mi)	1.0 km (0.6 mi)
2534	**119**	Methylchlorosilane	30 m (100 ft)	0.1 km (0.1 mi)	0.3 km (0.2 mi)	150 m (500 ft)	0.7 km (0.5 mi)	1.9 km (1.2 mi)

2548	**124**	Chlorine pentafluoride	100 m	(300 ft)	0.5 km	(0.3 mi)	2.5 km	(1.6 mi)	800 m	(2500 ft)	5.0 km	(3.1 mi)	11.0+ km	(7.0+ mi)
2605	**155**	Methoxymethyl isocyanate	30 m	(100 ft)	0.2 km	(0.1 mi)	0.2 km	(0.2 mi)	60 m	(200 ft)	0.6 km	(0.4 mi)	0.9 km	(0.6 mi)
2606	**155**	Methyl orthosilicate	30 m	(100 ft)	0.2 km	(0.1 mi)	0.3 km	(0.2 mi)	60 m	(200 ft)	0.7 km	(0.4 mi)	1.1 km	(0.7 mi)
2644	**151**	Methyl iodide	30 m	(100 ft)	0.1 km	(0.1 mi)	0.2 km	(0.1 mi)	100 m	(300 ft)	0.3 km	(0.2 mi)	0.7 km	(0.4 mi)
2646	**151**	Hexachlorocyclopentadiene	30 m	(100 ft)	0.1 km	(0.1 mi)	0.1 km	(0.1 mi)	30 m	(100 ft)	0.3 km	(0.2 mi)	0.3 km	(0.2 mi)
2668	**131**	Chloroacetonitrile	30 m	(100 ft)	0.1 km	(0.1 mi)	0.1 km	(0.1 mi)	30 m	(100 ft)	0.3 km	(0.2 mi)	0.4 km	(0.2 mi)
2676	**119**	Stibine	60 m	(200 ft)	0.3 km	(0.2 mi)	1.6 km	(1.0 mi)	200 m	(600 ft)	1.3 km	(0.8 mi)	4.1 km	(2.6 mi)
2691	**137**	Phosphorus pentabromide **(when spilled in water)**	30 m	(100 ft)	0.1 km	(0.1 mi)	0.1 km	(0.1 mi)	30 m	(100 ft)	0.1 km	(0.1 mi)	0.5 km	(0.3 mi)
2692	**157**	Boron tribromide **(when spilled on land)**	30 m	(100 ft)	0.1 km	(0.1 mi)	0.2 km	(0.1 mi)	30 m	(100 ft)	0.2 km	(0.1 mi)	0.4 km	(0.3 mi)
2692	**157**	Boron tribromide **(when spilled in water)**	30 m	(100 ft)	0.1 km	(0.1 mi)	0.2 km	(0.1 mi)	60 m	(200 ft)	0.5 km	(0.3 mi)	1.9 km	(1.2 mi)
2740	**155**	n-Propyl chloroformate	30 m	(100 ft)	0.1 km	(0.1 mi)	0.3 km	(0.2 mi)	60 m	(200 ft)	0.6 km	(0.4 mi)	1.0 km	(0.7 mi)
2742	**155**	sec-Butyl chloroformate	30 m	(100 ft)	0.1 km	(0.1 mi)	0.2 km	(0.1 mi)	30 m	(100 ft)	0.4 km	(0.2 mi)	0.5 km	(0.3 mi)
2742 2742	**155** **155**	Chloroformates, poisonous, corrosive, flammable, n.o.s. Chloroformates, toxic, corrosive, flammable, n.o.s.	30 m	(100 ft)	0.2 km	(0.1 mi)	0.2 km	(0.2 mi)	60 m	(200 ft)	0.5 km	(0.3 mi)	0.7 km	(0.5 mi)
2742	**155**	Isobutyl chloroformate	30 m	(100 ft)	0.1 km	(0.1 mi)	0.1 km	(0.1 mi)	30 m	(100 ft)	0.3 km	(0.2 mi)	0.5 km	(0.3 mi)
2743	**155**	n-Butyl chloroformate	30 m	(100 ft)	0.1 km	(0.1 mi)	0.1 km	(0.1 mi)	30 m	(100 ft)	0.3 km	(0.2 mi)	0.4 km	(0.3 mi)
2806	**139**	Lithium nitride **(when spilled in water)**	30 m	(100 ft)	0.1 km	(0.1 mi)	0.2 km	(0.2 mi)	60 m	(200 ft)	0.5 km	(0.3 mi)	1.9 km	(1.2 mi)
2826	**155**	Ethyl chlorothioformate	30 m	(100 ft)	0.2 km	(0.1 mi)	0.2 km	(0.2 mi)	60 m	(200 ft)	0.5 km	(0.3 mi)	0.7 km	(0.5 mi)
2845	**135**	Ethyl phosphonous dichloride, anhydrous	30 m	(100 ft)	0.3 km	(0.2 mi)	0.7 km	(0.5 mi)	100 m	(300 ft)	1.3 km	(0.8 mi)	2.3 km	(1.5 mi)

"+" means distance can be larger in certain atmospheric conditions

TABLE 1

TABLE 1 - INITIAL ISOLATION AND PROTECTIVE ACTION DISTANCES

ID No.	Guide	NAME OF MATERIAL	SMALL SPILLS (From a small package or small leak from a large package) First ISOLATE in all Directions Meters (Feet)	SMALL SPILLS Then PROTECT persons Downwind during DAY Kilometers (Miles)	SMALL SPILLS Then PROTECT persons Downwind during NIGHT Kilometers (Miles)	LARGE SPILLS (From a large package or from many small packages) First ISOLATE in all Directions Meters (Feet)	LARGE SPILLS Then PROTECT persons Downwind during DAY Kilometers (Miles)	LARGE SPILLS Then PROTECT persons Downwind during NIGHT Kilometers (Miles)
2845	**135**	Methyl phosphonous dichlor de	30 m (100 ft)	0.4 km (0.3 mi)	1.1 km (0.7 mi)	200 m (600 ft)	2.4 km (1.5 mi)	4.1 km (2.6 mi)
2901	**124**	Bromine chloride	100 m (300 ft)	0.5 km (0.3 mi)	1.8 km (1.1 mi)	1000 m (3000 ft)	5.4 km (3.4 mi)	11.0+ km (7.0+ mi)
2927	**154**	Ethyl phosphonothioic dichloride, anhydrous	30 m (100 ft)	0.1 km (0.1 mi)	0.1 km (0.1 mi)	30 m (100 ft)	0.2 km (0.1 mi)	0.2 km (0.1 mi)
2927	**154**	Ethyl phosphorodichloridate	30 m (100 ft)	0.1 km (0.1 mi)	0.1 km (0.1 mi)	30 m (100 ft)	0.3 km (0.2 mi)	0.3 km (0.2 mi)
2965	**139**	Boron trifluoride dimethyl etherate **(when spilled in water)**	30 m (100 ft)	0.1 km (0.1 mi)	0.3 km (0.2 mi)	100 m (300 ft)	1.2 km (0.8 mi)	3.6 km (2.2 mi)
2977 2977	**166** **166**	Radioactive material, Uranium hexafluoride, fissile **(when spilled in water)** Uranium hexafluoride, radioactive material, fissile **(when spilled in water)**	30 m (100 ft)	0.1 km (0.1 mi)	0.2 km (0.1 mi)	60 m (200 ft)	0.4 km (0.3 mi)	2.1 km (1.3 mi)
2978 2978	**166** **166**	Radioactive material, Uranium hexafluoride, non fissile or fissile-excepted **(when spilled in water)** Uranium hexafluoride, radioactive material, non fissile or fissile-excepted **(when spilled in water)**	30 m (100 ft)	0.1 km (0.1 mi)	0.2 km (0.1 mi)	60 m (200 ft)	0.4 km (0.3 mi)	2.1 km (1.3 mi)

2985	**155**	Chlorosilanes, flammable, corrosive, n.o.s. **(when spilled in water)**	30 m	(100 ft)	0.1 km	(0.1 mi)	0.2 km	(0.1 mi)	60 m	(200 ft)	0.5 km	(0.3 mi)	1.6 km	(1.0 mi)
2986	**155**	Chlorosilanes, corrosive, flammable, n.o.s. **(when spilled in water)**	30 m	(100 ft)	0.1 km	(0.1 mi)	0.2 km	(0.1 mi)	60 m	(200 ft)	0.5 km	(0.3 mi)	1.6 km	(1.0 mi)
2987	**156**	Chlorosilanes, corrosive, n.o.s. **(when spilled in water)**	30 m	(100 ft)	0.1 km	(0.1 mi)	0.2 km	(0.1 mi)	60 m	(200 ft)	0.5 km	(0.3 mi)	1.6 km	(1.0 mi)
2988	**139**	Chlorosilanes, water-reactive, flammable, corrosive, n.o.s. **(when spilled in water)**	30 m	(100 ft)	0.1 km	(0.1 mi)	0.2 km	(0.1 mi)	60 m	(200 ft)	0.5 km	(0.3 mi)	1.6 km	(1.0 mi)
3023	**131**	2-Methyl-2-heptanethiol	30 m	(100 ft)	0.2 km	(0.1 mi)	0.2 km	(0.1 mi)	60 m	(200 ft)	0.5 km	(0.4 mi)	0.8 km	(0.5 mi)
3048	**157**	Aluminum phosphide pesticide **(when spilled in water)**	30 m	(100 ft)	0.1 km	(0.1 mi)	0.7 km	(0.5 mi)	500 m	(1500 ft)	2.0 km	(1.3 mi)	6.5 km	(4.1 mi)
3057	**125**	Trifluoroacetyl chloride	30 m	(100 ft)	0.2 km	(0.1 mi)	0.9 km	(0.6 mi)	800 m	(2500 ft)	5.2 km	(3.3 mi)	11.0+ km	(7.0+ mi)
3079	**131P**	Methacrylonitrile, stabilized	30 m	(100 ft)	0.3 km	(0.2 mi)	0.7 km	(0.5 mi)	150 m	(500 ft)	1.6 km	(1.0 mi)	2.7 km	(1.7 mi)
3083	**124**	Perchloryl fluoride	30 m	(100 ft)	0.2 km	(0.2 mi)	1.1 km	(0.7 mi)	1000 m	(3000 ft)	5.5 km	(3.4 mi)	11.0+ km	(7.0+ mi)
3160 3160	**119** **119**	Liquefied gas, poisonous, flammable, n.o.s. Liquefied gas, poisonous, flammable, n.o.s. (Inhalation Hazard Zone A)	150 m	(500 ft)	1.0 km	(0.6 mi)	3.8 km	(2.4 mi)	1000 m	(3000 ft)	5.7 km	(3.6 mi)	10.1 km	(6.3 mi)
3160	**119**	Liquefied gas, poisonous, flammable, n.o.s. (Inhalation Hazard Zone B)	30 m	(100 ft)	0.1 km	(0.1 mi)	0.4 km	(0.2 mi)	300 m	(1000 ft)	1.3 km	(0.8 mi)	3.4 km	(2.1 mi)
3160	**119**	Liquefied gas, poisonous, flammable, n.o.s. (Inhalation Hazard Zone C)	30 m	(100 ft)	0.1 km	(0.1 mi)	0.3 km	(0.2 mi)	150 m	(500 ft)	1.0 km	(0.6 mi)	2.9 km	(1.8 mi)

"+" means distance can be larger in certain atmospheric conditions

TABLE 1

TABLE 1 - INITIAL ISOLATION AND PROTECTIVE ACTION DISTANCES

ID No.	Guide	NAME OF MATERIAL	SMALL SPILLS (From a small package or small leak from a large package) First ISOLATE in all Directions Meters (Feet)	SMALL SPILLS Then PROTECT persons Downwind during DAY Kilometers (Miles)	SMALL SPILLS Then PROTECT persons Downwind during NIGHT Kilometers (Miles)	LARGE SPILLS (From a large package or from many small packages) First ISOLATE in all Directions Meters (Feet)	LARGE SPILLS Then PROTECT persons Downwind during DAY Kilometers (Miles)	LARGE SPILLS Then PROTECT persons Downwind during NIGHT Kilometers (Miles)
3160	119	Liquefied gas, poisonous, flammable, n.o.s. (Inhalation Hazard Zone D)	30 m (100 ft)	0.1 km (0.1 mi)	0.2 km (0.1 mi)	150 m (500 ft)	0.8 km (0.5 mi)	2.0 km (1.3 mi)
3160 3160	119 119	Liquefied gas, toxic, flammable, n.o.s. Liquefied gas, toxic, flammable, n.o.s. (Inhalation Hazard Zone A)	150 m (500 ft)	1.0 km (0.6 mi)	3.8 km (2.4 mi)	1000 m (3000 ft)	5.7 km (3.6 mi)	10.1 km (6.3 mi)
3160	119	Liquefied gas, toxic, flammable, n.o.s. (Inhalation Hazard Zone B)	30 m (100 ft)	0.1 km (0.1 mi)	0.4 km (0.2 mi)	300 m (1000 ft)	1.3 km (0.8 mi)	3.4 km (2.1 mi)
3160	119	Liquefied gas, toxic, flammable, n.o.s. (Inhalation Hazard Zone C)	30 m (100 ft)	0.1 km (0.1 mi)	0.3 km (0.2 mi)	150 m (500 ft)	1.0 km (0.6 mi)	2.9 km (1.8 mi)
3160	119	Liquefied gas, toxic, flammable, n.o.s. (Inhalation Hazard Zone D)	30 m (100 ft)	0.1 km (0.1 mi)	0.2 km (0.1 mi)	150 m (500 ft)	0.8 km (0.5 mi)	2.0 km (1.3 mi)
3162 3162	123 123	Liquefied gas, poisonous, n.o.s. Liquefied gas, poisonous, n.o.s. (Inhalation Hazard Zone A)	100 m (300 ft)	0.5 km (0.3 mi)	2.5 km (1.6 mi)	1000 m (3000 ft)	5.7 km (3.6 mi)	10.1 km (6.3 mi)
3162	123	Liquefied gas, poisonous, n.o.s. (Inhalation Hazard Zone B)	30 m (100 ft)	0.2 km (0.1 mi)	0.9 km (0.6 mi)	400 m (1250 ft)	2.3 km (1.4 mi)	5.1 km (3.2 mi)
3162	123	Liquefied gas, poisonous, n.o.s. (Inhalation Hazard Zone C)	30 m (100 ft)	0.1 km (0.1 mi)	0.3 km (0.2 mi)	150 m (500 ft)	1.0 km (0.6 mi)	2.9 km (1.8 mi)

3162	**123**	Liquefied gas, poisonous, n.o.s. (Inhalation Hazard Zone D)	30 m	(100 ft)	0.1 km	(0.1 mi)	0.2 km	(0.1 mi)	150 m	(500 ft)	0.8 km	(0.5 mi)	2.0 km	(1.3 mi)
3162 3162	**123** **123**	Liquefied gas, toxic, n.o.s. Liquefied gas, toxic, n.o.s. (Inhalation Hazard Zone A)	100 m	(300 ft)	0.5 km	(0.3 mi)	2.5 km	(1.6 mi)	1000 m	(3000 ft)	5.7 km	(3.6 mi)	10.1 km	(6.3 mi)
3162	**123**	Liquefied gas, toxic, n.o.s. (Inhalation Hazard Zone B)	30 m	(100 ft)	0.2 km	(0.1 mi)	0.9 km	(0.6 mi)	400 m	(1250 ft)	2.3 km	(1.4 mi)	5.1 km	(3.2 mi)
3162	**123**	Liquefied gas, toxic, n.o.s. (Inhalation Hazard Zone C)	30 m	(100 ft)	0.1 km	(0.1 mi)	0.3 km	(0.2 mi)	150 m	(500 ft)	1.0 km	(0.6 mi)	2.9 km	(1.8 mi)
3162	**123**	Liquefied gas, toxic, n.o.s. (Inhalation Hazard Zone D)	30 m	(100 ft)	0.1 km	(0.1 mi)	0.2 km	(0.1 mi)	150 m	(500 ft)	0.8 km	(0.5 mi)	2.0 km	(1.3 mi)
3246 3246	**156** **156**	Methanesulfonyl chloride Methanesulphonyl chloride	30 m	(100 ft)	0.2 km	(0.2 mi)	0.3 km	(0.2 mi)	60 m	(200 ft)	0.7 km	(0.4 mi)	0.9 km	(0.6 mi)
3275 3275	**131** **131**	Nitriles, poisonous, flammable, n.o.s. Nitriles, toxic, flammable, n.o.s.	30 m	(100 ft)	0.3 km	(0.2 mi)	0.7 km	(0.5 mi)	150 m	(500 ft)	1.6 km	(1.0 mi)	2.7 km	(1.7 mi)
3276 3276 3276 3276	**151** **151** **151** **151**	Nitriles, liquid, poisonous, n.o.s. Nitriles, liquid, toxic, n.o.s. Nitriles, poisonous, liquid, n.o.s. Nitriles, toxic, liquid, n.o.s.	30 m	(100 ft)	0.3 km	(0.2 mi)	0.7 km	(0.5 mi)	150 m	(500 ft)	1.6 km	(1.0 mi)	2.7 km	(1.7 mi)
3278 3278 3278 3278	**151** **151** **151** **151**	Organophosphorus compound, liquid, poisonous, n.o.s. Organophosphorus compound, liquid, toxic, n.o.s. Organophosphorus compound, poisonous, liquid, n.o.s. Organophosphorus compound, toxic, liquid, n.o.s.	30 m	(100 ft)	0.4 km	(0.3 mi)	1.1 km	(0.7 mi)	200 m	(600 ft)	2.4 km	(1.5 mi)	4.1 km	(2.6 mi)

"+" means distance can be larger in certain atmospheric conditions

TABLE 1

TABLE 1 - INITIAL ISOLATION AND PROTECTIVE ACTION DISTANCES

ID No.	Guide	NAME OF MATERIAL	SMALL SPILLS (From a small package or small leak from a large package) First ISOLATE in all Directions Meters (Feet)	SMALL SPILLS Then PROTECT persons Downwind during DAY Kilometers (Miles)	SMALL SPILLS Then PROTECT persons Downwind during NIGHT Kilometers (Miles)	LARGE SPILLS (From a large package or from many small packages) First ISOLATE in all Directions Meters (Feet)	LARGE SPILLS Then PROTECT persons Downwind during DAY Kilometers (Miles)	LARGE SPILLS Then PROTECT persons Downwind during NIGHT Kilometers (Miles)
3279	**131**	Organophosphorus compound, poisonous, flammable, n.o.s.	30 m (100 ft)	0.4 km (0.3 mi)	1.1 km (0.7 mi)	200 m (600 ft)	2.4 km (1.5 mi)	4.1 km (2.6 mi)
3279	**131**	Organophosphorus compound, toxic, flammable, n.o.s.						
3280	**151**	Organoarsenic compound, liquid, n.o.s.	30 m (100 ft)	0.2 km (0.1 mi)	0.7 km (0.4 mi)	150 m (500 ft)	1.6 km (1.0 mi)	3.6 km (2.2 mi)
3281	**151**	Metal carbonyls, liquid, n.o.s.	100 m (300 ft)	1.3 km (0.8 mi)	5.0 km (3.1 mi)	1000 m (3000 ft)	10.8 km (6.8 mi)	11.0+ km (7.0+ mi)
3294	**131**	Hydrogen cyanide, solution in alcohol, with not more than 45% Hydrogen cyanide	30 m (100 ft)	0.1 km (0.1 mi)	0.3 km (0.2 mi)	200 m (600 ft)	0.5 km (0.3 mi)	1.9 km (1.2 mi)
3300	**119P**	Carbon dioxide and Ethylene oxide mixture, with more than 87% Ethylene oxide	30 m (100 ft)	0.1 km (0.1 mi)	0.2 km (0.2 mi)	150 m (500 ft)	0.8 km (0.5 mi)	2.2 km (1.4 mi)
3300	**119P**	Ethylene oxide and Carbon dioxide mixture, with more than 87% Ethylene oxide						
3303	**124**	Compressed gas, poisonous, oxidizing, n.o.s.	100 m (300 ft)	0.5 km (0.3 mi)	2.5 km (1.6 mi)	800 m (2500 ft)	5.0 km (3.1 mi)	11.0+ km (7.0+ mi)
3303	**124**	Compressed gas, poisonous, oxidizing, n.o.s. (Inhalation Hazard Zone A)						
3303	**124**	Compressed gas, poisonous, oxidizing, n.o.s. (Inhalation Hazard Zone B)	60 m (200 ft)	0.3 km (0.2 mi)	1.1 km (0.7 mi)	400 m (1250 ft)	2.5 km (1.5 mi)	6.7 km (4.2 mi)

3303	**124**	Compressed gas, poisonous, oxidizing, n.o.s. (Inhalation Hazard Zone C)	30 m	(100 ft)	0.1 km	(0.1 mi)	0.3 km	(0.2 mi)	150 m	(500 ft)	1.0 km	(0.6 mi)	2.9 km	(1.8 mi)
3303	**124**	Compressed gas, poisonous, oxidizing, n.o.s. (Inhalation Hazard Zone D)	30 m	(100 ft)	0.1 km	(0.1 mi)	0.2 km	(0.1 mi)	150 m	(500 ft)	0.8 km	(0.5 mi)	2.0 km	(1.3 mi)
3303 3303	**124** **124**	Compressed gas, toxic, oxidizing, n.o.s. Compressed gas, toxic, oxidizing, n.o.s. (Inhalation Hazard Zone A)	100 m	(300 ft)	0.5 km	(0.3 mi)	2.5 km	(1.6 mi)	800 m	(2500 ft)	5.0 km	(3.1 mi)	11.0+ km	(7.0+ mi)
3303	**124**	Compressed gas, toxic, oxidizing, n.o.s. (Inhalation Hazard Zone B)	60 m	(200 ft)	0.3 km	(0.2 mi)	1.1 km	(0.7 mi)	400 m	(1250 ft)	2.5 km	(1.5 mi)	6.7 km	(4.2 mi)
3303	**124**	Compressed gas, toxic, oxidizing, n.o.s. (Inhalation Hazard Zone C)	30 m	(100 ft)	0.1 km	(0.1 mi)	0.3 km	(0.2 mi)	150 m	(500 ft)	1.0 km	(0.6 mi)	2.9 km	(1.8 mi)
3303	**124**	Compressed gas, toxic, oxidizing, n.o.s. (Inhalation Hazard Zone D)	30 m	(100 ft)	0.1 km	(0.1 mi)	0.2 km	(0.1 mi)	150 m	(500 ft)	0.8 km	(0.5 mi)	2.0 km	(1.3 mi)
3304 3304	**125** **125**	Compressed gas, poisonous, corrosive, n.o.s. Compressed gas, poisonous, corrosive, n.o.s. (Inhalation Hazard Zone A)	100 m	(300 ft)	0.5 km	(0.3 mi)	2.5 km	(1.6 mi)	500 m	(1500 ft)	2.9 km	(1.8 mi)	9.2 km	(5.7 mi)
3304	**125**	Compressed gas, poisonous, corrosive, n.o.s. (Inhalation Hazard Zone B)	30 m	(100 ft)	0.2 km	(0.2 mi)	1.0 km	(0.7 mi)	400 m	(1250 ft)	2.3 km	(1.4 mi)	5.1 km	(3.2 mi)
3304	**125**	Compressed gas, poisonous, corrosive, n.o.s. (Inhalation Hazard Zone C)	30 m	(100 ft)	0.1 km	(0.1 mi)	0.5 km	(0.3 mi)	300 m	(1000 ft)	1.6 km	(1 0 mi)	3.2 km	(2.0 mi)

"+" means distance can be larger in certain atmospheric conditions

TABLE 1

TABLE 1 - INITIAL ISOLATION AND PROTECTIVE ACTION DISTANCES

ID No.	Guide	NAME OF MATERIAL	SMALL SPILLS (From a small package or small leak from a large package) First ISOLATE in all Directions Meters (Feet)	SMALL SPILLS Then PROTECT persons Downwind during DAY Kilometers (Miles)	SMALL SPILLS Then PROTECT persons Downwind during NIGHT Kilometers (Miles)	LARGE SPILLS (From a large package or from many small packages) First ISOLATE in all Directions Meters (Feet)	LARGE SPILLS Then PROTECT persons Downwind during DAY Kilometers (Miles)	LARGE SPILLS Then PROTECT persons Downwind during NIGHT Kilometers (Miles)
3304	**125**	Compressed gas, poisonous, corrosive, n.o.s. (Inhalation Hazard Zone D)	30 m (100 ft)	0.1 km (0.1 mi)	0.2 km (0.1 mi)	150 m (500 ft)	0.8 km (0.5 mi)	2.0 km (1.3 mi)
3304 3304	**125** **125**	Compressed gas, toxic, corrosive, n.o.s. Compressed gas, toxic, corrosive, n.o.s. (Inhalation Hazard Zone A)	100 m (300 ft)	0.5 km (0.3 mi)	2.5 km (1.6 mi)	500 m (1500 ft)	2.9 km (1.8 mi)	9.2 km (5.7 mi)
3304	**125**	Compressed gas, toxic, corrosive, n.o.s. (Inhalation Hazard Zone B)	30 m (100 ft)	0.2 km (0.2 mi)	1.0 km (0.7 mi)	400 m (1250 ft)	2.3 km (1.4 mi)	5.1 km (3.2 mi)
3304	**125**	Compressed gas, toxic, corrosive, n.o.s. (Inhalation Hazard Zone C)	30 m (100 ft)	0.1 km (0.1 mi)	0.5 km (0.3 mi)	300 m (1000 ft)	1.6 km (1.0 mi)	3.2 km (2.0 mi)
3304	**125**	Compressed gas, toxic, corrosive, n.o.s. (Inhalation Hazard Zone D)	30 m (100 ft)	0.1 km (0.1 mi)	0.2 km (0.1 mi)	150 m (500 ft)	0.8 km (0.5 mi)	2.0 km (1.3 mi)
3305 3305	**119** **119**	Compressed gas, poisonous, flammable, corrosive, n.o.s. Compressed gas, poisonous, flammable, corrosive, n.o.s. (Inhalation Hazard Zone A)	100 m (300 ft)	0.5 km (0.3 mi)	2.5 km (1.6 mi)	500 m (1500 ft)	2.9 km (1.8 mi)	9.2 km (5.7 mi)

3305	**119**	Compressed gas, poisonous, flammable, corrosive, n.o.s. (Inhalation Hazard Zone B)	30 m	(100 ft)	0.2 km	(0.2 mi)	1.0 km	(0.7 mi)	400 m	(1250 ft)	2.3 km	(1.4 mi)	5.1 km	(3.2 mi)
3305	**119**	Compressed gas, poisonous, flammable, corrosive, n.o.s. (Inhalation Hazard Zone C)	30 m	(100 ft)	0.1 km	(0.1 mi)	0.5 km	(0.3 mi)	300 m	(1000 ft)	1.6 km	(1.0 mi)	3.2 km	(2.0 mi)
3305	**119**	Compressed gas, poisonous, flammable, corrosive, n.o.s. (Inhalation Hazard Zone D)	30 m	(100 ft)	0.1 km	(0.1 mi)	0.2 km	(0.1 mi)	150 m	(500 ft)	0.8 km	(0.5 mi)	2.0 km	(1.3 mi)
3305 3305	**119** **119**	Compressed gas, toxic, flammable, corrosive, n.o.s. Compressed gas, toxic, flammable, corrosive, n.o.s. (Inhalation Hazard Zone A)	100 m	(300 ft)	0.5 km	(0.3 mi)	2.5 km	(1.6 mi)	500 m	(1500 ft)	2.9 km	(1.8 mi)	9.2 km	(5.7 mi)
3305	**119**	Compressed gas, toxic, flammable, corrosive, n.o.s. (Inhalation Hazard Zone B)	30 m	(100 ft)	0.2 km	(0.2 mi)	1.0 km	(0.7 mi)	400 m	(1250 ft)	2.3 km	(1.4 mi)	5.1 km	(3.2 mi)
3305	**119**	Compressed gas, toxic, flammable, corrosive, n.o.s. (Inhalation Hazard Zone C)	30 m	(100 ft)	0.1 km	(0.1 mi)	0.5 km	(0.3 mi)	300 m	(1000 ft)	1.6 km	(1.0 mi)	3.2 km	(2.0 mi)
3305	**119**	Compressed gas, toxic, flammable, corrosive, n.o.s. (Inhalation Hazard Zone D)	30 m	(100 ft)	0.1 km	(0.1 mi)	0.2 km	(0.1 mi)	150 m	(500 ft)	0.8 km	(0.5 mi)	2.0 km	(1.3 mi)
3306 3306	**124** **124**	Compressed gas, poisonous, oxidizing, corrosive, n.o.s. Compressed gas, poisonous, oxidizing, corrosive, n.o.s. (Inhalation Hazard Zone A)	100 m	(300 ft)	0.5 km	(0.3 mi)	2.5 km	(1.6 mi)	500 m	(1500 ft)	2.9 km	(1.8 mi)	9.2 km	(5.7 mi)
3306	**124**	Compressed gas, poisonous, oxidizing, corrosive, n.o.s. (Inhalation Hazard Zone B)	30 m	(100 ft)	0.2 km	(0.2 mi)	1.0 km	(0.7 mi)	400 m	(1250 ft)	2.3 km	(1.4 mi)	5.1 km	(3.2 mi)

"+" means distance can be larger in certain atmospheric conditions

TABLE 1

TABLE 1 - INITIAL ISOLATION AND PROTECTIVE ACTION DISTANCES

			SMALL SPILLS (From a small package or small leak from a large package)			LARGE SPILLS (From a large package or from many small packages)		
			First ISOLATE in all Directions	Then PROTECT persons Downwind during		First ISOLATE in all Directions	Then PROTECT persons Downwind during	
ID No.	Guide	NAME OF MATERIAL	Meters (Feet)	DAY Kilometers (Miles)	NIGHT Kilometers (Miles)	Meters (Feet)	DAY Kilometers (Miles)	NIGHT Kilometers (Miles)
3306	**124**	Compressed gas, poisonous, oxidizing, corrosive, n.o.s. (Inhalation Hazard Zone C)	30 m (100 ft)	0.1 km (0.1 mi)	0.5 km (0.3 mi)	300 m (1000 ft)	1.6 km (1.0 mi)	3.2 km (2.0 mi)
3306	**124**	Compressed gas, poisonous, oxidizing, corrosive, n.o.s. (Inhalation Hazard Zone D)	30 m (100 ft)	0.1 km (0.1 mi)	0.2 km (0.1 mi)	150 m (500 ft)	0.8 km (0.5 mi)	2.0 km (1.3 mi)
3306 3306	**124** **124**	Compressed gas, toxic, oxidizing, corrosive, n.o.s. Compressed gas, toxic, oxidizing, corrosive, n.o.s. (Inhalation Hazard Zone A)	100 m (300 ft)	0.5 km (0.3 mi)	2.5 km (1.6 mi)	500 m (1500 ft)	2.9 km (1.8 mi)	9.2 km (5.7 mi)
3306	**124**	Compressed gas, toxic, oxidizing, corrosive, n.o.s. (Inhalation Hazard Zone B)	30 m (100 ft)	0.2 km (0.2 mi)	1.0 km (0.7 mi)	400 m (1250 ft)	2.3 km (1.4 mi)	5.1 km (3.2 mi)
3306	**124**	Compressed gas, toxic, oxidizing, corrosive, n.o.s. (Inhalation Hazard Zone C)	30 m (100 ft)	0.1 km (0.1 mi)	0.5 km (0.3 mi)	300 m (1000 ft)	1.6 km (1.0 mi)	3.2 km (2.0 mi)
3306	**124**	Compressed gas, toxic, oxidizing, corrosive, n.o.s. (Inhalation Hazard Zone D)	30 m (100 ft)	0.1 km (0.1 mi)	0.2 km (0.1 mi)	150 m (500 ft)	0.8 km (0.5 mi)	2.0 km (1.3 mi)

3307 3307	**124** **124**	Liquefied gas, poisonous, oxidizing, n.o.s. Liquefied gas, poisonous, oxidizing, n.o.s. (Inhalation Hazard Zone A)	100 m	(300 ft)	0.5 km	(0.3 mi)	2.5 km	(1.6 mi)	800 m	(2500 ft)	5.0 km	(3.1 mi)	11.0+ km	(7.0+ mi)
3307	**124**	Liquefied gas, poisonous, oxidizing, n.o.s. (Inhalation Hazard Zone B)	60 m	(200 ft)	0.3 km	(0.2 mi)	1.1 km	(0.7 mi)	400 m	(1250 ft)	2.5 km	(1.5 mi)	6.7 km	(4.2 mi)
3307	**124**	Liquefied gas, poisonous, oxidizing, n.o.s. (Inhalation Hazard Zone C)	30 m	(100 ft)	0.1 km	(0.1 mi)	0.3 km	(0.2 mi)	150 m	(500 ft)	1.0 km	(0.6 mi)	2.9 km	(1.8 mi)
3307	**124**	Liquefied gas, poisonous, oxidizing, n.o.s. (Inhalation Hazard Zone D)	30 m	(100 ft)	0.1 km	(0.1 mi)	0.2 km	(0.1 mi)	150 m	(500 ft)	0.8 km	(0.5 mi)	2.0 km	(1.3 mi)
3307 3307	**124** **124**	Liquefied gas, toxic, oxidizing, n.o.s. Liquefied gas, toxic, oxidizing, n.o.s. (Inhalation Hazard Zone A)	100 m	(300 ft)	0.5 km	(0.3 mi)	2.5 km	(1.6 mi)	800 m	(2500 ft)	5.0 km	(3.1 mi)	11.0+ km	(7.0+ mi)
3307	**124**	Liquefied gas, toxic, oxidizing, n.o.s. (Inhalation Hazard Zone B)	60 m	(200 ft)	0.3 km	(0.2 mi)	1.1 km	(0.7 mi)	400 m	(1250 ft)	2.5 km	(1.5 mi)	6.7 km	(4.2 mi)
3307	**124**	Liquefied gas, toxic, oxidizing, n.o.s. (Inhalation Hazard Zone C)	30 m	(100 ft)	0.1 km	(0.1 mi)	0.3 km	(0.2 mi)	150 m	(500 ft)	1.0 km	(0.6 mi)	2.9 km	(1.8 mi)
3307	**124**	Liquefied gas, toxic, oxidizing, n.o.s. (Inhalation Hazard Zone D)	30 m	(100 ft)	0.1 km	(0.1 mi)	0.2 km	(0.1 mi)	150 m	(500 ft)	0.8 km	(0.5 mi)	2.0 km	(1.3 mi)

"+" means distance can be larger in certain atmospheric conditions

TABLE 1

TABLE 1 - INITIAL ISOLATION AND PROTECTIVE ACTION DISTANCES

ID No.	Guide	NAME OF MATERIAL	SMALL SPILLS (From a small package or small leak from a large package) First ISOLATE in all Directions Meters (Feet)	SMALL SPILLS Then PROTECT persons Downwind during DAY Kilometers (Miles)	SMALL SPILLS Then PROTECT persons Downwind during NIGHT Kilometers (Miles)	LARGE SPILLS (From a large package or from many small packages) First ISOLATE in all Directions Meters (Feet)	LARGE SPILLS Then PROTECT persons Downwind during DAY Kilometers (Miles)	LARGE SPILLS Then PROTECT persons Downwind during NIGHT Kilometers (Miles)
3308 3308	125 125	Liquefied gas, poisonous, corrosive, n.o.s. Liquefied gas, poisonous, corrosive, n.o.s. (Inhalation Hazard Zone A)	100 m (300 ft)	0.5 km (0.3 mi)	2.5 km (1.6 mi)	500 m (1500 ft)	2.9 km (1.8 mi)	9.2 km (5.7 mi)
3308	125	Liquefied gas, poisonous, corrosive, n.o.s. (Inhalation Hazard Zone B)	30 m (100 ft)	0.2 km (0.2 mi)	1.0 km (0.7 mi)	400 m (1250 ft)	2.3 km (1.4 mi)	5.1 km (3.2 mi)
3308	125	Liquefied gas, poisonous, corrosive, n.o.s. (Inhalation Hazard Zone C)	30 m (100 ft)	0.1 km (0.1 mi)	0.5 km (0.3 mi)	300 m (1000 ft)	1.6 km (1.0 mi)	3.2 km (2.0 mi)
3308	125	Liquefied gas, poisonous, corrosive, n.o.s. (Inhalation Hazard Zone D)	30 m (100 ft)	0.1 km (0.1 mi)	0.2 km (0.1 mi)	150 m (500 ft)	0.8 km (0.5 mi)	2.0 km (1.3 mi)
3308 3308	125 125	Liquefied gas, toxic, corrosive, n.o.s. Liquefied gas, toxic, corrosive, n.o.s. (Inhalation Hazard Zone A)	100 m (300 ft)	0.5 km (0.3 mi)	2.5 km (1.6 mi)	500 m (1500 ft)	2.9 km (1.8 mi)	9.2 km (5.7 mi)
3308	125	Liquefied gas, toxic, corrosive, n.o.s. (Inhalation Hazard Zone B)	30 m (100 ft)	0.2 km (0.2 mi)	1.0 km (0.7 mi)	400 m (1250 ft)	2.3 km (1.4 mi)	5.1 km (3.2 mi)

3308	**125**	Liquefied gas, toxic, corrosive, n.o.s. (Inhalation Hazard Zone C)	30 m	(100 ft)	0.1 km	(0.1 mi)	0.5 km	(0.3 mi)	300 m	(1000 ft)	1.6 km	(1.0 mi)	3.2 km	(2.0 mi)
3308	**125**	Liquefied gas, toxic, corrosive, n.o.s. (Inhalation Hazard Zone D)	30 m	(100 ft)	0.1 km	(0.1 mi)	0.2 km	(0.1 mi)	150 m	(500 ft)	0.8 km	(0.5 mi)	2.0 km	(1.3 mi)
3309 3309	**119** **119**	Liquefied gas, poisonous, flammable, corrosive, n.o.s. Liquefied gas, poisonous, flammable, corrosive, n.o.s. (Inhalation Hazard Zone A)	100 m	(300 ft)	0.5 km	(0.3 mi)	2.5 km	(1.6 mi)	500 m	(1500 ft)	2.9 km	(1.8 mi)	9.2 km	(5.7 mi)
3309	**119**	Liquefied gas, poisonous, flammable, corrosive, n.o.s. (Inhalation Hazard Zone B)	30 m	(100 ft)	0.2 km	(0.2 mi)	1.0 km	(0.7 mi)	400 m	(1250 ft)	2.3 km	(1.4 mi)	5.1 km	(3.2 mi)
3309	**119**	Liquefied gas, poisonous, flammable, corrosive, n.o.s. (Inhalation Hazard Zone C)	30 m	(100 ft)	0.1 km	(0.1 mi)	0.5 km	(0.3 mi)	300 m	(1000 ft)	1.6 km	(1.0 mi)	3.2 km	(2.0 mi)
3309	**119**	Liquefied gas, poisonous, flammable, corrosive, n.o.s. (Inhalation Hazard Zone D)	30 m	(100 ft)	0.1 km	(0.1 mi)	0.2 km	(0.1 mi)	150 m	(500 ft)	0.8 km	(0.5 mi)	2.0 km	(1.3 mi)
3309 3309	**119** **119**	Liquefied gas, toxic, flammable, corrosive, n.o.s. Liquefied gas, toxic, flammable, corrosive, n.o.s. (Inhalation Hazard Zone A)	100 m	(300 ft)	0.5 km	(0.3 mi)	2.5 km	(1.6 mi)	500 m	(1500 ft)	2.9 km	(1.8 mi)	9.2 km	(5.7 mi)
3309	**119**	Liquefied gas, toxic, flammable, corrosive, n.o.s. (Inhalation Hazard Zone B)	30 m	(100 ft)	0.2 km	(0.2 mi)	1.0 km	(0.7 mi)	400 m	(1250 ft)	2.3 km	(1.4 mi)	5.1 km	(3.2 mi)
3309	**119**	Liquefied gas, toxic, flammable, corrosive, n.o.s. (Inhalation Hazard Zone C)	30 m	(100 ft)	0.1 km	(0.1 mi)	0.5 km	(0.3 mi)	300 m	(1000 ft)	1.6 km	(1.0 mi)	3.2 km	(2.0 mi)

"+" means distance can be larger in certain atmospheric conditions

TABLE 1

TABLE 1 - INITIAL ISOLATION AND PROTECTIVE ACTION DISTANCES

ID No.	Guide	NAME OF MATERIAL	SMALL SPILLS (From a small package or small leak from a large package) First ISOLATE in all Directions Meters (Feet)	SMALL SPILLS Then PROTECT persons Downwind during DAY Kilometers (Miles)	SMALL SPILLS Then PROTECT persons Downwind during NIGHT Kilometers (Miles)	LARGE SPILLS (From a large package or from many small packages) First ISOLATE in all Directions Meters (Feet)	LARGE SPILLS Then PROTECT persons Downwind during DAY Kilometers (Miles)	LARGE SPILLS Then PROTECT persons Downwind during NIGHT Kilometers (Miles)
3309	**119**	Liquefied gas, toxic, flammable, corrosive, n.o.s. (Inhalation Hazard Zone D)	30 m (100 ft)	0.1 km (0.1 mi)	0.2 km (0.1 mi)	150 m (500 ft)	0.8 km (0.5 mi)	2.0 km (1.3 mi)
3310 3310	**124** **124**	Liquefied gas, poisonous, oxidizing, corrosive, n.o.s. Liquefied gas, poisonous, oxidizing, corrosive, n.o.s. (Inhalation Hazard Zone A)	100 m (300 ft)	0.5 km (0.3 mi)	2.5 km (1.6 mi)	500 m (1500 ft)	2.9 km (1.8 mi)	9.2 km (5.7 mi)
3310	**124**	Liquefied gas, poisonous, oxidizing, corrosive, n.o s. (Inhalation Hazard Zone B)	30 m (100 ft)	0.2 km (0.2 mi)	1.0 km (0.7 mi)	400 m (1250 ft)	2.3 km (1.4 mi)	5.1 km (3.2 mi)
3310	**124**	Liquefied gas, poisonous, oxidizing, corrosive, n.o.s. (Inhalation Hazard Zone C)	30 m (100 ft)	0.1 km (0.1 mi)	0.5 km (0.3 mi)	300 m (1000 ft)	1.6 km (1.0 mi)	3.2 km (2.0 mi)
3310	**124**	Liquefied gas, poisonous, oxidizing, corrosive, n.o.s. (Inhalation Hazard Zone D)	30 m (100 ft)	0.1 km (0.1 mi)	0.2 km (0.1 mi)	150 m (500 ft)	0.8 km (0.5 mi)	2.0 km (1.3 mi)
3310 3310	**124** **124**	Liquefied gas, toxic, oxidizing, corrosive, n.o.s. Liquefied gas, toxic, oxidizing, corrosive, n.o.s. (Inhalation Hazard Zone A)	100 m (300 ft)	0.5 km (0.3 mi)	2.5 km (1.6 mi)	500 m (1500 ft)	2.9 km (1.8 mi)	9.2 km (5.7 mi)

3310	**124**	Liquefied gas, toxic, oxidizing, corrosive, n.o.s. (Inhalation Hazard Zone B)	30 m (100 ft)	0.2 km (0.2 mi)	1.0 km (0.7 mi)	400 m (1250 ft)	2.3 km (1.4 mi)	5.1 km (3.2 mi)
3310	**124**	Liquefied gas, toxic, oxidizing, corrosive, n.o.s. (Inhalation Hazard Zone C)	30 m (100 ft)	0.1 km (0.1 mi)	0.5 km (0.3 mi)	300 m (1000 ft)	1.6 km (1.0 mi)	3.2 km (2.0 mi)
3310	**124**	Liquefied gas, toxic, oxidizing, corrosive, n.o.s. (Inhalation Hazard Zone D)	30 m (100 ft)	0.1 km (0.1 mi)	0.2 km (0.1 mi)	150 m (500 ft)	0.8 km (0.5 mi)	2.0 km (1.3 mi)
3318	**125**	Ammonia solution, with more than 50% Ammonia	30 m (100 ft)	0.1 km (0.1 mi)	0.2 km (0.1 mi)	150 m (500 ft)	0.8 km (0.5 mi)	2.1 km (1.3 mi)
3355 3355	**119** **119**	Insecticide gas, poisonous, flammable, n.o.s. Insecticide gas, poisonous, flammable, n.o.s. (Inhalation Hazard Zone A)	150 m (500 ft)	1.0 km (0.6 mi)	3.8 km (2.4 mi)	1000 m (3000 ft)	5.7 km (3.6 mi)	10.1 km (6.3 mi)
3355	**119**	Insecticide gas, poisonous, flammable, n.o.s. (Inhalation Hazard Zone B)	30 m (100 ft)	0.1 km (0.1 mi)	0.4 km (0.2 mi)	300 m (1000 ft)	1.3 km (0.8 mi)	3.4 km (2.1 mi)
3355	**119**	Insecticide gas, poisonous, flammable, n.o.s. (Inhalation Hazard Zone C)	30 m (100 ft)	0.1 km (0.1 mi)	0.3 km (0.2 mi)	150 m (500 ft)	1.0 km (0.6 mi)	2.9 km (1.8 mi)
3355	**119**	Insecticide gas, poisonous, flammable, n.o.s. (Inhalation Hazard Zone D)	30 m (100 ft)	0.1 km (0.1 mi)	0.2 km (0.1 mi)	150 m (500 ft)	0.8 km (0.5 mi)	2.0 km (1.3 mi)
3355 3355	**119** **119**	Insecticide gas, toxic, flammable, n.o.s. Insecticide gas, toxic, flammable, n.o.s. (Inhalation Hazard Zone A)	150 m (500 ft)	1.0 km (0.6 mi)	3.8 km (2.4 mi)	1000 m (3000 ft)	5.7 km (3.6 mi)	10.1 km (6.3 mi)

"+" means distance can be larger in certain atmospheric conditions

TABLE 1

TABLE 1 - INITIAL ISOLATION AND PROTECTIVE ACTION DISTANCES

ID No.	Guide	NAME OF MATERIAL	SMALL SPILLS (From a small package or small leak from a large package) First ISOLATE in all Directions Meters (Feet)	SMALL SPILLS Then PROTECT persons Downwind during DAY Kilometers (Miles)	SMALL SPILLS Then PROTECT persons Downwind during NIGHT Kilometers (Miles)	LARGE SPILLS (From a large package or from many small packages) First ISOLATE in all Directions Meters (Feet)	LARGE SPILLS Then PROTECT persons Downwind during DAY Kilometers (Miles)	LARGE SPILLS Then PROTECT persons Downwind during NIGHT Kilometers (Miles)
3355	**119**	Insecticide gas, toxic, flammable, n.o.s. (Inhalation Hazard Zone B)	30 m (100 ft)	0.1 km (0.1 mi)	0.4 km (0.2 mi)	300 m (1000 ft)	1.3 km (0.8 mi)	3.4 km (2.1 mi)
3355	**119**	Insecticide gas, toxic, flammable, n.o.s. (Inhalation Hazard Zone C)	30 m (100 ft)	0.1 km (0.1 mi)	0.3 km (0.2 mi)	150 m (500 ft)	1.0 km (0.6 mi)	2.9 km (1.8 mi)
3355	**119**	Insecticide gas, toxic, flammable, n.o.s. (Inhalation Hazard Zone D)	30 m (100 ft)	0.1 km (0.1 mi)	0.2 km (0.1 mi)	150 m (500 ft)	0.8 km (0.5 mi)	2.0 km (1.3 mi)
3361	**156**	Chlorosilanes, poisonous, corrosive, n.o.s. **(when spilled in water)**	30 m (100 ft)	0.1 km (0.1 mi)	0.2 km (0.1 mi)	60 m (200 ft)	0.5 km (0.3 mi)	1.6 km (1.0 mi)
3361	**156**	Chlorosilanes, toxic, corrosive, n.o.s. **(when spilled in water)**						
3362	**155**	Chlorosilanes, poisonous, corrosive, flammable, n.o.s. **(when spilled in water)**	30 m (100 ft)	0.1 km (0.1 mi)	0.2 km (0.1 mi)	60 m (200 ft)	0.5 km (0.3 mi)	1.6 km (1.0 mi)
3362	**155**	Chlorosilanes, toxic, corrosive, flammable, n.o.s. **(when spilled in water)**						
3381	**151**	Poisonous by inhalation liquid, n.o.s. (Inhalation Hazard Zone A)	60 m (200 ft)	0.6 km (0.4 mi)	1.2 km (0.8 mi)	200 m (600 ft)	2.2 km (1.4 mi)	4.2 km (2.6 mi)
3381	**151**	Toxic by inhalation liquid, n.o.s. (Inhalation Hazard Zone A)						

3382 3382	**151** **151**	Poisonous by inhalation liquid, n.o.s. (Inhalation Hazard Zone B) Toxic by inhalation liquid, n.o.s. (Inhalation Hazard Zone B)	30 m	(100 ft)	0.2 km	(0.1 mi)	0.2 km	(0.2 mi)	60 m	(200 ft)	0.5 km	(0.3 mi)	0.7 km	(0.5 mi)
3383 3383	**131** **131**	Poisonous by inhalation liquid, flammable, n.o.s. (Inhalation Hazard Zone A) Toxic by inhalation liquid, flammable, n.o.s. (Inhalation Hazard Zone A)	60 m	(200 ft)	0.5 km	(0.3 mi)	1.5 km	(0.9 mi)	300 m	(1000 ft)	3.1 km	(2.0 mi)	5.8 km	(3.6 mi)
3384 3384	**131** **131**	Poisonous by inhalation liquid, flammable, n.o.s. (Inhalation Hazard Zone B) Toxic by inhalation liquid, flammable, n.o.s. (Inhalation Hazard Zone B)	30 m	(100 ft)	0.2 km	(0.1 mi)	0.3 km	(0.2 mi)	60 m	(200 ft)	0.6 km	(0.4 mi)	1.0 km	(0.6 mi)
3385 3385	**139** **139**	Poisonous by inhalation liquid, water-reactive, n.o.s. (Inhalation Hazard Zone A) Toxic by inhalation liquid, water-reactive, n.o.s. (Inhalation Hazard Zone A)	60 m	(200 ft)	0.6 km	(0.4 mi)	1.2 km	(0.8 mi)	200 m	(600 ft)	2.2 km	(1.4 mi)	4.2 km	(2.6 mi)
3386 3386	**139** **139**	Poisonous by inhalation liquid, water-reactive, n.o.s. (Inhalation Hazard Zone B) Toxic by inhalation liquid, water-reactive, n.o.s. (Inhalation Hazard Zone B)	30 m	(100 ft)	0.2 km	(0.1 mi)	0.2 km	(0.2 mi)	60 m	(200 ft)	0.5 km	(0.3 mi)	0.7 km	(0.5 mi)

"+" means distance can be larger in certain atmospheric conditions

TABLE 1

TABLE 1 - INITIAL ISOLATION AND PROTECTIVE ACTION DISTANCES

ID No.	Guide	NAME OF MATERIAL	SMALL SPILLS (From a small package or small leak from a large package) First ISOLATE in all Directions Meters (Feet)	SMALL SPILLS Then PROTECT persons Downwind during DAY Kilometers (Miles)	SMALL SPILLS Then PROTECT persons Downwind during NIGHT Kilometers (Miles)	LARGE SPILLS (From a large package or from many small packages) First ISOLATE in all Directions Meters (Feet)	LARGE SPILLS Then PROTECT persons Downwind during DAY Kilometers (Miles)	LARGE SPILLS Then PROTECT persons Downwind during NIGHT Kilometers (Miles)
3387	**142**	Poisonous by inhalation liquid, oxidizing, n.o.s. (Inhalation Hazard Zone A)	60 m (200 ft)	0.6 km (0.4 mi)	1.2 km (0.8 mi)	200 m (600 ft)	2.2 km (1.4 mi)	4.2 km (2.6 mi)
3387	**142**	Toxic by inhalation liquid, oxidizing, n.o.s. (Inhalation Hazard Zone A)						
3388	**142**	Poisonous by inhalation liquid, oxidizing, n.o.s. (Inhalation Hazard Zone B)	30 m (100 ft)	0.1 km (0.1 mi)	0.1 km (0.1 mi)	30 m (100 ft)	0.3 km (0.2 mi)	0.4 km (0.3 mi)
3388	**142**	Toxic by inhalation liquid, oxidizing, n.o.s. (Inhalation Hazard Zone B)						
3389	**154**	Poisonous by inhalation liquid, corrosive, n.o.s. (Inhalation Hazard Zone A)	100 m (300 ft)	0.3 km (0.2 mi)	0.8 km (0.5 mi)	400 m (1250 ft)	1.4 km (0.9 mi)	3.3 km (2.1 mi)
3389	**154**	Toxic by inhalation liquid, corrosive, n.o.s. (Inhalation Hazard Zone A)						
3390	**154**	Poisonous by inhalation liquid, corrosive, n.o.s (Inhalation Hazard Zone B)	30 m (100 ft)	0.2 km (0.1 mi)	0.2 km (0.1 mi)	30 m (100 ft)	0.4 km (0.3 mi)	0.6 km (0.4 mi)
3390	**154**	Toxic by inhalation liquid, corrosive, n.o.s. (Inhalation Hazard Zone B)						

3456	**157**	Nitrosylsulfuric acid, solid **(when spilled in water)**	30 m	(100 ft)	0.1 km	(0.1 mi)	0.3 km	(0.2 mi)	300 m	(1000 ft)	1.0 km	(0.6 mi)	2.9 km	(1.8 mi)
3456	**157**	Nitrosylsulphuric acid, solid **(when spilled in water)**												
3488	**131**	Poisonous by inhalation liquid, flammable, corrosive, n.o.s. (Inhalation Hazard Zone A)	100 m	(300 ft)	0.9 km	(0.6 mi)	2.0 km	(1.2 mi)	400 m	(1250 ft)	4.8 km	(3.0 mi)	7.5 km	(4.7 mi)
3488	**131**	Toxic by inhalation liquid, flammable, corrosive, n.o.s. (Inhalation Hazard Zone A)												
3489	**131**	Poisonous by inhalation liquid, flammable, corrosive, n.o.s. (Inhalation Hazard Zone B)	30 m	(100 ft)	0.2 km	(0.1 mi)	0.3 km	(0.2 mi)	60 m	(200 ft)	0.6 km	(0.4 mi)	1.0 km	(0.6 mi)
3489	**131**	Toxic by inhalation liquid, flammable, corrosive, n.o.s. (Inhalation Hazard Zone B)												
3490	**155**	Poisonous by inhalation liquid, water-reactive, flammable, n.o.s. (Inhalation Hazard Zone A)	60 m	(200 ft)	0.5 km	(0.3 mi)	1.5 km	(0.9 mi)	300 m	(1000 ft)	3.1 km	(2.0 mi)	5.8 km	(3.6 mi)
3490	**155**	Toxic by inhalation liquid, water-reactive, flammable, n.o.s. (Inhalation Hazard Zone A)												
3491	**155**	Poisonous by inhalation liquid, water-reactive, flammable, n.o.s. (Inhalation Hazard Zone B)	30 m	(100 ft)	0.2 km	(0.1 mi)	0.3 km	(0.2 mi)	60 m	(200 ft)	0.6 km	(0.4 mi)	1.0 km	(0.6 mi)
3491	**155**	Toxic by inhalation liquid, water-reactive, flammable, n.o.s. (Inhalation Hazard Zone B)												

"+" means distance can be larger in certain atmospheric conditions

TABLE 1

TABLE 1 - INITIAL ISOLATION AND PROTECTIVE ACTION DISTANCES

			SMALL SPILLS (From a small package or small leak from a large package)			LARGE SPILLS (From a large package or from many small packages)		
			First ISOLATE in all Directions	Then PROTECT persons Downwind during		First ISOLATE in all Directions	Then PROTECT persons Downwind during	
ID No.	Guide	NAME OF MATERIAL	Meters (Feet)	DAY Kilometers (Miles)	NIGHT Kilometers (Miles)	Meters (Feet)	DAY Kilometers (Miles)	NIGHT Kilometers (Miles)
3492	**131**	Poisonous by inhalation liquid, corrosive, flammable, n.o.s. (Inhalation Hazard Zone A)	100 m (300 ft)	0.9 km (0.6 mi)	2.0 km (1.2 mi)	400 m (1250 ft)	4.8 km (3.0 mi)	7.5 km (4.7 mi)
3492	**131**	Toxic by inhalation liquid, corrosive, flammable, n.o.s. (Inhalation Hazard Zone A)						
3493	**131**	Poisonous by inhalation liquid, corrosive, flammable, n.o.s. (Inhalation Hazard Zone B)	30 m (100 ft)	0.2 km (0.1 mi)	0.3 km (0.2 mi)	60 m (200 ft)	0.6 km (0.4 mi)	1.0 km (0.6 mi)
3493	**131**	Toxic by inhalation liquid, corrosive, flammable, n.o.s. (Inhalation Hazard Zone B)						
3494	**131**	Petroleum sour crude oil, flammable, poisonous	30 m (100 ft)	0.2 km (0.1 mi)	0.2 km (0.2 mi)	60 m (200 ft)	0.5 km (0.3 mi)	0.7 km (0.5 mi)
3494	**131**	Petroleum sour crude oil, flammable, toxic						
3507	**166**	Uranium hexafluoride, radioactive material, excepted package, less than 0.1 kg per package, non-fissile or fissile-excepted **(when spilled in water)**	30 m (100 ft)	0.1 km (0.1 mi)	0.1 km (0.1 mi)	30 m (100 ft)	0.1 km (0.1 mi)	0.1 km (0.1 mi)

3512 3512	173 173	Adsorbed gas, poisonous, n.o.s. Adsorbed gas, poisonous, n.o.s. (Inhalation hazard zone A)	30 m	(100 ft)	0.1 km	(0.1 mi)	0.1 km	(0.1 mi)	30 m	(100 ft)	0.1 km	(0.1 mi)	0.2 km	(0.2 mi)
3512 3512 3512	173 173 173	Adsorbed gas, poisonous, n.o.s. (Inhalation hazard zone B) Adsorbed gas, poisonous, n.o.s. (Inhalation hazard zone C) Adsorbed gas, poisonous, n.o.s. (Inhalation hazard zone D)	30 m	(100 ft)	0.1 km	(0.1 mi)	0.1 km	(0.1 mi)	30 m	(100 ft)	0.1 km	(0.1 mi)	0.1 km	(0.1 mi)
3512 3512	173 173	Adsorbed gas, toxic, n.o.s. Adsorbed gas, toxic, n.o.s. (Inhalation hazard zone A)	30 m	(100 ft)	0.1 km	(0.1 mi)	0.1 km	(0.1 mi)	30 m	(100 ft)	0.1 km	(0.1 mi)	0.2 km	(0.2 mi)
3512 3512 3512	173 173 173	Adsorbed gas, toxic, n.o.s. (Inhalation hazard zone B) Adsorbed gas, toxic, n.o.s. (Inhalation hazard zone C) Adsorbed gas, toxic, n.o.s. (Inhalation hazard zone D)	30 m	(100 ft)	0.1 km	(0.1 mi)	0.1 km	(0.1 mi)	30 m	(100 ft)	0.1 km	(0.1 mi)	0.1 km	(0.1 mi)
3514 3514	173 173	Adsorbed gas, poisonous, flammable, n.o.s. Adsorbed gas, poisonous, flammable, n.o.s. (Inhalation hazard zone A)	30 m	(100 ft)	0.1 km	(0.1 mi)	0.1 km	(0.1 mi)	30 m	(100 ft)	0.1 km	(0.1 mi)	0.2 km	(0.2 mi)

"+" means distance can be larger in certain atmospheric conditions

TABLE 1

TABLE 1 - INITIAL ISOLATION AND PROTECTIVE ACTION DISTANCES

			SMALL SPILLS (From a small package or small leak from a large package)			LARGE SPILLS (From a large package or from many small packages)		
			First ISOLATE in all Directions	Then PROTECT persons Downwind during		First ISOLATE in all Directions	Then PROTECT persons Downwind during	
ID No.	Guide	NAME OF MATERIAL	Meters (Feet)	DAY Kilometers (Miles)	NIGHT Kilometers (Miles)	Meters (Feet)	DAY Kilometers (Miles)	NIGHT Kilometers (Miles)
3514	173	Adsorbed gas, poisonous, flammable, n.o.s. (Inhalation hazard zone B)						
3514	173	Adsorbed gas, poisonous, flammable, n.o.s. (Inhalation hazard zone C)	30 m (100 ft)	0.1 km (0.1 mi)	0.1 km (0.1 mi)	30 m (100 ft)	0.1 km (0.1 mi)	0.1 km (0.1 mi)
3514	173	Adsorbed gas, poisonous, flammable, n.o.s. (Inhalation hazard zone D)						
3514	173	Adsorbed gas, toxic, flammable, n.o.s.						
3514	173	Adsorbed gas, toxic, flammable, n.o.s. (Inhalation hazard zone A)	30 m (100 ft)	0.1 km (0.1 mi)	0.1 km (0.1 mi)	30 m (100 ft)	0.1 km (0.1 mi)	0.2 km (0.2 mi)
3514	173	Adsorbed gas, toxic, flammable, n.o.s. (Inhalation hazard zone B)						
3514	173	Adsorbed gas, toxic, flammable, n.o.s. (Inhalation hazard zone C)	30 m (100 ft)	0.1 km (0.1 mi)	0.1 km (0.1 mi)	30 m (100 ft)	0.1 km (0.1 mi)	0.1 km (0.1 mi)
3514	173	Adsorbed gas, toxic, flammable, n.o.s. (Inhalation hazard zone D)						

3515	**173**	Adsorbed gas, poisonous, oxidizing, n.o.s.												
3515	**173**	Adsorbed gas, poisonous, oxidizing, n.o.s. (Inhalation hazard zone A)	30 m	(100 ft)	0.1 km	(0.1 mi)	0.1 km	(0.1 mi)	30 m	(100 ft)	0.1 km	(0.1 mi)	0.2 km	(0.2 mi)
3515	**173**	Adsorbed gas, poisonous, oxidizing, n.o.s. (Inhalation hazard zone B)												
3515	**173**	Adsorbed gas, poisonous, oxidizing, n.o.s. (Inhalation hazard zone C)	30 m	(100 ft)	0.1 km	(0.1 mi)	0.1 km	(0.1 mi)	30 m	(100 ft)	0.1 km	(0.1 mi)	0.1 km	(0.1 mi)
3515	**173**	Adsorbed gas, poisonous, oxidizing, n.o.s. (Inhalation hazard zone D)												
3515	**173**	Adsorbed gas, toxic, oxidizing, n.o.s.												
3515	**173**	Adsorbed gas, toxic, oxidizing, n.o.s. (Inhalation hazard zone A)	30 m	(100 ft)	0.1 km	(0.1 mi)	0.1 km	(0.1 mi)	30 m	(100 ft)	0.1 km	(0.1 mi)	0.2 km	(0.2 mi)
3515	**173**	Adsorbed gas, toxic, oxidizing, n.o.s. (Inhalation hazard zone B)												
3515	**173**	Adsorbed gas, toxic, oxidizing, n.o.s. (Inhalation hazard zone C)	30 m	(100 ft)	0.1 km	(0.1 mi)	0.1 km	(0.1 mi)	30 m	(100 ft)	0.1 km	(0.1 mi)	0.1 km	(0.1 mi)
3515	**173**	Adsorbed gas, toxic, oxidizing, n.o.s. (Inhalation hazard zone D)												
3516	**173**	Adsorbed gas, poisonous, corrosive, n.o.s.												
3516	**173**	Adsorbed gas, poisonous, corrosive, n.o.s. (Inhalation hazard zone A)	30 m	(100 ft)	0.1 km	(0.1 mi)	0.1 km	(0.1 mi)	30 m	(100 ft)	0.1 km	(0.1 mi)	0.2 km	(0.2 mi)

"+" means distance can be larger in certain atmospheric conditions

TABLE 1 - INITIAL ISOLATION AND PROTECTIVE ACTION DISTANCES

ID No.	Guide	NAME OF MATERIAL	SMALL SPILLS (From a small package or small leak from a large package) First ISOLATE in all Directions Meters	(Feet)	Then PROTECT persons Downwind during DAY Kilometers	(Miles)	NIGHT Kilometers	(Miles)	LARGE SPILLS (From a large package or from many small packages) First ISOLATE in all Directions Meters	(Feet)	Then PROTECT persons Downwind during DAY Kilometers	(Miles)	NIGHT Kilometers	(Miles)
3516	173	Adsorbed gas, poisonous, corrosive, n.o.s. (Inhalation hazard zone B)												
3516	173	Adsorbed gas, poisonous, corrosive, n.o.s. (Inhalation hazard zone C)	30 m	(100 ft)	0.1 km	(0.1 mi)	0.1 km	(0.1 mi)	30 m	(100 ft)	0.1 km	(0.1 mi)	0.1 km	(0.1 mi)
3516	173	Adsorbed gas, poisonous, corrosive, n.o.s. (Inhalation hazard zone D)												
3516	173	Adsorbed gas, toxic, corrosive, n.o.s.												
3516	173	Adsorbed gas, toxic, corrosive, n.o.s. (Inhalation hazard zone A)	30 m	(100 ft)	0.1 km	(0.1 mi)	0.1 km	(0.1 mi)	30 m	(100 ft)	0.1 km	(0.1 mi)	0.2 km	(0.2 mi)
3516	173	Adsorbed gas, toxic, corrosive, n.o.s. (Inhalation hazard zone B)												
3516	173	Adsorbed gas, toxic, corrosive, n.o.s. (Inhalation hazard zone C)	30 m	(100 ft)	0.1 km	(0.1 mi)	0.1 km	(0.1 mi)	30 m	(100 ft)	0.1 km	(0.1 mi)	0.1 km	(0.1 mi)
3516	173	Adsorbed gas, toxic, corrosive, n.o.s. (Inhalation hazard zone D)												
3517	173	Adsorbed gas, poisonous, flammable, corrosive, n.o.s.	30 m	(100 ft)	0.1 km	(0.1 mi)	0.1 km	(0.1 mi)	30 m	(100 ft)	0.1 km	(0.1 mi)	0.2 km	(0.2 mi)
3517	173	Adsorbed gas, poisonous, flammable, corrosive, n.o.s. (Inhalation hazard zone A)												

3517	**173**	Adsorbed gas, poisonous, flammable, corrosive, n.o.s. (Inhalation hazard zone B) Adsorbed gas, poisonous, flammable, corrosive, n.o.s. (Inhalation hazard zone C) Adsorbed gas, poisonous, flammable, corrosive, n.o.s. (Inhalation hazard zone D)	30 m	(100 ft)	0.1 km	(0.1 mi)	0.1 km	(0.1 mi)	30 m	(100 ft)	0.1 km	(0.1 mi)	0.1 km	(0.1 mi)
3517 3517	**173** **173**	Adsorbed gas, toxic, flammable, corrosive, n.o.s Adsorbed gas, toxic, flammable, corrosive, n.o.s. (Inhalation hazard zone A)	30 m	(100 ft)	0.1 km	(0.1 mi)	0.1 km	(0.1 mi)	30 m	(100 ft)	0.1 km	(0.1 mi)	0.2 km	(0.2 mi)
3517 3517 3517	**173** **173** **173**	Adsorbed gas, toxic, flammable, corrosive, n.o.s. (Inhalation hazard zone B) Adsorbed gas, toxic, flammable, corrosive, n.o.s. (Inhalation hazard zone C) Adsorbed gas, toxic, flammable, corrosive, n.o.s. (Inhalation hazard zone D)	30 m	(100 ft)	0.1 km	(0.1 mi)	0.1 km	(0.1 mi)	30 m	(100 ft)	0.1 km	(0.1 mi)	0.1 km	(0.1 mi)
3518 3518	**173** **173**	Adsorbed gas, poisonous, oxidizing, corrosive, n.o.s Adsorbed gas, poisonous, oxidizing, corrosive, n.o.s. (Inhalation hazard zone A)	30 m	(100 ft)	0.1 km	(0.1 mi)	0.1 km	(0.1 mi)	30 m	(100 ft)	0.1 km	(0.1 mi)	0.2 km	(0.2 mi)

"+" means distance can be larger in certain atmospheric conditions

TABLE 1 - INITIAL ISOLATION AND PROTECTIVE ACTION DISTANCES

ID No.	Guide	NAME OF MATERIAL	SMALL SPILLS (From a small package or small leak from a large package) First ISOLATE in all Directions Meters (Feet)	SMALL SPILLS Then PROTECT persons Downwind during DAY Kilometers (Miles)	SMALL SPILLS Then PROTECT persons Downwind during NIGHT Kilometers (Miles)	LARGE SPILLS (From a large package or from many small packages) First ISOLATE in all Directions Meters (Feet)	LARGE SPILLS Then PROTECT persons Downwind during DAY Kilometers (Miles)	LARGE SPILLS Then PROTECT persons Downwind during NIGHT Kilometers (Miles)
3518	173	Adsorbed gas, poisonous, oxidizing, corrosive, n.o.s. (Inhalation hazard zone B)	30 m (100 ft)	0.1 km (0.1 mi)	0.1 km (0.1 mi)	30 m (100 ft)	0.1 km (0.1 mi)	0.1 km (0.1 mi)
3518	173	Adsorbed gas, poisonous, oxidizing, corrosive, n.o.s (Inhalation hazard zone C)	30 m (100 ft)	0.1 km (0.1 mi)	0.1 km (0.1 mi)	30 m (100 ft)	0.1 km (0.1 mi)	0.1 km (0.1 mi)
3518	173	Adsorbed gas, poisonous, oxidizing, corrosive, n.o.s. (Inhalation hazard zone D)	30 m (100 ft)	0.1 km (0.1 mi)	0.1 km (0.1 mi)	30 m (100 ft)	0.1 km (0.1 mi)	0.1 km (0.1 mi)
3518	173	Adsorbed gas, toxic, oxidizing, corrosive, n.o.s.	30 m (100 ft)	0.1 km (0.1 mi)	0.1 km (0.1 mi)	30 m (100 ft)	0.1 km (0.1 mi)	0.2 km (0.2 mi)
3518	173	Adsorbed gas, toxic, oxidizing, corrosive, n.o.s. (Inhalation hazard zone A)	30 m (100 ft)	0.1 km (0.1 mi)	0.1 km (0.1 mi)	30 m (100 ft)	0.1 km (0.1 mi)	0.2 km (0.2 mi)
3518	173	Adsorbed gas, toxic, oxidizing, corrosive, n.o.s. (Inhalation hazard zone B)	30 m (100 ft)	0.1 km (0.1 mi)	0.1 km (0.1 mi)	30 m (100 ft)	0.1 km (0.1 mi)	0.1 km (0.1 mi)
3518	173	Adsorbed gas, toxic, oxidizing, corrosive, n.o.s. (Inhalation hazard zone C)	30 m (100 ft)	0.1 km (0.1 mi)	0.1 km (0.1 mi)	30 m (100 ft)	0.1 km (0.1 mi)	0.1 km (0.1 mi)
3518	173	Adsorbed gas, toxic, oxidizing, corrosive, n.o.s. (Inhalation hazard zone D)	30 m (100 ft)	0.1 km (0.1 mi)	0.1 km (0.1 mi)	30 m (100 ft)	0.1 km (0.1 mi)	0.1 km (0.1 mi)
3519	173	Boron trifluoride, adsorbed	30 m (100 ft)	0.1 km (0.1 mi)	0.1 km (0.1 mi)	30 m (100 ft)	0.1 km (0.1 mi)	0.1 km (0.1 mi)
3520	173	Chlorine, adsorbed	30 m (100 ft)	0.1 km (0.1 mi)	0.1 km (0.1 mi)	30 m (100 ft)	0.1 km (0.1 mi)	0.1 km (0.1 mi)

3521	**173**	Silicon tetrafluoride, adsorbed	30 m	(100 ft)	0.1 km	(0.1 mi)	0.1 km	(0.1 mi)	30 m	(100 ft)	0.1 km	(0.1 mi)	0.1 km	(0.1 mi)
3522	**173**	Arsine, adsorbed	30 m	(100 ft)	0.1 km	(0.1 mi)	0.1 km	(0.1 mi)	30 m	(100 ft)	0.1 km	(0.1 mi)	0.2 km	(0.2 mi)
3523	**173**	Germane, adsorbed	30 m	(100 ft)	0.1 km	(0.1 mi)	0.1 km	(0.1 mi)	30 m	(100 ft)	0.1 km	(0.1 mi)	0.2 km	(0.2 mi)
3524	**173**	Phosphorus pentafluoride, adsorbed	30 m	(100 ft)	0.1 km	(0.1 mi)	0.1 km	(0.1 mi)	30 m	(100 ft)	0.1 km	(0.1 mi)	0.1 km	(0.1 mi)
3525	**173**	Phosphine, adsorbed	30 m	(100 ft)	0.1 km	(0.1 mi)	0.1 km	(0.1 mi)	30 m	(100 ft)	0.1 km	(0.1 mi)	0.1 km	(0.1 mi)
3526	**173**	Hydrogen selenide, adsorbed	30 m	(100 ft)	0.1 km	(0.1 mi)	0.1 km	(0.1 mi)	30 m	(100 ft)	0.1 km	(0.1 mi)	0.4 km	(0.3 mi)
3539	**123**	Articles containing toxic gas, n.o.s.	30 m	(100 ft)	0.1 km	(0.1 mi)	0.1 km	(0.1 mi)	30 m	(100 ft)	0.1 km	(0.1 mi)	0.4 km	(0.3 mi)
9191	**143**	Chlorine dioxide, hydrate, frozen (**when spilled in water**)	30 m	(100 ft)	0.1 km	(0.1 mi)	0.1 km	(0.1 mi)	30 m	(100 ft)	0.2 km	(0.1 mi)	0.5 km	(0.3 mi)
9202	**168**	Carbon monoxide, refrigerated liquid (cryogenic liquid)	30 m	(100 ft)	0.1 km	(0.1 mi)	0.2 km	(0.1 mi)	200 m	(600 ft)	1.2 km	(0.7 mi)	4.3 km	(2.7 mi)
9206	**137**	Methyl phosphonic dichloride	30 m	(100 ft)	0.1 km	(0.1 mi)	0.2 km	(0.1 mi)	30 m	(100 ft)	0.4 km	(0.3 mi)	0.6 km	(0.4 mi)
9263	**156**	Chloropivaloyl chloride	30 m	(100 ft)	0.1 km	(0.1 mi)	0.1 km	(0.1 mi)	30 m	(100 ft)	0.2 km	(0.2 mi)	0.3 km	(0.2 mi)
9264	**151**	3,5-Dichloro-2,4,6-trifluoropyridine	30 m	(100 ft)	0.1 km	(0.1 mi)	0.1 km	(0.1 mi)	30 m	(100 ft)	0.2 km	(0.2 mi)	0.3 km	(0.2 mi)
9269	**132**	Trimethoxysilane	30 m	(100 ft)	0.2 km	(0.2 mi)	0.6 km	(0.4 mi)	100 m	(300 ft)	1.3 km	(0.8 mi)	2.3 km	(1.5 mi)

See Next Page for Table of Water-Reactive Materials Which Produce Toxic Gases

"+" means distance can be larger in certain atmospheric conditions

HOW TO USE TABLE 2 – WATER-REACTIVE MATERIALS THAT PRODUCE TOXIC GASES

Table 2 lists materials that produce large amounts of Toxic Inhalation Hazard (TIH) (PIH in the US) gases when spilled in water, and identifies the TIH gases produced.

The materials are listed by order of ID number.

These Water-Reactive materials are easily identified in Table 1 as their name is immediately followed by **(when spilled in water)**.

Note 1: The TIH gases indicated in Table 2 are for information purposes only. In Table 1, the initial isolation and protective action distances have already taken into consideration the TIH gases produced.

For example: Table 2 indicates that UN1689 sodium cyanide, when spilled in water, will generate hydrogen cyanide gas (HCN). In Table 1, you must refer to the distances for sodium cyanide and not the distances for hydrogen cyanide gas.

Note 2: Some Water-Reactive materials are also TIH materials themselves (e.g., UN1746 (Bromine trifluoride), UN1836 (Thionyl chloride)). In these instances, two entries are provided in Table 1 for land-based and water-based spills. If a water-reactive material only has one entry in Table 1 for **(when spilled in water)**, and the product is **NOT** spilled in water, Tables 1 and 2 do **NOT** apply. Refer only to the appropriate orange-bordered guide.

Note 3: Materials classified as a Division 4.3 are substances that, on contact with water, are liable to become spontaneously **FLAMMABLE** or give off **FLAMMABLE** or sometimes **TOXIC** gases in dangerous quantities. For the purpose of this table, water-reactive materials are materials that generate substantial quantities of **TOXIC** gases rapidly after a spill into water; therefore, a material classified as a Division 4.3 will not always be included in Table 2.

Materials Which Produce Large Amounts of Toxic-by-Inhalation (TIH) (PIH in the US) Gas(es) When Spilled in Water

ID No.	Guide No.	Name of Material	TIH Gas(es) Produced
1162	**155**	Dimethyldichlorosilane	HCl
1183	**139**	Ethyldichlorosilane	HCl
1196	**155**	Ethyltrichlorosilane	HCl
1242	**139**	Methyldichlorosilane	HCl
1250	**155**	Methyltrichlorosilane	HCl
1295	**139**	Trichlorosilane	HCl
1298	**155**	Trimethylchlorosilane	HCl
1305	**155P**	Vinyltrichlorosilane	HCl
1305	**155P**	Vinyltrichlorosilane, stabilized	HCl
1340	**139**	Phosphorus pentasulfide, free from yellow and white Phosphorus	H_2S
1340	**139**	Phosphorus pentasulphide, free from yellow and white Phosphorus	H_2S
1360	**139**	Calcium phosphide	PH_3
1384	**135**	Sodium dithionite	H_2S SO_2
1384	**135**	Sodium hydrosulfite	H_2S SO_2
1384	**135**	Sodium hydrosulphite	H_2S SO_2
1390	**139**	Alkali metal amides	NH_3
1397	**139**	Aluminum phosphide	PH_3
1419	**139**	Magnesium aluminum phosphide	PH_3
1432	**139**	Sodium phosphide	PH_3
1541	**155**	Acetone cyanohydrin, stabilized	HCN
1680	**157**	Potassium cyanide, solid	HCN
1689	**157**	Sodium cyanide, solid	HCN

Chemical Symbols for TIH (PIH in the US) Gases:

Br_2	Bromine	HF	Hydrogen fluoride	NO_2	Nitrogen dioxide
Cl_2	Chlorine	HI	Hydrogen iodide	PH_3	Phosphine
HBr	Hydrogen bromide	H_2S	Hydrogen sulfide	SO_2	Sulfur dioxide
HCl	Hydrogen chloride	H_2S	Hydrogen sulphide	SO_2	Sulphur dioxide
HCN	Hydrogen cyanide	NH_3	Ammonia		

Use this list only when material is spilled in water.

TABLE 2 - WATER-REACTIVE MATERIALS WHICH PRODUCE TOXIC GASES

Materials Which Produce Large Amounts of Toxic-by-Inhalation (TIH) (PIH in the US) Gas(es) When Spilled in Water

ID No.	Guide No.	Name of Material	TIH Gas(es) Produced
1716	**156**	Acetyl bromide	HBr
1717	**155**	Acetyl chloride	HCl
1724	**155**	Allyltrichlorosilane, stabilized	HCl
1725	**137**	Aluminum bromide, anhydrous	HBr
1726	**137**	Aluminum chloride, anhydrous	HCl
1728	**155**	Amyltrichlorosilane	HCl
1732	**157**	Antimony pentafluoride	HF
1741	**125**	Boron trichloride	HCl
1745	**144**	Bromine pentafluoride	HF Br_2
1746	**144**	Bromine trifluoride	HF Br_2
1747	**155**	Butyltrichlorosilane	HCl
1752	**156**	Chloroacetyl chloride	HCl
1753	**156**	Chlorophenyltrichlorosilane	HCl
1754	**137**	Chlorosulfonic acid (with or without sulfur trioxide)	HCl
1754	**137**	Chlorosulphonic acid (with or without sulphur trioxide)	HCl
1758	**137**	Chromium oxychloride	HCl
1762	**156**	Cyclohexenyltrichlorosilane	HCl
1763	**156**	Cyclohexyltrichlorosilane	HCl
1765	**156**	Dichloroacetyl chloride	HCl
1766	**156**	Dichlorophenyltrichlorosilane	HCl
1767	**155**	Diethyldichlorosilane	HCl
1769	**156**	Diphenyldichlorosilane	HCl
1771	**156**	Dodecyltrichlorosilane	HCl

Chemical Symbols for TIH (PIH in the US) Gases:

Br_2	Bromine	HF	Hydrogen fluoride	NO_2	Nitrogen dioxide
Cl_2	Chlorine	HI	Hydrogen iodide	PH_3	Phosphine
HBr	Hydrogen bromide	H_2S	Hydrogen sulfide	SO_2	Sulfur dioxide
HCl	Hydrogen chloride	H_2S	Hydrogen sulphide	SO_2	Sulphur dioxide
HCN	Hydrogen cyanide	NH_3	Ammonia		

Use this list only when material is spilled in water.

Materials Which Produce Large Amounts of Toxic-by-Inhalation (TIH) (PIH in the US) Gas(es) When Spilled in Water

ID No.	Guide No.	Name of Material	TIH Gas(es) Produced
1777	**137**	Fluorosulfonic acid	HF
1777	**137**	Fluorosulphonic acid	HF
1781	**156**	Hexadecyltrichlorosilane	HCl
1784	**156**	Hexyltrichlorosilane	HCl
1799	**156**	Nonyltrichlorosilane	HCl
1800	**156**	Octadecyltrichlorosilane	HCl
1801	**156**	Octyltrichlorosilane	HCl
1804	**156**	Phenyltrichlorosilane	HCl
1806	**137**	Phosphorus pentachloride	HCl
1808	**137**	Phosphorus tribromide	HBr
1809	**137**	Phosphorus trichloride	HCl
1810	**137**	Phosphorus oxychloride	HCl
1815	**132**	Propionyl chloride	HCl
1816	**155**	Propyltrichlorosilane	HCl
1818	**157**	Silicon tetrachloride	HCl
1828	**137**	Sulfur chlorides	HCl SO_2 H_2S
1828	**137**	Sulphur chlorides	HCl SO_2 H_2S
1834	**137**	Sulfuryl chloride	HCl
1834	**137**	Sulphuryl chloride	HCl
1836	**137**	Thionyl chloride	HCl SO_2
1838	**137**	Titanium tetrachloride	HCl
1898	**156**	Acetyl iodide	HI
1923	**135**	Calcium dithionite	H_2S SO_2

Chemical Symbols for TIH (PIH in the US) Gases:

Br_2	Bromine	HF	Hydrogen fluoride	NO_2	Nitrogen dioxide
Cl_2	Chlorine	HI	Hydrogen iodide	PH_3	Phosphine
HBr	Hydrogen bromide	H_2S	Hydrogen sulfide	SO_2	Sulfur dioxide
HCl	Hydrogen chloride	H_2S	Hydrogen sulphide	SO_2	Sulphur dioxide
HCN	Hydrogen cyanide	NH_3	Ammonia		

Use this list only when material is spilled in water.

TABLE 2

TABLE 2 - WATER-REACTIVE MATERIALS WHICH PRODUCE TOXIC GASES

Materials Which Produce Large Amounts of Toxic-by-Inhalation (TIH) (PIH in the US) Gas(es) When Spilled in Water

ID No.	Guide No.	Name of Material	TIH Gas(es) Produced
1923	**135**	Calcium hydrosulfite	H_2S SO_2
1923	**135**	Calcium hydrosulphite	H_2S SO_2
1929	**135**	Potassium dithionite	H_2S SO_2
1929	**135**	Potassium hydrosulfite	H_2S SO_2
1929	**135**	Potassium hydrosulphite	H_2S SO_2
1931	**171**	Zinc dithionite	H_2S SO_2
1931	**171**	Zinc hydrosulfite	H_2S SO_2
1931	**171**	Zinc hydrosulphite	H_2S SO_2
2004	**135**	Magnesium diamide	NH_3
2011	**139**	Magnesium phosphide	PH_3
2012	**139**	Potassium phosphide	PH_3
2013	**139**	Strontium phosphide	PH_3
2308	**157**	Nitrosylsulfuric acid, liquid	NO_2
2308	**157**	Nitrosylsulphuric acid, liquid	NO_2
2353	**132**	Butyryl chloride	HCl
2395	**132**	Isobutyryl chloride	HCl
2434	**156**	Dibenzyldichlorosilane	HCl
2435	**156**	Ethylphenyldichlorosilane	HCl
2437	**156**	Methylphenyldichlorosilane	HCl
2495	**144**	Iodine pentafluorlde	HF
2691	**137**	Phosphorus pentabromide	HBr
2692	**157**	Boron tribromide	HBr
2806	**139**	Lithium nitride	NH_3

Chemical Symbols for TIH (PIH in the US) Gases:

Br_2	Bromine	HF	Hydrogen fluoride	NO_2	Nitrogen dioxide
Cl_2	Chlorine	HI	Hydrogen iodide	PH_3	Phosphine
HBr	Hydrogen bromide	H_2S	Hydrogen sulfide	SO_2	Sulfur dioxide
HCl	Hydrogen chloride	H_2S	Hydrogen sulphide	SO_2	Sulphur dioxide
HCN	Hydrogen cyanide	NH_3	Ammonia		

Use this list only when material is spilled in water.

Materials Which Produce Large Amounts of Toxic-by-Inhalation (TIH) (PIH in the US) Gas(es) When Spilled in Water

ID No.	Guide No.	Name of Material	TIH Gas(es) Produced
2965	**139**	Boron trifluoride dimethyl etherate	HF
2977	**166**	Radioactive material, Uranium hexafluoride, fissile	HF
2977	**166**	Uranium hexafluoride, radioactive material, fissile	HF
2978	**166**	Radioactive material, Uranium hexafluoride, non fissile or fissile-excepted	HF
2978	**166**	Uranium hexafluoride, radioactive material, non fissile or fissile-excepted	HF
2985	**155**	Chlorosilanes, flammable, corrosive, n.o.s	HCl
2986	**155**	Chlorosilanes, corrosive, flammable, n.o.s	HCl
2987	**156**	Chlorosilanes, corrosive, n.o.s	HCl
2988	**139**	Chlorosilanes, water-reactive, flammable, corrosive, n.o.s.	HCl
3048	**157**	Aluminum phosphide pesticide	PH_3
3361	**156**	Chlorosilanes, poisonous, corrosive, n.o.s.	HCl
3361	**156**	Chlorosilanes, toxic, corrosive, n.o.s.	HCl
3362	**155**	Chlorosilanes, poisonous, corrosive, flammable, n.o.s.	HCl
3362	**155**	Chlorosilanes, toxic, corrosive, flammable, n.o.s.	HCl
3456	**157**	Nitrosylsulfuric acid, solid	NO_2
3456	**157**	Nitrosylsulphuric acid, solid	NO_2
3507	**166**	Uranium hexafluoride, radioactive material, excepted package, less than 0.1 kg per package, non-fissile or fissile-excepted	HF
9191	**143**	Chlorine dioxide, hydrate, frozen	Cl_2

Chemical Symbols for TIH (PIH in the US) Gases:

Br_2	Bromine	HF	Hydrogen fluoride	NO_2	Nitrogen dioxide
Cl_2	Chlorine	HI	Hydrogen iodide	PH_3	Phosphine
HBr	Hydrogen bromide	H_2S	Hydrogen sulfide	SO_2	Sulfur dioxide
HCl	Hydrogen chloride	H_2S	Hydrogen sulphide	SO_2	Sulphur dioxide
HCN	Hydrogen cyanide	NH_3	Ammonia		

Use this list only when material is spilled in water.

HOW TO USE TABLE 3 – INITIAL ISOLATION AND PROTECTIVE ACTION DISTANCES FOR LARGE SPILLS FOR DIFFERENT QUANTITIES OF SIX COMMON TIH (PIH in the US) GASES

Table 3 lists Toxic Inhalation Hazard (TIH) materials that may be more commonly encountered.

The selected materials are:

- UN1005 - Ammonia, anhydrous
- UN1017 - Chlorine
- UN1040 - Ethylene oxide and UN1040 – Ethylene oxide with nitrogen
- UN1050 - Hydrogen chloride, anhydrous and UN2186 - and Hydrogen chloride, refrigerated liquid
- UN1052 - Hydrogen fluoride, anhydrous
- UN1079 - Sulfur dioxide/Sulphur dioxide

The materials are presented in numerical order of ID number and provide Initial Isolation and Protective Action Distances **FOR LARGE SPILLS** (more than 208 liters or 55 US gallons) involving different container types (therefore different volume capacities, see below) for day time and night time situations and different wind speeds.

- Rail tank car: 80 000 kg (176 368 lbs.)
- Highway tank truck or trailer: 20 000 – 25 000 kg (44 092 – 55 115 lbs.)
- Agricultural nurse tank: 3785 L (1000 gallons)
- Small cylinder: 72 L (19 gallons)
- Ton cylinder: 757 - 1135 L (200 - 300 gallons)

Estimating Wind Speed from Environmental Clues

mph	km/h	Wind Description	Specifications
< 6	< 10	Low wind	Wind felt on face; leaves rustle; ordinary vane moved by wind
6 - 12	10 - 20	Moderate wind	Raises dust, loose paper; small branches are moved
> 12	> 20	High wind	Large branches in motion; whistling heard in telephone wires; umbrellas used with difficulty

(Data taken from the Beaufort Wind Scale has been reworked in order to create 3 categories of wind speed: Low, Moderate and High)

TABLE 3 - INITIAL ISOLATION AND PROTECTIVE ACTION DISTANCES FOR LARGE SPILLS FOR DIFFERENT QUANTITIES OF SIX COMMON TIH (PIH in the US) GASES

	First **ISOLATE** in all Directions		Then **PROTECT** persons Downwind during											
			DAY						NIGHT					
			Low wind (< 6 mph = < 10 km/h)		Moderate wind (6-12 mph = 10 - 20 km/h)		High wind (> 12 mph = > 20 km/h)		Low wind (< 6 mph = < 10 km/h)		Moderate wind (6-12 mph = 10 - 20 km/h)		High wind (> 12 mph = > 20 km/h)	
	Meters	(Feet)	km	(Miles)	km	(Miles)	km	(Miles)	km	(Miles)	km	(Miles)	km	(Miles)
TRANSPORT CONTAINER	**UN1005 Ammonia, anhydrous: Large Spills**													
Rail tank car	300	(1000)	1.9	(1.2)	1.5	(0.9)	1.1	(0.6)	4.5	(2.8)	2.5	(1.5)	1.4	(0.9)
Highway tank truck or trailer	150	(500)	0.9	(0.6)	0.5	(0.3)	0.4	(0.3)	2.0	(1.3)	0.8	(0.5)	0.6	(0.4)
Agricultural nurse tank	60	(200)	0.5	(0.3)	0.3	(0.2)	0.3	(0.2)	1.4	(0.9)	0.3	(0.2)	0.3	(0.2)
Multiple small cylinders	30	(100)	0.3	(0.2)	0.2	(0.1)	0.1	(0.1)	0.7	(0.5)	0.3	(0.2)	0.2	(0.1)
TRANSPORT CONTAINER	**UN1017 Chlorine: Large Spills**													
Rail tank car	1000	(3000)	10.1	(6.3)	6.8	(4.2)	5.3	(3.3)	11+	(7+)	9.2	(5.7)	6.9	(4.3)
Highway tank truck or trailer	600	(2000)	5.8	(3.6)	3.4	(2.1)	2.9	(1.8)	6.7	(4.3)	5.0	(3.1)	4.1	(2.5)
Multiple ton cylinders	300	(1000)	2.1	(1.3)	1.3	(0.8)	1.0	(0.6)	4.0	(2.5)	2.4	(1.5)	1.3	(0.8)
Multiple small cylinders or single ton cylinder	150	(500)	1.5	(0.9)	0.8	(0.5)	0.5	(0.3)	2.9	(1.8)	1.3	(0.8)	0.6	(0.4)

"+" means distance can be larger in certain atmospheric conditions

TABLE 3 - INITIAL ISOLATION AND PROTECTIVE ACTION DISTANCES FOR LARGE SPILLS FOR DIFFERENT QUANTITIES OF SIX COMMON TIH (PIH in the US) GASES

	First **ISOLATE** in all Directions		Then **PROTECT** persons Downwind during											
			DAY						NIGHT					
			Low wind (< 6 mph = < 10 km/h)		Moderate wind (6-12 mph = 10 - 20 km/h)		High wind (> 12 mph = > 20 km/h)		Low wind (< 6 mph = < 10 km/h)		Moderate wind (6-12 mph = 10 - 20 km/h)		High wind (> 12 mph = > 20 km/h)	
	Meters	(Feet)	km	(Miles)	km	(Miles)	km	(Miles)	km	(Miles)	km	(Miles)	km	(Miles)
TRANSPORT CONTAINER	**UN1040 Ethylene oxide: Large Spills** **UN1040 Ethylene oxide with Nitrogen: Large Spills**													
Rail tank car	200	(600)	1.6	(1.0)	0.8	(0.5)	0.7	(0.5)	3.3	(2.1)	1.4	(0.9)	0.8	(0.5)
Highway tank truck or trailer	100	(300)	0.9	(0.6)	0.5	(0.3)	0.4	(0.3)	2.0	(1.3)	0.7	(0.4)	0.4	(0.3)
Multiple small cylinders or single ton cylinder	30	(100)	0.4	(0.3)	0.2	(0.1)	0.1	(0.1)	0.9	(0.6)	0.3	(0.2)	0.2	(0.1)
TRANSPORT CONTAINER	**UN1050 Hydrogen chloride, anhydrous: Large Spills** **UN2186 Hydrogen chloride, refrigerated liquid: Large Spills**													
Rail tank car	500	(1500)	3.9	(2.5)	2.1	(1.2)	1.8	(1.2)	10.1	(6.3)	3.5	(2.2)	2.3	(1.5)
Highway tank truck or trailer	200	(600)	1.5	(0.9)	0.8	(0.5)	0.6	(0.4)	3.9	(2.5)	1.5	(0.9)	0.8	(0.5)
Multiple ton cylinders	30	(100)	0.4	(0.3)	0.2	(0.1)	0.1	(0.1)	1.1	(0.7)	0.3	(0.2)	0.2	(0.1)
Multiple small cylinders or single ton cylinder	30	(100)	0.3	(0.2)	0.2	(0.1)	0.1	(0.1)	0.9	(0.6)	0.3	(0.2)	0.2	(0.1)

TABLE 3 - INITIAL ISOLATION AND PROTECTIVE ACTION DISTANCES FOR LARGE SPILLS FOR DIFFERENT QUANTITIES OF SIX COMMON TIH (PIH in the US) GASES

	First **ISOLATE** in all Directions		Then **PROTECT** persons Downwind during											
			DAY						NIGHT					
			Low wind (< 6 mph = < 10 km/h)		Moderate wind (6-12 mph = 10 - 20 km/h)		High wind (> 12 mph = > 20 km/h)		Low wind (< 6 mph = < 10 km/h)		Moderate wind (6-12 mph = 10 - 20 km/h)		High wind (> 12 mph = > 20 km/h)	
	Meters	(Feet)	km	(Miles)	km	(Miles)	km	(Miles)	km	(Miles)	km	(Miles)	km	(Miles)
TRANSPORT CONTAINER	**UN1052 Hydrogen fluoride, anhydrous: Large Spills**													
Rail tank car	500	(1500)	3.5	(2.2)	2.1	(1.3)	1.8	(1.2)	6.6	(4.1)	3.1	(1.9)	2.0	(1.2)
Highway tank truck or trailer	200	(700)	2.0	(1.2)	1.0	(0.7)	0.9	(0.6)	3.7	(2.3)	1.6	(1.0)	0.9	(0.6)
Multiple small cylinders or single ton cylinder	100	(300)	0.8	(0.5)	0.4	(0.2)	0.3	(0.2)	1.7	(1.1)	0.5	(0.3)	0.3	(0.2)
TRANSPORT CONTAINER	**UN1079 Sulfur dioxide/Sulphur dioxide: Large Spills**													
Rail tank car	1000	(3000)	11+	(7+)	11+	(7+)	7.2	(4.5)	11+	(7+)	11+	(7+)	10.1	(6.3)
Highway tank truck or trailer	1000	(3000)	11+	(7+)	6.2	(3.8)	5.3	(3.3)	11+	(7+)	8.2	(5.1)	6.2	(3.9)
Multiple ton cylinders	500	(1500)	5.4	(3.4)	2.4	(1.5)	1.8	(1.1)	7.8	(4.8)	4.2	(2.6)	2.9	(1.8)
Multiple small cylinders or single ton cylinder	200	(600)	3.2	(2.0)	1.5	(0.9)	1.1	(0.7)	5.8	(3.6)	2.5	(1.6)	1.5	(0.9)

"+" means distance can be larger in certain atmospheric conditions

ERG2020 USER'S GUIDE

For the purposes of this guidebook, the terms hazardous materials/dangerous goods are synonymous.

The 2020 Emergency Response Guidebook (ERG2020) was developed jointly by Transport Canada (TC), the U.S. Department of Transportation (DOT), and the Secretariat of Communications and Transport of Mexico (SCT), with help from CIQUIME (Centro de Información Química para Emergencias) of Argentina.

This guidebook is for firefighters, police and other emergency services personnel who may be first to arrive at the scene of a transportation incident involving dangerous goods.

It is primarily a guide to help first responders to quickly:

- **identify the specific or generic hazards of material(s) involved in a transportation incident**
- **protect themselves and the general public during the initial response phase of the incident**

For the purposes of this guidebook, "initial response phase" is the period after first responders arrive at the scene of an incident. During this phase, responders:

- confirm the presence and/or identification of dangerous goods
- start taking protective action and securing the area
- request the help of qualified personnel

This guide is designed for use at a dangerous goods incident on a highway or railroad. It may have limited value at fixed-facility locations, or onboard aircrafts or vessels.

This guide **does not**:

- provide information on the physical or chemical properties of dangerous goods
- replace emergency response training, knowledge, or sound judgment
- address all possible circumstances that may be associated with a dangerous goods incident

ERG2020 incorporates dangerous goods lists from the most recent United Nations Recommendations, and from other international and national regulations.

Explosives are not listed individually (by either proper shipping name or ID number) but, under the general heading "Explosives", they do appear:

- on the first page of the ID Number index (yellow-bordered pages)
- alphabetically in the Name of Material index (blue-bordered pages)

Chemical warfare agents do not have an assigned ID number because they are not commercially transported. In an emergency situation, the assigned guide (orange-bordered pages) will provide guidance for the initial response.

The letter **(P)** following the guide number in the yellow and blue bordered pages identifies materials that present a polymerization hazard under certain conditions. For example: UN1092 - Acrolein, stabilized GUIDE **131P**.

First responders at the scene of a dangerous goods incident should not solely rely on this guidebook. Always seek specific information about any material in question as soon as possible. To do so:

- Contact the appropriate emergency response agency listed on the inside back cover.
- Call the emergency response telephone number on the shipping paper.
- Consult information on or accompanying the shipping paper.

BEFORE AN EMERGENCY – BECOME FAMILIAR WITH THIS GUIDEBOOK! In the U.S., according to the requirements of the U.S. Department of Labor's Occupational Safety and Health Administration (OSHA, 29 CFR 1910.120) and regulations issued by the U.S. Environmental Protection Agency (EPA, 40 CFR Part 311), first responders must be trained in how to use this guidebook.

GUIDEBOOK CONTENTS

1- Yellow-bordered pages: Index list of dangerous goods in order of ID number. The list displays the 4-digit ID followed by its assigned emergency response guide and material name.

For example:	ID No.	GUIDE No.	Name of Material
	1090	127	Acetone

2- Blue-bordered pages: Index list of dangerous goods in alphabetical order of material name. The list displays the name followed by its assigned emergency response guide and 4-digit ID number.

For example:	Name of Material	GUIDE No.	ID No.
	Sulfuric acid	137	1830

3- Orange-bordered pages: All safety recommendations are provided here. It is made up of 62 individual guides in a 2-page format. Each guide recommends safety and emergency response procedures to protect yourself and the public. The left-hand page gives safety-related information and evacuation distances. The right-hand page gives emergency response guidance for fires, spills or leaks, and first aid. Each guide applies to a group of materials with similar chemical and toxicological characteristics. The guide title identifies the general hazards of the dangerous goods.

For example: GUIDE 124 - **Gases - Toxic and/or Corrosive - Oxidizing**.

Each guide is divided into 3 main sections:

POTENTIAL HAZARDS:

- Displays the hazards in terms of **FIRE OR EXPLOSION** and **HEALTH** effects upon exposure.
- Primary potential hazard is listed first.
- Consult this section first to help you make decisions about how to protect the emergency response team and surrounding population.

PUBLIC SAFETY:

- Provides general information on initial precautionary measures to be taken by those first on scene.
- Provides general guidance on **PROTECTIVE CLOTHING** requirements and respiratory protection.
- Lists suggested **EVACUATION** distances for immediate precautionary measures, spills, and for fires (fragmentation hazard).
- When the material is highlighted in green in the yellow and blue bordered pages, it directs the reader to consult Table 1, which lists Toxic Inhalation Hazard (TIH) (PIH in the U.S.) materials, water-reactive materials and chemical warfare agents (green-bordered pages).

EMERGENCY RESPONSE:

- Outlines special precautions for incidents that involve **FIRE**, **SPILL OR LEAK** or chemical exposure.
- Lists several recommendations under each part to further assist your decision-making process.
- Provides general **FIRST AID** guidance to use before seeking medical care.

4- Green-bordered pages: This section has 3 tables.

Table 1 - Initial Isolation and Protective Action Distances

Lists, by order of ID number:

- TIH (PIH in the U.S.) materials
- water-reactive materials that produce toxic gases upon contact with water
- certain chemical warfare agents

These materials are highlighted in green in the yellow and blue bordered pages so you can easily identify them.

Table 1 provides two types of recommended safety distances: **"initial isolation distances"** and **"protective action distances"** for:

- **small spills**: 208 liters (55 US gallons) or less
- **large spills**: more than 208 liters (55 US gallons)
- Exception: For entries marked **(when used as a weapon)**, volumes vary, but in most cases, small spills include releases up to 2 kg (4.4 lbs.), and large spills include releases up to 25 kg (55 lbs.).

Within the **"initial isolation distance"**, protective clothing and respiratory protection is required. You should consider evacuating all people **in all directions** from the spill or leak source. This distance defines the radius of the "initial isolation zone" surrounding the spill in which people may be exposed to:

- dangerous concentrations upwind of the source
- life-threatening concentrations downwind of the source

The **"protective action distances"** are downwind distances from the spill or leak source, within which responders could carry out protective actions to:

- preserve the health and safety of emergency responders and the public
- evacuate and/or shelter-in-place people in this area (For more information, consult pp. 289 to 291)

The "protective action distance" is divided into **daytime** and **nighttime** incidents because varying atmospheric conditions affect a hazardous area's size. In fact, the quantity or concentration of the material's vapor poses problems, not its mere presence. During the night, the air is generally calmer. This causes the vapor to disperse less and therefore creates a greater toxic zone. In daytime, the atmosphere is more active, so the vapor disperses more. As a result, there is a lower concentration of vapor in the surrounding air and the area that reaches toxic levels is smaller. Daytime is after sunrise and before sunset. Nighttime is between sunset and sunrise.

For example, in the case of a small spill of UN1955 - compressed gas, toxic, n.o.s., the **"initial isolation distance"** is 100 meters (300 feet); therefore its "initial isolation zone" is 200 meters (600 feet) in diameter. Its **"protective action distance"** is 0.5 kilometers (0.3 miles) for daytime and 2.5 kilometers (1.6 miles) for nighttime.

Note 1: Some water-reactive materials have 2 entries in Table 1. They are identified by **(when spilled on land)** since they are TIH products and **(when spilled in water)** because they produce additional toxic gases when spilled in water.

For example: UN1746 - Bromine trifluoride and UN1836 - Thionyl chloride.

Note 2: If a water-reactive material only has one entry in Table 1 for **(when spilled in water)** and the product is NOT spilled in water, Table 1 and Table 2 do not apply. You will find safe distances in the appropriate orange-bordered guide.

For example: UN1183 - Ethyldichlorosilane and UN1898 – Acetyl iodide.

Table 2 - Water-Reactive Materials Which Produce Toxic Gases

Lists:

- by order of ID number, materials that produce large amounts of Toxic Inhalation Hazard (TIH) gases when spilled in water; and
- TIH gases produced by these materials.

You can easily identify water-reactive materials in **Table 1,** as their names are immediately followed by **(when spilled in water).**

NOTE: The TIH gases indicated in Table 2 are for information purposes only. These TIH gases have already been taken into consideration in the distances of Table 1.

For example, Table 2 indicates that UN1689 sodium cyanide, when spilled in water, will generate hydrogen cyanide gas (HCN). In Table 1, you must refer to the distances for sodium cyanide, solid and not the distances for hydrogen cyanide gas.

Table 3 - Initial Isolation and Protective Action Distances for Large Spills for Different Quantities of Six Common TIH Gases

Lists the following 6 most common TIH materials:

- UN1005 - Ammonia, anhydrous
- UN1017 - Chlorine
- UN1040 - Ethylene oxide and UN1040 - Ethylene oxide with nitrogen
- UN1050 - Hydrogen chloride, anhydrous and UN2186 - Hydrogen chloride, refrigerated liquid
- UN1052 - Hydrogen fluoride, anhydrous
- UN1079 - Sulfur dioxide/Sulphur dioxide

Table 3 shows:

- initial isolation and protective action distances for large spills (more than 208 liters or 55 US gallons)
- different container types (therefore different volume capacities) for daytime and nighttime, and for three different wind speeds (low, moderate and high)

HOW TO CHOOSE THE APPROPRIATE ISOLATION AND PROTECTIVE ACTION DISTANCES

ERG2020 lists isolation or evacuation distances in 2 places:

- the individual guides (orange-bordered pages)
- Table 1 – Initial Isolation and Protective Action Distances (green-bordered pages)

If you are dealing with a **non-TIH material** (not highlighted in green in the yellow-bordered or blue-bordered pages),

- Go to the assigned guide for the material (orange-bordered pages).
- Under **EVACUATION**, you will find:
  - initial isolation distance as an immediate precautionary measure
  - specific distances for spill or fire situations (fragmentation hazard)
  - **Please note** that certain guides may also refer to Table 1. This is just a reminder for green highlighted materials only.

If you are dealing with a **TIH, water-reactive** or **chemical warfare** material (green highlighted entries in the yellow or blue bordered pages):

If there is no fire:

- Go directly to Table 1 – Initial Isolation and Protective Action Distances (green-bordered pages).
- Also, consult the assigned guide for the material (orange-bordered pages).

If a fire is involved:

- Go directly to the assigned guide (orange-bordered pages) and apply the distances found under **EVACUATION** - Fire.
- Also, consult Table 1 distances for residual material release.

PROTECTIVE CLOTHING

STREET CLOTHING AND WORK UNIFORMS

These garments, such as uniforms worn by police and emergency medical services personnel, provide almost no protection from the harmful effects of hazardous materials/dangerous goods.

STRUCTURAL FIREFIGHTERS' PROTECTIVE CLOTHING (SFPC)

This category of clothing, often called turnout or bunker gear, is the protective clothing firefighters normally wear during structural firefighting operations. It includes a helmet, coat, pants, boots, gloves and a hood to cover parts of the head that are not protected by the helmet and facepiece. It can be used with full-facepiece positive pressure self-contained breathing apparatus (SCBA). It should, at minimum, meet the OSHA Fire Brigades Standard (29 CFR 1910.156) or NFPA 1851.

Structural firefighters' protective clothing provides limited protection from heat and cold. It may not provide adequate protection from harmful vapors or liquids encountered during hazardous materials/dangerous goods incidents.

Each guide includes a statement about the use of SFPC in incidents involving the materials referenced by that guide. Some guides state that SFPC provides limited protection. In those cases, the responder wearing SFPC and SCBA may be able to perform a quick "in-and-out" operation. However, this type of operation can place the responder at risk of exposure, injury or death. The incident commander makes the decision to do this only if there is an overriding benefit (for example, to perform an immediate rescue, turn off a valve to control a leak, etc.).

Please note that the coverall-type protective clothing customarily worn to fight fires in forests or wildlands is not SFPC and **is not** recommended nor referred to elsewhere in this guidebook.

POSITIVE PRESSURE SELF-CONTAINED BREATHING APPARATUS (SCBA)

This apparatus provides a constant, positive pressure flow of air within the facepiece.

You should always use an SCBA certified by NIOSH and the Department of Labor/Mine Safety and Health Administration, in accordance with:

- 42 CFR Part 84
- requirements for respiratory protection specified in OSHA 29 CFR 1910.134 (Respiratory Protection) and/or 29 CFR 1910.156 (f) (Fire Brigades Standard)
- NFPA 1852

Chemical-cartridge respirators or other filtering masks are not acceptable substitutes for positive pressure SCBA. Demand-type SCBA does not meet the OSHA 29 CFR 1910.156 (f)(1)(i) of the Fire Brigades Standard.

RESPIRATORS

If you suspect a chemical warfare agent is involved in an incident, use NIOSH-certified respirators with CBRN protection.

N95 respirators are the most common of the seven types of particulate filtering facepiece respirators. This product filters at least 95% of airborne particles (0.3 microns), but is not resistant to oil. N95 filtering facepiece respirators do not protect against gases and vapors.

Powered air-purifying respirators (PAPR) force ambient air through the air-purifying cartridge or filter into the facepiece. A PAPR does not supply oxygen or air from a separate source (e.g., cylinders).

CHEMICAL PROTECTIVE CLOTHING AND EQUIPMENT

For you to safely use this type of protective clothing and equipment, you need specific skills developed through training and experience. This type of special clothing may protect against one chemical but be readily permeated by chemicals for which it was not designed. Therefore, do not use this type of protective clothing unless it is compatible with the released material. Also, be aware that it offers little or no protection against heat and/or cold.

Examples of this type of equipment have been described as:

(1) Vapor Protective Suits (NFPA 1991), also known as Totally-Encapsulating Chemical Protective Suits or Level A* protection (OSHA 29 CFR 1910.120, Appendix A & B)

(2) Liquid-Splash Protective Suits (NFPA 1992), also known as Level B* or C* protection (OSHA 29 CFR 1910.120, Appendix A & B), or suits for chemical/biological terrorism incidents (NFPA 1994), class 1, 2 or 3 Ensembles and Standard CAN/CGSB/CSA-Z1610-11 – Protection of first responders from chemical, biological, radiological, and nuclear (CBRN) events

No single protective clothing material will protect you from all hazardous materials/dangerous goods. Do not assume any protective clothing is resistant to cold and/or heat or flame exposure, unless certified by the manufacturer (NFPA 1991 5-3 Flammability Resistance Test and 5-6 Cold Temperature Performance Test).

*Consult the glossary for more information about protection levels under the heading "Protective Clothing."

DECONTAMINATION

The ways to decontaminate people and equipment can vary. If you need help with decontamination, contact the emergency response telephone number provided on the shipping papers or the agencies listed on the inside back cover. These resources may be able to put you in contact with the chemical manufacturer to determine the appropriate procedure if not otherwise available.

Decontamination is the process of removing or neutralizing hazardous materials/dangerous goods that have contaminated people and equipment during an incident.

Contamination happens in the area generally referred to as the Hot Zone. Everything and everyone entering this zone should be decontaminated when leaving, including emergency response personnel. This reduces the chances that more contamination will occur.

There are two main types of contamination:

- **Direct contamination** happens in the Hot Zone.
- **Cross contamination** happens when someone or something outside the Hot Zone was not properly decontaminated and comes in contact with another object or person, usually in the Warm or Cold Zone.

To decontaminate, you must:

- physically remove contaminants; and/or
- chemically neutralize contaminants*.

The NFPA 472, Chapter 3, describes the following four kinds of decontamination.

(1) **Gross decontamination:** Quickly removing surface contamination, which usually happens by mechanically removing the contaminant or rinsing with water from handheld hose lines, emergency showers, or other nearby water sources.

(2) **Technical decontamination:** Reducing contamination to a level as low as possible by chemical or physical methods. A hazmat team will perform this kind of decontamination.

(3) **Mass decontamination:** Reducing or removing surface contaminants as fast as possible from a large number of people in potentially life-threatening situations.

(4) **Emergency decontamination:** Immediately reducing contamination of people in potentially life-threatening situations with or without formally setting up a decontamination corridor. This process should be performed upwind and uphill from victims. Responders should avoid contact with victims, runoff or spray from the decontamination process.

Emergency and mass decontamination can be done with firefighting and rescue operations equipment. Nozzles can be put on wide-angle fog patterns and sprayed towards the ground to create a decontamination shower. Responders can also place nozzles on the discharge ports of engines.

Contaminated clothing and equipment must be removed after use and stored in a controlled area (Warm Zone) until cleanup procedures can begin. Sometimes protective clothing and equipment cannot be decontaminated and must be disposed of properly.

*Chemical neutralization releases heat. DO NOT PERFORM on a victim.

FIRE AND SPILL CONTROL

FIRE CONTROL

Water is the most common and generally most available fire extinguishing agent. Use caution in selecting a fire extinguishing method, as there are many factors to consider. Water may be ineffective in fighting fires that involve some materials.

Fires Involving a Spill of Flammable Liquids

These fires are usually controlled by applying a firefighting foam to the surface of the burning material.

Fighting flammable liquid fires requires:

- foam concentrate that is chemically compatible with the burning material
- correct mixing of the foam concentrate with water and air
- careful application and maintenance of the foam blanket

There are two general types of firefighting foam: regular and alcohol-resistant. Examples of regular foam are protein-base, fluoroprotein, and aqueous film-forming foam (AFFF).

You can control some flammable liquid fires, including many petroleum products, by applying regular foam. Other flammable liquids, including polar solvents (flammable liquids that are water soluble), such as alcohols and ketones, have different chemical properties. You cannot easily control a fire that involves these materials with regular foam, and should use alcohol-resistant foam instead.

Polar solvent fires may be difficult to control and require a higher foam application rate than other flammable liquid fires (see NFPA Standards 11 for further information). Refer to the appropriate guide to determine which type of foam to use. For flammable liquids which have subsidiary corrosive or toxic hazards, it is difficult to make specific recommendations. However, alcohol-resistant foam may be effective for many of these materials.

Contact the emergency response telephone number on the shipping paper, or the appropriate emergency response agency, as soon as possible for guidance on the proper fire extinguishing agent to use.

How you decide to control the fire depends on factors such as:

- incident location
- exposure hazards
- size of the fire
- environmental concerns
- availability of extinguishing agents and equipment at the scene

WATER-REACTIVE MATERIALS

Water is sometimes used to flush spills and reduce or direct vapors in spill situations. Some of the materials covered by this guidebook can react violently or even explosively with water. In these cases, consider letting the fire burn or leaving the spill alone (except to prevent its spreading by diking) until you can get more technical advice.

The applicable guides clearly warn you of these potentially dangerous reactions. Technical advice is required for these materials since:

- Water getting inside a ruptured or leaking container may cause an explosion.
- You may need to cool adjoining containers with water to prevent them from rupturing (exploding), or to prevent the fire spreading further.
- Water may be effective in mitigating an incident involving a water-reactive material, but only if you can apply it at a **sufficient flooding rate for a long period**.
- Products from the reaction with water may be more toxic, corrosive or undesirable than the product that caused the fire.

When you respond to an incident involving water-reactive materials, take into account:

- existing conditions, such as wind, precipitation, location and accessibility to the incident
- availability of agents to control the fire or spill

Because there are variables to consider, base your decision to use water on fires or spills involving water-reactive materials on information from a reliable source. For example, consult the material's manufacturer through the emergency response telephone number or the appropriate emergency response agency listed on the inside back cover.

VAPOR CONTROL

Limiting the amount of vapor released from a pool of flammable or corrosive liquids is an operational concern. It requires proper protective clothing, specialized equipment, appropriate chemical agents and skilled personnel. Before you engage in vapor control, seek advice on tactics to be used from qualified personnel.

There are several ways to minimize the amount of vapors escaping from pools of spilled liquids, such as special foams, adsorbing agents, absorbents, and neutralizing agents. To be effective, you must select a method for the specific material involved, and use it in a way that mitigates, not worsens, the incident.

Where specific materials are known, such as at a manufacturing or storage facilities, the hazardous materials/dangerous goods response team should prearrange with the facility operators to select and stockpile these control agents before a spill.

In the field, first responders may not have the most effective vapor control agent for the material available. They will be more likely to have only water, and only one type of firefighting foam on their vehicles. If the available foam is not appropriate, they will probably use water spray. Because water is being used to form a vapor seal, care must be taken not to churn or further spread the spill during application. Vapors that do not react with water may be directed away from the site using the air currents surrounding the water spray. Before using water spray or other methods to safely control vapor emission or suppress ignition, get technical advice based on a specific chemical name.

BLEVE AND HEAT INDUCED TEAR

BLEVE (BOILING LIQUID EXPANDING VAPOR EXPLOSION)

The following pages present important safety-related information on BLEVEs, including a table, to consider in a situation involving Liquefied Petroleum Gases (LPG), UN1075.

LPGs include the following flammable gases:

- UN1011 - Butane
- UN1012 - Butylene
- UN1055 - Isobutylene
- UN1077 - Propylene
- UN1969 - Isobutane
- UN1978 - Propane

A BLEVE occurs when a fire impinged or damaged tank car fails to contain its internal pressure and explodes with a sudden product release. This catastrophic failure is more likely to occur with damaged pressure tank cars, even in the absence of an active fire.

The **main hazards** from a LPG BLEVE are:

- Fire: If the released substance is ignited, there is an immediate fireball.
- Thermal radiation: At a distance of about 4 times the radius of a fireball, the heat radiated from a fireball is enough to burn exposed skin in 2 seconds. Wearing protective clothing limits the thermal radiation dose.
- Blast: A concussive force caused by the sudden release of the pressurized substance. For a BLEVE occurring out in the open, the blast strength at a distance of 4 times the radius of a fireball can break window glass and may cause minor damage to buildings.
- Projectiles: Tank failure can throw metal fragments over large distances. These fragments can and have been deadly.

The danger decreases as you move away from the BLEVE centre. The furthest-reaching hazard is projectiles.

For a video with information on critical safety issues concerning BLEVEs, please visit *http://www.tc.gc.ca/eng/tdg/publications-menu-1238.html.*

HEAT INDUCED TEAR (HIT)

A heat induced tear (HIT) is a rupture of a NON-PRESSURE tank car containing flammable liquids when exposed to the intense heat of a fire. The metal will soften and the pressure in the tank car will increase which can lead to containment failure. The tear generally occurs at the vapor space (upper side) of the container, venting large quantities of flammable liquid and vapors at high speed. A fireball and an intense heat wave will occur.

Compared to BLEVEs, HITs rarely result in the projection of tank car fragments. Heat induced tearing has occurred within 20 minutes of the derailment and as long as 10+ hours following the initial fire.

Responding to these types of incidents (BLEVE and HIT) requires specialized training, equipment and a tactical approach.

BLEVE – SAFETY PRECAUTIONS

Use with caution. The following table gives a summary of tank properties, critical times, critical distances and cooling water flow rates for various tank sizes. This table is provided to give responders some guidance but it should be used with caution.

Tank dimensions are approximate and can vary depending on the tank design and application.

Minimum time to failure is based on ***severe torch fire impingement*** on the vapor space of a tank in good condition, and is approximate. Tanks may fail earlier if they are damaged or corroded. Tanks may fail minutes or hours later than these minimum times depending on the conditions. It has been assumed here that the tanks are not equipped with thermal barriers or water spray cooling.

Minimum time to empty is based on an engulfing fire with a properly sized pressure relief valve. If the tank is only partially engulfed, then time to empty will increase (i.e., if tank is 50% engulfed, then the tanks will take twice as long to empty). Once again, it has been assumed that the tank is not equipped with a thermal barrier or water spray.

Tanks equipped with thermal barriers or water spray cooling significantly increase the times to failure and the times to empty. A thermal barrier can reduce the heat input to a tank by a factor of ten or more. This means it could take ten times as long to empty the tank through the Pressure Relief Valve (PRV).

Fireball radius and emergency response distance is based on mathematical equations and is approximate. They assume spherical fireballs and this is not always the case.

Two safety distances for public evacuation. The minimum distance is based on tanks that are launched with a small elevation angle (i.e., a few degrees above horizontal). This is most common for horizontal cylinders. The preferred evacuation distance has more margin of safety since it assumes the tanks are launched at a 45 degree angle to the horizontal. This might be more appropriate if a vertical cylinder is involved.

It is understood that these distances are very large and may not be practical in a highly populated area. However, it should be understood that the risks increase rapidly the closer you are to a BLEVE. Keep in mind that the furthest reaching projectiles tend to come off in the zones 45 degrees on each side of the tank ends.

Water flow rate is based on 5 ($\sqrt{\text{capacity (USgal)}}$) = USgal/min needed to cool tank metal.

Warning: the data given are approximate and should only be used with extreme caution. For example, where times are given for tank failure or tank emptying through the pressure relief valve – these times are typical but they can vary from situation to situation. Therefore, never risk life based on these times.

WARNING: The data given are approximate and should only be used with extreme caution. These times can vary from situation to situation. LPG tanks have been known to BLEVE within minutes. Therefore, never risk life based on these times.

BLEVE
(USE WITH CAUTION)

Capacity		Diameter		Length		Propane Mass		Minimum time to failure for severe torch	Approximate time to empty for engulfing fire	Fireball radius		Emergency response distance		Minimum evacuation distance		Preferred evacuation distance		Cooling water flow rate	
Litres	(Gallons)	Meters	(Feet)	Meters	(Feet)	Kilograms	(Pounds)	Minutes	Minutes	Meters	(Feet)	Meters	(Feet)	Meters	(Feet)	Meters	(Feet)	Litres/min	USgal/min
100	(26.4)	0.3	(1)	1.5	(4.9)	40	(88)	4	8	10	(33)	90	(295)	154	(505)	307	(1007)	97	26
400	(106)	0.61	(2)	1.5	(4.9)	160	(353)	4	12	16	(53)	90	(295)	244	(801)	488	(1601)	195	51
2000	(528)	0.96	(3.2)	3	(9.8)	800	(1764)	5	18	28	(92)	111	(364)	417	(1368)	834	(2736)	435	115
4000	(1057)	1	(3.3)	4.9	(16.1)	1600	(3527)	5	20	35	(115)	140	(459)	525	(1722)	1050	(3445)	615	163
8000	(2113)	1.25	(4.1)	6.5	(21.3)	3200	(7055)	6	22	44	(144)	176	(577)	661	(2169)	1323	(4341)	870	230
22000	(5812)	2.1	(6.9)	6.7	(22)	8800	(19400)	7	28	62	(203)	247	(810)	926	(3038)	1852	(6076)	1443	381
42000	(11095)	2.1	(6.9)	11.8	(38.7)	16800	(37037)	7	32	77	(253)	306	(1004)	1149	(3770)	2200	(7218)	1994	527
82000	(21662)	2.75	(9)	13.7	(45)	32800	(72310)	8	40	96	(315)	383	(1257)	1435	(4708)	2200	(7218)	2786	736
140000	(36984)	3.3	(10.8)	17.2	(56.4)	56000	(123457)	9	45	114	(374)	457	(1499)	1715	(5627)	2200	(7218)	3640	962

CRIMINAL OR TERRORIST USE OF CHEMICAL, BIOLOGICAL AND RADIOLOGICAL AGENTS

If you suspect an intentional release of a chemical, biological or radiological agent (CBRN), you should immediately contact your local emergency response authorities (911). Additionally, for CBRN incidents occurring:

- within the United States, call the National Response Center at 1-800-424-8802
- within Canada, call CANUTEC at 613-996-6666 (1-888-226-8832)
- within Mexico, call CENACOM at 555128-0000 extensions 36428, 36422, 36469, 37807, 37810
- in other countries, consult page 392

The following is general guidance and does not serve as specialized incident response training. Do not enter the scene without appropriate training and equipment.

First responders can use the following information to make an initial assessment of a situation they suspect involves criminal or terrorist use of chemical agents, biological agents and/or radioactive materials (CBRN). To help with this, the following paragraphs have a list of observable indicators that a CB agent or radioactive material has been used or is present. This section ends with a Safe Stand-Off Distance Chart for various threats when improvised explosive devices (IEDs) are involved.

DIFFERENCES BETWEEN A CHEMICAL, BIOLOGICAL AND RADIOLOGICAL AGENT

Chemical and biological agents as well as radioactive materials can be dispersed in the air we breathe, the water we drink, or on surfaces we physically contact. Dispersion methods may be as simple as opening a container or using conventional (garden) spray devices, or as elaborate as detonating an improvised explosive device.

Chemical incidents are characterized by the rapid onset of medical symptoms (in minutes to hours) and easily observed signatures (colored residue, dead foliage, pungent odor, dead insects and animals).

Biological incidents are characterized by the onset of symptoms in hours to days. Typically, there will be no characteristic signatures because biological agents are usually odorless and colorless. Because of the delayed onset of symptoms, the affected area may be greater due to the movement of infected people.

Radiological incidents are characterized by the onset of symptoms, if any, in days to weeks or longer. Typically, there will be no characteristic signatures because radioactive materials are usually odorless and colorless. Specialized equipment is needed to determine the size of the affected area, and if the level of radioactivity is an immediate or long-term health hazard. Because it is impossible to detect radioactivity without special equipment, the affected area may be greater due to the migration of contaminated people.

The most probable sources would not generate enough radiation to kill people or cause severe illness. In a radiological incident generated by a "dirty bomb," or radiological dispersal device (RDD), in which a conventional explosive is detonated to spread radioactive contamination, the primary hazard is from the explosion. However, certain radioactive materials dispersed in the air could contaminate up to several city blocks, creating fear and possibly panic, and needing potentially costly cleanup.

INDICATORS OF A POSSIBLE CHEMICAL INCIDENT

Dead animals/birds/fish	Not just an occasional road kill, but numerous animals (wild and domestic, small and large), birds, and fish in the same area.
Lack of insect life	If normal insect activity (ground, air, and/or water) is missing, check the ground, water surface or shore line for dead insects. If near water, check for dead fish and/or aquatic birds.
Unexplained odors	Possible odors include fruity, flowery, sharp, pungent, garlic, horseradish-like, bitter almonds, peach kernels, or newly mown hay. The odor is completely out of character with its surroundings.
Unusual numbers of dying or sick people (mass casualties)	Health problems including nausea, disorientation, difficulty in breathing, convulsions, localized sweating, conjunctivitis (reddening of eyes), erythema (reddening of skin) and death.
Pattern of casualties	Casualties will likely be distributed downwind, or if indoors, by the air ventilation system.
Blisters or rashes	Numerous people experiencing unexplained water-like blisters, weals (like bee stings), and/or rashes.
Illness in confined area	Different casualty rates for people working indoors versus outdoors dependent on where the agent was released.
Unusual liquid droplets	Numerous surfaces show oily droplets or film; numerous water surfaces have an oily film (no recent rain).
Different-looking areas	Not just a patch of dead weeds, but trees, shrubs, bushes, food crops, and/or lawns that are dead, discolored, or withered (no current drought).
Low-lying clouds	Low-lying cloud or fog-like condition not consistent with its surroundings.
Unusual metal debris	Unexplained bomb or munitions-like material, especially if it contains a liquid.

INDICATORS OF A POSSIBLE BIOLOGICAL INCIDENT

Unusual numbers of sick or dying people or animals	Any number of symptoms may occur. Casualties may occur hours to days after an incident has occurred. The time required before symptoms are observed is dependent on the agent.
Unscheduled and unusual spray being disseminated	Especially if outdoors during periods of darkness.
Abandoned spray devices	Devices may not have distinct odors.

INDICATORS OF A POSSIBLE RADIOLOGICAL INCIDENT

Radiation Symbols	Containers may display a "propeller" radiation symbol.
Unusual metal debris	Unexplained bomb or munitions-like material.
Heat-emitting material	Material that is hot or seems to emit heat without any sign of an external heat source.
Glowing material	Strongly radioactive material may emit or cause radioluminescence.
Sick people/animals	In very improbable scenarios there may be unusual numbers of sick or dying people or animals. Casualties may occur hours to days or weeks after an incident has occurred. The time required before symptoms are observed is dependent on the radioactive material used, and the dose received. Possible symptoms include skin reddening or vomiting.

PERSONAL SAFETY CONSIDERATIONS

When you approach a scene that may involve CB agents or radioactive materials, the most critical thing to consider is your safety and that of other responders.

Use protective clothing and respiratory protection of an appropriate level of safety. In incidents where you suspect that CBRN materials have been used as weapons, NIOSH-certified respirators with CBRN protection are highly recommended. Be aware that you may not be able to verify or identify CB agents or radioactive materials, especially in the case of biological or radiological agents.

The following actions apply to a chemical, biological or radiological incident. This guidance is general. Responders will need to apply it on a case-by-case basis.

Approach and response strategies:

- Minimize exposure time.
- Maximize the distance between you and the item that is likely to harm you.
- Use cover as protection.

- Wear appropriate personal protective equipment and respiratory protection.
- Identify and estimate the hazard by using the indicators above.
- Isolate the area and secure the scene.
- Isolate and decontaminate potentially contaminated people as soon as possible.
- To the extent possible, take measures to limit the spread of contamination.

In the event of a **chemical** incident, the fading of chemical odors does not necessarily indicate reduced vapor concentrations. Some chemicals deaden the senses, giving you the false perception that the chemical is no longer present.

If there is any indication that an area may be contaminated with **radioactive** materials, including the site of any non-accidental explosion, responders:

- should be equipped with radiation detection equipment
- should have adequate training in how to use this equipment

This equipment should be designed to also alert responders when an unacceptable ambient dose rate or ambient dose has been reached.

Initial actions to consider in a potential CBRN/terrorism event:

- Avoid using cell phones, radios, etc. within 100 meters (300 feet) of a suspect device.
- Notify your local police by calling 911.
- Set up incident command upwind and uphill of the area.
- Do **not** touch or move suspicious packages or containers.
- Be cautious about the potential presence of secondary devices (e.g., improvised explosive devices (IEDs)).
- Avoid contamination.
- Limit access to only those responsible for rescue of victims or assessment of unknown materials or devices.
- Evacuate and isolate people who were potentially exposed to hazardous materials/ dangerous goods.
- Isolate contaminated areas and secure the scene for analysis of material.

DECONTAMINATION MEASURES

For chemical and biological agents: Emergency responders should follow standard decontamination procedures (flush-strip-flush). Mass casualty decontamination should begin as soon as possible by stripping all clothing, and flushing with soap and water. For further information, contact the agencies listed on the inside back cover of this guidebook.

For people contaminated with radioactive material: Take care to minimize the spread of the contamination to the extent possible. Move them to a low radiation area if necessary, and if it can be done safely. Remove their clothing and place it in a clearly marked and sealed receptacle, such as a plastic bag, for later testing. Use decontamination methods described above, but avoid breaking the skin (e.g., vigorous brushing). External radiological contamination on intact skin rarely causes a high enough dose to be a hazard, to either the contaminated individual or the first responders. For this reason, prioritize medical stabilization for a contaminated injured individual.

NOTE: The above information was developed in part by the Department of National Defence (Canada), the U.S. Department of the Army, Aberdeen Proving Ground and the Federal Bureau of Investigation (FBI).

IMPROVISED EXPLOSIVE DEVICE (IED)

An IED is a "homemade" bomb and/or destructive device used to destroy, incapacitate, harass, or distract. Because they are improvised, IEDs can come in many forms, ranging from a small pipe bomb to a sophisticated device capable of causing massive damage and loss of life.

The following table predicts the damage radius based on the volume or weight of explosive (TNT equivalent) and the type of bomb.

Improvised Explosive Device (IED)
SAFE STAND-OFF DISTANCE

	Threat Description		Explosives Capacity[1]		Mandatory Evacuation Distance[2]		Shelter-in-Place Zone		Preferred Evacuation Distance[3]	
High Explosives (TNT Equivalent)		Pipe Bomb	5 lbs	2.3 kg	70 ft	21 m	71 - 1,199 ft	22 - 365 m	+1,200 ft	366 m
		Suicide Bomber	20 lbs	9 kg	110 ft	34 m	111 - 1,699 ft	35 - 518 m	+1,700 ft	519 m
		Briefcase/Suitcase	50 lbs	23 kg	150 ft	46 m	151 - 1,849 ft	47 - 563 m	+1,850 ft	564 m
	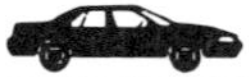	Car	500 lbs	227 kg	320 ft	98 m	321 - 1,899 ft	99 - 579 m	+1,900 ft	580 m
	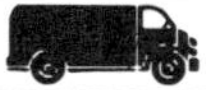	SUV/Van	1,000 lbs	454 kg	400 ft	122 m	401 - 2,399 ft	123 - 731 m	+2,400 ft	732 m
	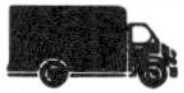	Small Delivery Truck	4,000 lbs	1,814 kg	640 ft	195 m	641 - 3,799 ft	196 - 1,158 m	+3,800 ft	1,159 m
		Container/Water Truck	10,000 lbs	4,536 kg	860 ft	263 m	861 - 5,099 ft	264 - 1,554 m	+5,100 ft	1,555 m
		Semi-Trailer	60,000 lbs	27,216 kg	1,570 ft	475 m	1,571 - 9,299 ft	476 - 2,834 m	+9,300 ft	2,835 m

[1] Based on the maximum amount of material that could reasonably fit into a container or vehicle. Variations possible.

[2] Governed by the ability of an unreinforced building to withstand severe damage or collapse.

[3] Governed by the greater of fragment throw distance or glass breakage/falling glass hazard distance. These distances can be reduced for personnel wearing ballistic protection. Note that the pipe bomb, suicide bomb, and briefcase/suitcase bomb are assumed to have a fragmentation characteristic that requires greater stand-off distances than an equal amount of explosives in a vehicle.

Improvised Explosive Device (IED)
SAFE STAND-OFF DISTANCE

	Threat Description	LPG Mass / Volume[1]		Fireball Diameter[2]		Safe Distance[3, 4]	
LPG - Butane or Propane	Small LPG Tank	20 lbs / 5 gal	9 kg / 19 L	40 ft	12 m	160 ft	48 m
	Large LPG Tank	100 lbs / 25 gal	45 kg / 95 L	69 ft	21 m	276 ft	84 m
	Commercial/Residential LPG Tank	2,000 lbs / 500 gal	907 kg / 1,893 L	184 ft	56 m	736 ft	224 m
	Small LPG Truck	8,000 lbs / 2,000 gal	3,630 kg / 7,570 L	292 ft	89 m	1,168 ft	356 m
	Semitanker LPG	40,000 lbs / 10,000 gal	18,144 kg / 37,850 L	499 ft	152 m	1,996 ft	608 m

1 Based on the maximum amount of LPG that could reasonably fit into a container or vehicle. Variations possible.

2 Assuming efficient mixing of the flammable gas with ambient air.

3 Determined by U.S. firefighting practices wherein safe distances are approximately 4 times the flame height.

4 This table is for a loaded LPG tank with explosives on the exterior. Note that an LPG tank filled with high explosives would require a significantly greater stand-off distance than if it were filled with LPG.

GLOSSARY

Adsorbed gas — A gas which sticks (adsorbs) to the surface of a solid and porous material (such as activated charcoal) contained within a metal cylinder. This results in an internal cylinder pressure of less than 101.3 kPa at 20°C (14 psi at 68°F) and less than 300 kPa at 50°C (43 psi at 122°F). These pressures are much lower than those of conventional cylinders containing compressed or liquefied gases.

AEGL(s) — Acute Exposure Guideline Level(s), AEGLs represent threshold exposure limits for the general public after a once-in-a-lifetime, or rare, exposure and are applicable to emergency exposure periods ranging from 10 minutes to 8 hours. Three levels AEGL-1, AEGL-2 and AEGL-3 are developed for each of five exposure periods (10 and 30 minutes, 1 hour, 4 hours, and 8 hours) and are distinguished by varying degrees of severity of toxic effects; see AEGL-1, AEGL-2 and AEGL-3.

AEGL-1 — AEGL-1 is the airborne concentration (expressed as parts per million or milligrams per cubic meter [ppm or mg/m^3]) of a substance above which it is predicted that the general population, including susceptible individuals, could experience notable discomfort, irritation, or certain asymptomatic, non-sensory effects. However, the effects are not disabling and are transient and reversible upon cessation of exposure.

AEGL-2 — AEGL-2 is the airborne concentration (expressed as ppm or mg/m^3) of a substance above which it is predicted that the general population, including susceptible individuals, could experience irreversible or other serious, long-lasting adverse health effects or an impaired ability to escape.

AEGL-3 — AEGL-3 is the airborne concentration (expressed as ppm or mg/m^3) of a substance above which it is predicted that the general population, including susceptible individuals, could experience life-threatening health effects or death.

Alcohol-resistant foam — A foam that is resistant to polar chemicals such as ketones and esters which may break down other types of foam.

Biological agents — Pathogens (bacteria, viruses, etc.) or the toxins they produce (such as anthrax) that are dispersed with criminal intent. They can cause disease or death in otherwise healthy humans. **Refer to GUIDE 158**.

BLEVE — Boiling Liquid Expanding Vapor Explosion

GLOSSARY

Blister agents (vesicants)
Substances that cause blistering of the skin. Exposure is through liquid or vapor contact with any exposed tissue (eyes, skin, lungs). Mustard (H), Distilled Mustard (HD), Nitrogen Mustard (HN) and Lewisite (L) are blister agents.

Symptoms: Red eyes, skin irritation, burning of skin, blisters, upper respiratory damage, cough, hoarseness.

Blood agents
Substances that injure a person by interfering with cell respiration (the exchange of oxygen and carbon dioxide between blood and tissues). Hydrogen cyanide (AC) and Cyanogen chloride (CK) are blood agents.

Symptoms: Respiratory distress, headache, unresponsiveness, seizures, coma.

Boil over
A sudden increase in fire intensity associated with the expulsion of burning flammable liquid caused by the boiling of water that has accumulated in the bottom of a tank car.

Burn
Refers to either a chemical or thermal burn, the former may be caused by corrosive substances and the latter by liquefied cryogenic gases, hot molten substances, or flames.

Carcinogen
A substance or mixture which induces cancer or increases its incidence.

Category A
An infectious substance that poses a high risk to the health of individuals and/or animals or public health. These substances can cause serious disease and can lead to death. Effective treatment and preventative measures may not be available.

Category B
An infectious substance that poses a low to moderate risk to individuals and/or animals and/or public health. These substances are unlikely to cause serious disease. Effective treatment and preventative measures are available.

CBRN
Chemical, biological, radiological or nuclear agent.

Choking agents
Substances that cause physical injury to the lungs. Exposure is through inhalation. In extreme cases, membranes swell and lungs become filled with liquid (pulmonary edema). Death results from lack of oxygen; hence, the victim is "choked". Phosgene (CG) is a choking agent.

Symptoms: Irritation to eyes/nose/throat, respiratory distress, nausea and vomiting, burning of exposed skin.

CO_2
Carbon dioxide gas.

GLOSSARY

Cold zone Area where the command post and support functions that are necessary to control the incident are located. This is also referred to as the clean zone, green zone or support zone in other documents. (EPA Standard Operating Safety Guidelines, OSHA 29 CFR 1910.120, NFPA 472).

Combustible liquid Liquids which have a flash point greater than 60°C (140°F) and below 93°C (200°F). U.S. regulations permit a flammable liquid with a flash point between 38°C (100°F) and 60°C (140°F) to be reclassed as a combustible liquid.

Compatibility Group Letters identify explosives that are deemed to be compatible. The definition of these Compatibility Groups in this Glossary are intended to be descriptive. Please consult the transportation of hazardous materials/dangerous goods or explosives regulations of your jurisdiction for the exact wording of the definitions. Class 1 materials are considered to be "compatible" if they can be transported together without significantly increasing either the probability of an incident or, for a given quantity, the magnitude of the effects of such an incident.

A Substances which are expected to mass detonate very soon after fire reaches them.

B Articles which are expected to mass detonate very soon after fire reaches them.

C Substances or articles which may be readily ignited and burn violently without necessarily exploding.

D Substances or articles which may mass detonate (with blast and/or fragment hazard) when exposed to fire.

E & F Articles which may mass detonate in a fire.

G Substances and articles which may mass explode and give off smoke or toxic gases.

H Articles which in a fire may eject hazardous projectiles and dense white smoke.

J Articles which may mass explode.

K Articles which in a fire may eject hazardous projectiles and toxic gases.

L Substances and articles which present a special risk and could be activated by exposure to air or water.

Compatibility Group (continued)

N — Articles which contain only extremely insensitive detonating substances and demonstrate a negligible probability of accidental ignition or propagation.

S — Packaged substances or articles which, if accidentally initiated, produce effects that are usually confined to the immediate vicinity.

Control zones — Designated areas at hazardous materials/dangerous goods incidents, based on safety and the degree of hazard. Many terms are used to describe control zones; however, in this guidebook, these zones are defined as the hot/exclusion/red/restricted zone, warm/contamination reduction/yellow/limited access zone, and cold/support/green/clean zone. (EPA Standard Operating Safety Guidelines, OSHA 29 CFR 1910.120, NFPA 472).

Cryogenic liquid — A refrigerated, liquefied gas that has a boiling point colder than -90°C (-130°F) at atmospheric pressure or is handled or transported at a temperature equal to or less than -100°C (-148°F).

Decomposition products — Products of a chemical or thermal break-down of a substance.

Decontamination — The removal of hazardous materials/dangerous goods from personnel and equipment to the extent necessary to prevent potential adverse health effects. See "Decontamination", page 362.

Dry chemical — A preparation designed for fighting fires involving flammable liquids, pyrophoric substances and electrical equipment. Common types contain sodium bicarbonate or potassium bicarbonate.

Edema — The accumulation of an excessive amount of watery fluid in cells and tissues. Pulmonary edema is an excessive buildup of water in the lungs, for instance, after inhalation of a gas that is corrosive to lung tissue.

ERPG(s) — Emergency Response Planning Guideline(s). Values intended to provide estimates of concentration ranges above which one could reasonably anticipate observing adverse health effects; see ERPG-1, ERPG-2 and ERPG-3.

ERPG-1 — The maximum airborne concentration below which it is believed nearly all individuals could be exposed for up to 1 hour without experiencing more than mild, transient adverse health effects or without perceiving a clearly defined objectionable odor.

GLOSSARY

ERPG-2	The maximum airborne concentration below which it is believed nearly all individuals could be exposed for up to 1 hour without experiencing or developing irreversible or other serious health effects or symptoms that could impair an individual's ability to take protective action.
ERPG-3	The maximum airborne concentration below which it is believed nearly all individuals could be exposed for up to 1 hour without experiencing or developing life-threatening health effects.
Flammable liquid	A liquid that has a flash point of 60°C (140°F) or lower.
Flash point	Lowest temperature at which a liquid or solid gives off vapor in such a concentration that, when the vapor combines with air near the surface of the liquid or solid, a flammable mixture is formed. Hence, the lower the flash point, the more flammable the material.
Flooding quantities	Minimum of 1900 L/min (500 US gal/min) of water.
Hazard zones (Inhalation Hazard Zones)	**HAZARD ZONE A:** Gases: LC50 of less than or equal to 200 ppm, Liquids: V equal to or greater than 500 LC50 and LC50 less than or equal to 200 ppm. **HAZARD ZONE B:** Gases: LC50 greater than 200 ppm and less than or equal to 1000 ppm, Liquids: V equal to or greater than 10 LC50; LC50 less than or equal to 1000 ppm and criteria for Hazard Zone A are not met. **HAZARD ZONE C:** LC50 greater than 1000 ppm and less than or equal to 3000 ppm. **HAZARD ZONE D:** LC50 greater than 3000 ppm and less than or equal to 5000 ppm. Please note: even though the term "zone" is used, hazard zones are not an actual area or distance. How zones are assigned is strictly a function of the lethal concentration 50 (LC50) of the product. For example, TIH Zone A is more toxic than Zone D.
High expansion foam	Foams that have a high expansion ratio (over 1:200) with a low water content.
Hot zone	Area immediately surrounding a hazardous materials/dangerous goods incident which extends far enough to prevent adverse effects from the released product to personnel outside the zone. This zone is also referred to as exclusion zone, red zone or restricted zone in other documents. (EPA Standard Operating Safety Guidelines, OSHA 29 CFR 1910.120, NFPA 472).
IED	See "Improvised Explosive Device".

GLOSSARY

Immiscible	In this guidebook, means that a material does not mix readily with water.
Improvised Explosive Device	A bomb that is manufactured from commercial, military or homemade explosives.
Large spill	A spill that involves quantities that are greater than 208 liters (55 US gallons). This usually involves a spill from a large package, or multiple spills from many small packages.
LC50	Lethal concentration 50. The concentration of a material administered by inhalation that is expected to cause the death of 50% of an experimental animal population within a specified time. (Concentration is reported in either ppm or mg/m^3).
Mass explosion	Explosion which affects almost the entire load virtually instantaneously.
MAWP	Maximum Allowable Working Pressure: The maximum allowable internal pressure that the tank may experience during normal operations.
mg/m^3	Milligrams of a material per cubic meter of air.
Miscible	In this guidebook, means that a material mixes readily with water.
mL/m^3	Milliliters of a material per cubic meter of air. (1 mL/m^3 equals 1 ppm).
Mutagen	An agent giving rise to an increased occurrence of mutations in populations of cells and/or organisms. Mutation means a permanent change in the amount or structure of the genetic material in a cell.
Narcotic	A substance which acts as a central nervous system depressor producing effects such as drowsiness, narcosis, reduced alertness, loss of reflexes, lack of coordination, and vertigo. These effects can also be manifested as severe headache or nausea, and can lead to reduced judgment, dizziness, irritability, fatigue, impaired memory function, deficit in perception and coordination, reaction time, or sleepiness.
Nerve agents	Substances that interfere with the central nervous system. Exposure is primarily through contact with the liquid (via skin and eyes) and secondarily through inhalation of the vapor. Tabun (GA), Sarin (GB), Soman (GD) and VX are nerve agents. **Symptoms:** Pinpoint pupils, extreme headache, severe tightness in the chest, dyspnea, runny nose, coughing, salivation, unresponsiveness, seizures.

GLOSSARY

n.o.s.	These letters refer to "not otherwise specified". The entries which use this description are generic names such as "Corrosive liquid, n.o.s." This means that the actual chemical name for that corrosive liquid is not listed in the regulations; therefore, a generic name must be used to describe it on shipping papers.
Noxious	In this guidebook, means that a material may be harmful or injurious to health or physical well-being.
Organic Peroxide	An organic (carbon-containing) compound having two oxygen atoms joined together. Organic peroxides are thermally unstable chemicals. They may have one or more of the following properties: be liable to explosive decomposition; burn rapidly; be sensitive to impact or friction; react dangerously with other substances.
Oxidizer	A chemical which supplies its own oxygen and which helps other combustible material burn more readily.
P	See "Polymerization".
Packing Group	The Packing Group (PG) is assigned based on the degree of danger presented by the hazardous material/dangerous good: PG I : Great danger PG II : Medium danger PG III : Minor danger
PG	See "Packing Group".
pH	pH is a value that represents the acidity or alkalinity of a water solution. Pure water has a pH of 7. A pH value below 7 indicates an acid solution (a pH of 1 is extremely acidic). A pH above 7 indicates an alkaline solution (a pH of 14 is extremely alkaline). Acids and alkalies (bases) are commonly referred to as corrosive materials.
PIH	Poison Inhalation Hazard. See "TIH".
Polar	See "Miscible".
Polymerization	A chemical reaction that often produces heat and pressure. Once initiated, the reaction is accelerated by the heat that it produces. The uncontrolled buildup of heat and pressure can cause a fire or an explosion, or can rupture closed containers. The letter (**P**) following a guide number in the yellow-bordered and blue-bordered pages identifies a material that may polymerize violently under high temperature conditions or contamination with other products during a transportation incident. It is also used to identify materials that have a strong potential for polymerization in the absence of an inhibitor due to depletion of this inhibitor caused by accident conditions.

GLOSSARY

ppm	Parts per million. (1 ppm equals 1 mL/m^3).
Protective clothing	In this guidebook, protective clothing includes both respiratory and physical protection. One cannot assign a level of protection to clothing or respiratory devices separately. These levels were accepted and defined by response organizations such as U.S. Coast Guard, NIOSH, and U.S. EPA. Level A: SCBA plus totally encapsulating chemical resistant clothing (permeation resistant). Level B: SCBA plus hooded chemical resistant clothing (splash suit). Level C: Full or half-face respirator plus hooded chemical resistant clothing (splash suit). Level D: Coverall, including structural firefighters' protective clothing (SFPC), with no respiratory protection. SCBA: Self-contained breathing apparatus. Consult "Protective Clothing", pages 360-361
Pyrophoric	A material which ignites spontaneously upon exposure to air (or oxygen).
Radiation Authority	As referred to in GUIDES 161 through 166 for radioactive materials, the Radiation Authority is either a Federal, state/provincial agency or state/province designated official. The responsibilities of this authority include evaluating radiological hazard conditions during normal operations and during emergencies. If the identity and telephone number of the authority are not known by emergency responders, or included in the local response plan, the information can be obtained from the agencies listed on the inside back cover. They maintain a periodically updated list of radiation authorities.
Radioactivity	The property of some substances to emit invisible and potentially harmful radiation.
Refrigerated liquid	See "Refrigerated liquefied gas".
Refrigerated liquefied gas	A gas which when packaged for transport is made partially liquid because of its low temperature. See "Cryogenic liquid".
Respiratory sensitizer	A substance that induces hypersensitivity of the airways following inhalation of the substance.
Right-of-way	A defined area on a property containing one or more high-pressure natural gas pipelines.

GLOSSARY

Shelter-in-place People should seek shelter inside a building and remain inside until the danger passes. **Sheltering-in-place is used when evacuating the public would cause greater risk than staying where they are, or when an evacuation cannot be performed.** Direct the people inside to **close all doors and windows** and to **shut off all ventilating, heating and cooling systems.** In-place protection (shelter-in-place) may not be the best option if (a) the vapors are flammable; (b) if it will take a long time for the gas to clear the area; or (c) if buildings cannot be closed tightly. Vehicles can offer some protection for a short period if the windows are closed and the ventilating systems are shut off. Vehicles are not as effective as buildings for in-place protection.

Skin corrosion The production of irreversible damage to the skin following the application of a test substance for up to 4 hours.

Skin irritation The production of reversible damage to the skin following the application of a test substance for up to 4 hours.

Skin sensitizer A substance that will induce an allergic response following skin contact.

Small spill A spill that involves quantities that are 208 liters (55 US gallons) or less. This generally corresponds to a spill from a single small package (for example, a drum), a small cylinder, or a small leak from a large package.

Specific gravity Weight of a substance compared to the weight of an equal volume of water at a given temperature. Specific gravity less than 1 indicates a substance is lighter than water; specific gravity greater than 1 indicates a substance is heavier than water.

Straight (solid) stream Method used to apply or distribute water from the end of a hose. The water is delivered under pressure for penetration. In an efficient straight (solid) stream, approximately 90% of the water passes through an imaginary circle 38 cm (15 inches) in diameter at the breaking point. Hose (solid or straight) streams are frequently used to cool tanks and other equipment exposed to flammable liquid fires, or for washing burning spills away from danger points. However, straight streams will cause a spill fire to spread if improperly used or when directed into open containers of flammable and combustible liquids.

TIH Toxic Inhalation Hazard. Term used to describe gases and volatile liquids that are toxic when inhaled (same as PIH). These materials pose a known hazard to human health during transport or is presumed to be toxic to humans because of animal-based studies.

GLOSSARY

V	Saturated vapor concentration in air of a material in mL/m^3 (ppm) at 20°C and standard atmospheric pressure.
Vapor density	Weight of a volume of pure vapor or gas (with no air present) compared to the weight of an equal volume of dry air at the same temperature and pressure. A vapor density less than 1 (one) indicates that the vapor is lighter than air and will tend to rise. A vapor density greater than 1 (one) indicates that the vapor is heavier than air and may travel along the ground
Vapor pressure	Pressure at which a liquid and its vapor are in equilibrium at a given temperature. Liquids with high vapor pressures evaporate rapidly.
Viscosity	Measure of a liquid's internal resistance to flow. This property is important because it indicates how fast a material will leak out through holes in containers or tanks.
Warm zone	Area between Hot and Cold zones where personnel and equipment decontamination and hot zone support take place. It includes control points for the access corridor and thus assists in reducing the spread of contamination. Also referred to as the contamination reduction corridor (CRC), contamination reduction zone (CRZ), yellow zone or limited access zone in other documents. (EPA Standard Operating Safety Guidelines, OSHA 29 CFR 1910.120, NFPA 472).
Water Reactive Material	In this guidebook, materials which produce significant toxic gas when it comes in contact with water.
Water-sensitive	Substances which may produce flammable and/or toxic decomposition products upon contact with water.

Water spray (fog)

Method or way to apply or distribute water. The water is finely divided to provide for high heat absorption. Water spray patterns can range from about 10 to 90 degrees. Water spray streams can be used to extinguish or control the burning of a fire or to provide exposure protection for personnel, equipment, buildings, etc. **(This method can be used to absorb vapors, knock-down vapors or disperse vapors. Direct a water spray (fog), rather than a straight (solid) stream, into the vapor cloud to accomplish any of the above).**

Water spray is particularly effective on fires of flammable liquids and volatile solids having flash points above 37.8°C (100°F).

Regardless of the above, water spray can be used successfully on flammable liquids with low flash points. The effectiveness depends particularly on the method of application. With proper nozzles, even gasoline spill fires of some types have been extinguished when coordinated hose lines were used to sweep the flames off the surface of the liquid. Furthermore, water spray carefully applied has frequently been used with success in extinguishing fires involving flammable liquids with high flash points (or any viscous liquids) by causing frothing to occur only on the surface, and this foaming action blankets and extinguishes the fire.

PUBLICATION DATA

The 2020 Emergency Response Guidebook (ERG2020) was prepared by the staff of Transport Canada, the U.S. Department of Transportation, and the Secretariat of Communications and Transport of Mexico with the assistance of many interested parties from government and industry including the collaboration of CIQUIME of Argentina. Printing and publication services are provided through U.S. DOT's Pipeline and Hazardous Materials Safety Administration (PHMSA), Outreach, Engagement, and Grants Division.

ERG2020 is based on earlier Transport Canada, U.S. DOT, and Secretariat of Communications and Transport emergency response guidebooks. ERG2020 is published in three languages: English, French and Spanish. The Emergency Response Guidebook has been translated and printed in other languages, including Chinese, German, Hebrew, Japanese, Portuguese, Korean, Hungarian, Polish, Turkish and Thai.

We encourage countries that wish to translate this Guidebook to please contact any of the websites or telephone numbers in the next paragraph.

DISTRIBUTION OF THIS GUIDEBOOK

The primary objective is to place one copy of the ERG2020 in each publicly owned emergency service vehicle through distribution to Federal, state, provincial and local public safety authorities. The distribution of this guidebook is being accomplished through the voluntary cooperation of a network of key agencies. Emergency service organizations that have not yet received copies of ERG2020 should contact the respective distribution center in their country, state or province. In the U.S., information about the distribution center for your location may be obtained from the Office of Hazardous Materials Safety website at https://www.phmsa.dot.gov/hazmat/erg/emergency-response-guidebook-erg or call 202-366-4900. In Canada, contact CANUTEC at 613-992-4624 or via the website at https://www.tc.gc.ca/canutec for information. In Mexico, call SCT at +52 55-57-23-93-00 ext. 20010 or 20577, or via email at cserrano@sct.gob.mx. In Argentina, call CIQUIME at +54-11-5199-1409, or via the website at http://www.ciquime.org or via email at gre@ciquime.org.

REPRODUCTION AND RESALE

Constructive comments concerning ERG2020 are solicited; in particular, comments concerning its use in handling incidents involving hazardous materials/dangerous goods. Comments should be addressed to:

In Canada:

Director, CANUTEC
Transport Dangerous Goods
Transport Canada
Ottawa, Ontario
Canada K1A 0N5

Phone: 613-992-4624 (information)
Fax: 613-954-5101
Email: canutec@tc.gc.ca

In the U.S.:

U. S. Department of Transportation
Pipeline and Hazardous Materials Safety Administration
Outreach, Engagement, and Grants Division (PHH-50)
Washington, DC 20590-0001

Phone: 202-366-4900
Fax: 202-366-7342
Email: ERGComments@dot.gov

In Mexico:

Secretaría de Comunicaciones y Transportes
Dirección General de Autotransporte Federal
Dirección General Adjunta de Normas y Especificaciones
Técnicas y de Seguridad en el Autotransporte
Calzada de las Bombas No. 411-2 piso,
Col. Los Girasoles,
Alcaldía de Coyoacán,
Código Postal 04920,
Ciudad de México
Phone: +52 55-57-23-93-00 ext. 20010 or 20577
Email: cserrano@sct.gob.mx

In Argentina:

Centro de Información Química para Emergencias (CIQUIME)
Av. Alvarez Thomas 636
C1427CCT Buenos Aires, Argentina
Phone: +54-11-5199-1409
Email: gre@ciquime.org

The Emergency Response Guidebook is normally revised and reissued every four years. However, in the event of a significant mistake, omission or change in the state of knowledge, special instructions to change the guidebook (in pen-and-ink, with paste-over stickers, or with a supplement) may be issued.

Users of this guidebook should check periodically (about every 6 months) to make sure their version is current. Changes should be annotated below. Contact:

DOT/PHMSA
https://www.phmsa.dot.gov/hazmat/erg/emergency-response-guidebook-erg

TRANSPORT CANADA
https://www.tc.gc.ca/eng/canutec/menu.htm

CIQUIME
http://www.ciquime.org

This guidebook incorporates changes dated:

____

____

____

CANADA AND UNITED STATES NATIONAL RESPONSE CENTERS

For the purposes of this guidebook, the terms hazardous materials/dangerous goods are synonymous.

CANADA

1. **CANUTEC**

CANUTEC is the **Canadian Transport Emergency Centre** operated by the Transportation of Dangerous Goods Directorate of Transport Canada.
CANUTEC provides a national bilingual (French and English) advisory service and is staffed by professional scientists experienced and trained in interpreting technical information and providing emergency response advice.

In an emergency, CANUTEC may be called at 1-888-CANUTEC (226-8832)
or collect at 613-996-6666 (24 hours)
***666 cellular (Press Star 666, Canada only)**

In a non-emergency situation, please call the information line at 613-992-4624 (24 hours).

2. **PROVINCIAL/TERRITORIAL AGENCIES**

Although technical information and emergency response assistance can be obtained from **CANUTEC**, there are federal, provincial and territorial regulations requiring the reporting of dangerous goods incidents to certain authorities.

The following list of provincial/territorial agencies is supplied for your convenience.

Province	Emergency Authority and/or Telephone Number
Alberta	Local Police and Provincial Authorities 1-800-272-9600 or 780-422-9600
British Columbia	Local Police and Provincial Authorities 1-800-663-3456
Manitoba	Provincial Authority 204-945-4888 and Local Police or fire brigade, as appropriate
New Brunswick	Local Police or 1-800-565-1633
Newfoundland and Labrador	Local Police and 709-772-2083
Northwest Territories	867-920-8130
Nova Scotia	Local Police or 1-800-565-1633
Nunavut	Local Police and 867-920-8130
Ontario	Local Police
Prince Edward Island	Local Police or 1-800-565-1633
Quebec	Local Police
Saskatchewan	Local Police or 1-800-667-7525
Yukon Territory	867-667-7244

NOTE:

1. The appropriate federal agency must be notified in the case of rail, air or marine incidents.
2. The nearest police department must be notified in the case of lost, stolen or misplaced explosives, radioactive materials or infectious substances.
3. **CANUTEC must** be notified in the case of:
    a. lost, stolen or unlawfully interfered with dangerous goods (except Class 9)
    b. an incident involving infectious substances
    c. an accidental release from a cylinder that has suffered a catastrophic failure
    d. an incident where the shipping papers display **CANUTEC**'s telephone number 1-888-CANUTEC (226-8832) or 613-996-6666 as the emergency telephone number or
    e. a dangerous goods incident in which a railway vehicle, a ship, an aircraft, an aerodrome or an air cargo facility is involved

3. EMERGENCY RESPONSE ASSISTANCE PLANS (Applies in Canada ONLY)

An ERAP or Emergency Response Assistance Plan is an approved plan that describes what is to be done in the event of a transportation accident involving certain higher risk dangerous goods. The ERAP is required by the Canadian *Transportation of Dangerous Goods Act* for dangerous goods that require special expertise and response equipment to respond to an incident. The plan is intended to assist local emergency responders by providing them with technical experts and specially trained and equipped emergency response personnel at the scene of a dangerous goods incident.

The ERAP will describe the specialized response capabilities, equipment and procedures that will be used to support a response to incidents involving high risk dangerous goods. The plan will also address emergency preparedness, including personnel training, response exercises and equipment maintenance. The ERAP plans supplement those of the carrier and of the local and provincial authorities, and must be integrated with other organizations to help mitigate the consequences of an accident.

For shipments that require an ERAP, the ERAP number and the phone number to activate the ERAP will be included on the shipping paper. If additional information is required, or to determine if the product involved in the emergency requires an ERAP, contact **CANUTEC**.

CANUTEC may be called at 1-888-CANUTEC (226-8832)
or collect at 613-996-6666 (24 hours)
666 on cellular phone (Press star 666) *In Canada Only

UNITED STATES

NATIONAL RESPONSE CENTER (NRC)

The NRC, which is operated by the U.S. Coast Guard, receives reports required when hazardous materials are spilled. After receiving notification of an incident, the NRC will immediately notify the appropriate Federal On-Scene Coordinator and concerned Federal agencies. Federal law requires that anyone who releases into the environment a reportable quantity of a hazardous material (including oil when water is, or may be affected) or a material identified as a marine pollutant, must **immediately** notify the NRC. When in doubt as to whether the amount released equals the required reporting levels for these materials, the NRC should be notified.

CALL **NRC** (24 hours)

1-800-424-8802

(Toll-free in the U.S., Canada, and the U.S. Virgin Islands)

202-267-2675 in the District of Columbia

Calling the emergency response telephone number, CHEMTREC®, CHEMTEL, INC., INFOTRAC or 3E COMPANY, does not constitute compliance with regulatory requirements to call the NRC.

24-HOUR EMERGENCY RESPONSE TELEPHONE NUMBERS

MEXICO

1. CENACOM
   555128-0000 extensions 36428, 36422, 36469, 37807, 37810

2. CONASENUSA
   800-11-131-68 in the Republic of Mexico

3. SETIQ
   800-00-21-400 or **55-5559-1588**
   For calls originating elsewhere, call: **+52-55-5559-1588**

ARGENTINA

1. CIQUIME
   0-800-222-2933 in the Republic of Argentina
   For calls originating elsewhere, call: **+54-11-4552-8747***

BRAZIL

1. PRÓ-QUÍMICA
   0-800-118270 in Brazil
   For calls originating elsewhere, call: **+55-19-3833-5310***

COLOMBIA

1. CISPROQUIM
   01-800-091-6012 in Colombia
   For calls originating in Bogotá, Colombia call: **288-6012**
   For calls originating elsewhere call: **+57-1-288-6012**

CHILE

1. CITUC QUÍMICO
   2-2247-3600 in the Republic of Chile
   For calls originating elsewhere call **+56-2-2247-3600**

* Collect calls are accepted